INHIBITION OF MEMORY FORMATION

M. E. Gibbs

Lecturer in Psychology
School of Behavioural Sciences
La Trobe University
Melbourne, Australia

and

R. F. Mark

Reader in Physiology
Monash University
Melbourne, Australia

PLENUM PRESS • NEW YORK — LONDON • 1973

INHIBITION OF
MEMORY FORMATION

Library of Congress Catalog Card Number 73-82140

ISBN-13: 978-1-4684-2063-0   e-ISBN-13: 978-1-4684-2061-6
DOI: 10.1007/978-1-4684-2061-6

A Division of Plenum Publishing Corporation
227 West 17th Street, New York, N.Y. 10011

United Kingdom edition published by Plenum Press, London
A Division of Plenum Publishing Company, Ltd.
Davis House (4th Floor), 8 Scrubs Lane, Harlesden, London, NW10 6SE, England

ACKNOWLEDGMENTS

This book was made possible by the help of Professor
A.K. McIntyre, Department of Physiology, Monash University
and Professor G. Singer, Psychology Department, La Trobe
University.
The authors wish to thank Mrs. Margaret Lodge and
Miss Barbara Genat for help with the manuscript.
A La Trobe University Research Grant covered the costs
incurred in the preparation of the manuscript.
A portion of this book formed part of a Ph.D. thesis
submitted to the Department of Physiology, Monash University,
by M.E. Gibbs in 1972.

CONTENTS

ABBREVIATIONS

Type of Task

CER	conditioned emotional response
PA	passive avoidance
AA	active avoidance
DA	discriminative avoidance
D	discrimination e.g. pattern discrimination

Associated with Learning and Incentive Conditions

FS	foot shock
MS	mouth shock
RS	reminder shock
NCFS	non contingent foot shock
CS	conditional stimulus
UCS	unconditional stimulus
FAM	familiarization trials
NFAM	no familiarization trials
ITE	inter trial environment
T_0	original training trial
T_1	first retention test
T_2	second retention test
CRF	continuous reinforcement schedule
FR	fixed ratio schedule
VR	variable ratio schedule

Amnesic Treatments

ECS	electroconvulsive shock
NECS	no electroconvulsive shock
EC	electroconvulsive e.g. threshold or treatment
ES	electrical stimulation
SCC	subconvulsive current
EEG	electroencephalogram
ECoG	electrocorticogram

PAD	primary after discharge
SAD	secondary or spontaneous after discharge
REM	rapid eye movement sleep
REMD	rapid eye movement sleep deprivation
AXM	acetoxycycloheximide
CXM	cycloheximide
T	bilateral temporal cortical injections
V	bilateral ventricular injections
F	bilateral frontal cortical injections
i.p.	intraperitoneal injection
sub.cut.	subcutaneous injection
E	ether
NE	no ether

Retention

RA	retrograde amnesia
SDL	step-down latencies
STL	step-through latencies
PAR	passive avoidance response
AAR	active avoidance response
STM	short-term memory
LTM	long-term memory

INTRODUCTION

All animals show longlasting changes in behaviour as a result of individual experience and this adaptability is one of their most striking features. The changes may be abrupt, radical and permanent. In higher animals it seems reasonable to ascribe their ability to change behaviour to the same physiological process that underlies human behavioural change and memory.

The known physiology of the brain gives no clues as to the mechanism. On the contrary, physiological research on the nervous system has relied upon the fact that the reactions of nerve cells studied were stereotyped and could be repeated frequently without modification. Only recently has the deliberate search for modifiable nerve cells begun but nothing yet discovered shows the rapidity, certainty and permanence of a behavioural change in intact animal. (Kandel and Spencer, 1968).

Research on memory therefore must combine the accurate observation of animal behaviour, in very well understood situations, and a knowledge of the biology of the brain and of the kind of physiological processes likely to be involved in memory storage. If one is sure that a certain behavioural change does depend uniquely on memories gained during an experiment it is possible, by using likely inhibitors of brain physiology to test the susceptibility of memories to disruption. A long list of those treatments or chemical substances that affect memory more than other functions of the brain, coupled with a knowledge of how the same treatments affect nerve cell metabolism should enable the sequence of cellular events in memory formation to be pieced together.

This manuscript is a detailed tabulation of all or most of the experiments on memory disruption published in English from 1949 to 1972. Experiments are grouped according to the kind of treatment or drug used in the attempt to alter memory and sub-grouped according to the main author and his collaborators. All the points of likely significance in the interpretation of the experimental results are noted. A critical summary and appraisal of the effects of each treatment goes with each table, and an alphabetical list of

1

all the references cited is provided. There are 8 sections covering
electroconvulsive shock, presumed neurotransmitters, anaesthetics,
barbiturates, tranquilizers and convulsants, changes in body
temperature, changes in oxygen tension, potassium chloride and
lastly antibiotic inhibitors of protein synthesis.

We have tried to be scholarly and reasonably exhaustive in
our search of the literature and we have tried to be realistic in
our assessment of results. We are forced to conclude we know almost
nothing about the likely physiology of memory but since these
experiments are in fact the only source of information on the
physical nature of memory, a knowledge of this literature is
necessary for further research.

Background to Experiments on the Physical Nature of Memory

Early this century, theories of perseveration arose in
attempts to understand the phenomena of learning and forgetting.
A neural fixation process was assumed to continue after the organism
was no longer confronted with the stimuli to be learned. Interference with perseveration was presumed to have an adverse effect on
an organism's ability to remember the stimuli to which it has been
exposed. Müller and Pilzecker (1900) produced the first clear
statement of such a perseveration theory in an attempt to account for
retroactive inhibition but it met with many difficulties as an
explanation of this and was replaced by the current concepts of
associative interference. However, this type of theory was favourable
to the explanation of clinically observed retrograde amnesia in
humans produced by concussion, anoxia, brain damage or anaesthesia
(Russell and Nathan, 1946).

The modern concept of a two stage theory of memory arose
from this with Hebb (1949) who reformulated the perseveration theory
in terms of neurophysiological substrates of memory. In his theory,
the memory trace was assumed to be held initially in the form of
reverberatory electrical activity of the central nervous system
whilst a permanent structural change was effected. The massive
interference of for example, electroconvulsive shock (ECS)
initially, followed by a near cessation of electrical activity
during the comatose phase, would presumably disrupt the memory trace
whilst it was in the form of electrical activity but not after it
was structurally fixed. Many animal studies have now been done
using a number of agents to produce retrograde amnesia (RA) - ECS,
anaesthetics and chemical convulsants, temperature changes, potassium
chloride application, transmitters and their analogues and antagonists,
anoxia and antibiotics. Generally, an animal is given one or more
learning trials and at various times after the last learning trial is
given the treatment to interrupt memory formation. Retention is
measured by the animal's performance on trials usually 24 hours
later. The greater the interval between the learning trial and the

treatment, the less is the retrograde amnesia, as shown in the lack of retention compared with controls receiving no treatment. These treatments therefore appear to have in common the ability to block recently acquired memories, whereas other memories are retained, which is also the case with retrograde amnesia after head injury or electroconvulsive therapy in man. The amnesia shrinks with time but special vulnerability of memories for events within the ten minutes leading up to the amnesic treatment suggests that memory processes through a labile stage in which it may strongly influence behaviour but is lost when brain function is interrupted. Later on memory becomes resistant to similar treatments and therefore must have now become incorporated in some way into the brain structure rather than into activity patterns by a process known as consolidation.

The importance of some structural change was affired when it was discovered that antibiotics which block DNA - dependent RNA synthesis or ribosomal protein synthesis will also block the form- ation of permanent memory. Acquisition of new behavioural patterns is still possible when brain protein synthesis is inhibited to a considerable extent but the responses are lost within a few hours. Blocking protein synthesis a few minutes after learning also blocks memory. Effects are even seen even when the injection is delayed for a day although these are weaker and may not be due to the action of the drug on new protein synthesis (Roberts and Flexner, 1969).

Since 1949, most workers have accepted the two-stage consolidation theory at least as the starting point for their experiments. However any treatment to the brain interferes to some extent with the behavioural situation used to test memory, either by the treatment acquiring stimulus value of its own which subsequently directs behaviour in the memory tests in unexpected ways, or by damaging the brain so that recognition, recall or motivational factors do not remain constant during the recovery and test period.

Many other hypotheses have been developed to explain the interactions of the various treatments with the behavioural situation and with memory formation. In examining in detail the evidence for the consolidation hypothesis of long-term memory, therefore it is necessary to collect together all the relevant experiments and to analyse critically the behavioural methods, the care with control groups together with legitimacy of conclusions as to the physiological mechanisms of memory. It is the first time all this work has been brought together, so the different agents can be directly compared. In a final short discussion we try to evaluate how much information all this work has yielded about the physiology of memory.

Note on references

The figures in brackets in the text (e.g.(1.1)) refer
to the number of the table and the number of the entry
in the table. The complete bibliographical reference
can be found by looking up the alphabetical list of
references for the appropriate table. Table numbers
are listed on the right of each entry in the
alphabetical list.

The work of a particular author can be found by starting with the author index which refers to page numbers
in the alphabetical reference lists. The table numbers
beside the reference will lead to the tabular summary
of the paper and the relevant text may be found from
this.

ELECTROCONVULSIVE SHOCK

Five major hypotheses have been advanced to explain the retrograde effect of ECS on learned responses. The earliest and most widely accepted hypothesis is that the ECS disrupts a temporally graded memory consolidation process which continues for an hour or more after learning. An alternative hypothesis is that the ECS is a highly aversive stimulus so that it acts as an unconditioned stimulus (UCS) in Pavlovian (classical) conditioning. A partial convulsion response, conditioned to situational cues as conditioned stimulus (CS) comes to complete with the learned response. A third alternative is that the effects of ECS given at post-learning intervals longer than a few seconds were on a non-discriminative conditioned emotional response (CER). Finally, it has been suggested that the retrograde effects of ECS were due to an increase in the strength of the avoidance response with time following an aversive simulus rather than due to the disruption of the memory process.

The Consolidation Hypothesis

The first experimenter to attempt to systematically use ECS for working out the physiological basis of the perseverating memory trace was C.P. Duncan (1.1, 1.2, 1.3). The procedure involved training rats to avoid shock in a shuttle box (1.3). A light, turned on 10 seconds prior to a grid shock to the feet served as CS and the rat had to run into a second compartment on presentation of the CS to avoid the footshock (FS). The ECS was delivered through electrodes attached to the rats' pinnae, with the current of sufficient intensity and duration to elicit convulsions. An ECS was given after each daily trial for 18 days. Animals in different groups were given ECS either 20, 40, 60 seconds, 4, 15 minutes, 1, 4 or 14 hours after each of the daily trails. Control subjects were given no ECS. The results indicated that in the groups administered ECS within 15 min after each training trial, learning was markedly slower than in the other ECS and nonconvulsed control groups. The effect was graded; the magnitude decreased as the trial-ECS interval was increased to produce a negatively accelerated curve. Animals given ECS 20 seconds after each training trial showed almost no learning, and the longer the interval between training and ECS treatment, the better was the learning.

These results were interpreted in terms of a consolidation theory. It was considered that the memory traces were labile and destructible shortly after being laid down, these memory traces were temporarily graded becoming increasingly invulnerable due to changing state or consolidating. If the time taken for consolidation could be measured then it was thought that some clue as to the physical identity of the trace might be found. The consolidation time can be defined as the minimum learning-ECS interval where the ECS no longer causes a loss in retention on retraining or testing. The intermediate intervals will produce a negatively accelerated response decrement, the closer the ECS is to the learning trial the greater is the loss in retention. The consolidation hypothesis infers that the time course of RA reflects the kinetics of the rate determining step of the fixation process.

Duncan's study raised a number of important questions, some of which are not yet resolved. The primary question concerns the basis of the retrograde amnesia produced by ECS. Are the learning deficits observed in animals administered ECS shortly after each trial the result of retroactive interference with memory processes, or are they caused by the punishing effects of ECS or by some other general effect of the treatment? Are the ECS-produced deficits in learning permanent, or are they merely transient effects? Are they due to the accompanying behavioural convulsion or to interference with neural, electrical, or biochemical activity? Does the graded amnesic effect obtained by Duncan reflect the "true course" of the consolidation process, or were these results specific to the particular conditions of his study? These are only a few of the issues raised by Duncan's findings (McGaugh and Herz, 1972).

During the 10 years following the publication of this study, Thompson and his colleagues (1.10 - 1.16) conducted a systematic and detailed series of investigations into the generality of the amnesic effects in rats. Thompson gave animals only one ECS at various intervals after a series of training trials and he suggested that multiple convulsions as used by Duncan might have a cumulative effect on behaviour. Thompson looked at the effect of ECS on rats of different ages (1.12, 1.13); distribution of practice in training (1.14); amount of practice and task difficulty (1.15). Different gradients of ECS-induced RA were found with different manipulations of these variables.

One problem for the consolidation theory has been the large range of reported consolidation times and this has contributed to the formulation of conflicting interpretations for retrograde amnesic experiments. Consolidation times vary from seconds (e.g. 1.21, 1.103, 1.140, 1.162, 1.173) to minutes (e.g. 1.62, 1.88, 1.116) and even hours (e.g. 1.35, 1.128, 1.129). Probit analysis by Cherkin (1966) of the results of four comparable studies (1.21, 1.88, 1.103, 1.116) revealed that there was a normal distribution of memory against

the logarithm of the consolidation interval. The probit regression
lines of 3 of these studies in rats had similar slopes suggesting
a consolidation process working at similar rates. Many of the
conflicts in published consolidation times arise from differences in
learning strength and artefacts of data handling and other variables
in experimental design.

Alternative Interpretations of ECS-induced RA

The findings of Duncan, Thompson and others in the late
1940's and 1950's provided strong evidence that memory-storage
processes are time dependent. However, it was apparent at that time
that there might be other interpretations of the data. There seem
to be two general alternative explanations: ECS does have an affect
on memory processes, but the graded amnesic effects are not due to
effects of the treatment on time-dependent consolidation processes;
or ECS does not impair memory consolidation at all but proactive
effects on behaviour are seen that are mistakenly regarded as
evidence of memory impairment.

Development of Fear

It has been suggested that fear develops for the ECS and
this is a punishing stimulus. Coons and Miller (1.20) argued that
the poor learning observed when ECS treatment closely followed
learning trials could also be explained in terms of an ECS-induced
fear of the goal, with a resulting conflict that interfered with
performance. In Duncan's active avoidance situation, animals
received an ECS on entry into the safe chamber and a failure to avoid
could have been because the ECS was more aversive than the FS.
Duncan had used control rats which received a shock through the
hindlimbs of equal intensity to the ECS (but which did not produce
convulsions). These control animals showed a greater avoidance, but
the two shocks were not necessarily equally aversive. Coons and
Miller confirmed most of Duncan's findings but also found that rats
given ECS soon after learning trials showed increased fear, with
increased urination and defaecation.

A second experiment was designed to distinguish between
the aversive and amnesic effects of ECS. The animals were first
trained, in an active-avoidance task, to avoid the shocked side of
a grid, and then the conditions were reversed with the shock
introduced on the previously 'safe' side of the grid, so the
animals now had to passively avoid the shock. Under these conditions
the sooner ECS followed each learning trial, the faster was the rate
of learning. If ECS did produce amnesia then ECS animals should
require more trials to acquire the reversal task than animals not
receiving the ECS. But animals receiving FS plus ECS learned the
reversal task faster than those only receiving the FS, indicating
that FS plus ECS was more aversive than FS alone.

Competing Response Hypothesis

Another interpretation of the effects of ECS is the conditioned-inhibition hypothesis proposed by Lewis and Maher (1965). They said that ECS interferes with the performance of a response by causing the subject to be less active in the experimental situation. Adams and Lewis (1.63, 1.64) proposed that loss of consciousness is an unconditioned response produced by ECS, and that a weakened version of this loss of consciousness - relaxation and lowered activity level - becomes conditioned to the cues present at the time of ECS administration. They suggest further that the conditioned inhibition is a function of the nearness in time and space of the cues associated with the convulsion. This supposition can account for the graded amnesic effect commonly observed when ECS is administered to different groups of subjects at increasing intervals after the learning trial. They showed that animals given a series of ECS treatments inside the start compartment of an active avoidance box prior to training showed slower acquisition than those not given ECS. The competing responses - crouching and freezing - extinguished normally and were weaker when ECS was administered outside the apparatus. In another experiment (1.65), ECS followed 3 daily trials either in the start compartment, safe compartment or outside the apparatus. Performance was best in the group given ECS outside the apparatus and poorest in the group convulsed in the shock compartment.

This conditioned-inhibition interpretation can be used to interpret the results of Duncan's study (1.3) as well as those of Adams and Lewis (1.63, 1.65). However, it is extremely difficult to explain the findings of the one-trial inhibitory or passive avoidance experiments in these terms. The experiments cited show the disadvantage of using an active avoidance learning task where the aversive or competing responses (conditioned suppression) and the possible amnesic effects of ECS have the same behavioural consequences. These tasks also have required more than one trial to acquire the learned response and the time of learning cannot be accurately specified.

Madsen and McGaugh (1.28) developed a passive avoidance procedure avoiding both of these complications. The animal was placed on a small platform suspended a few centimeters above a grid floor. On stepping down from the platform, a mild shock was delivered to the feet. The animal learned in this one trial to stay on the platform on subsequent tests and avoid the footshock. Using a one-trial passive avoidance task (1.30, 1.31, 1.103, 1.175) the amnesic properties of ECS were demonstrated after only one trial; whereas the aversive properties of ECS alone appeared after at least three treatment trials.

Similar experiments using one-trial passive avoidance (PA) paradigms also indicate that the effect of ECS on the performance of a learned response is a negatively accelerated function of the learning-ECS interval (1.58, 1.87, 1.116, 1.187). The results of these experiments do not appear to be adequately accounted for either by the aversive effects of ECS or by competing responses conditioned by the ECS.

Lewis and Maher (1965, 1966) also proposed that any procedure that eliminates the behavioural convulsion produced by ECS should prevent the conditioned inhibition. However, retrograde amnesia is readily obtained when convulsions are prevented by light ether anaesthesia prior to ECS treatment (1.33, 1.44, 1.46, 1.51, 1.89, 1.217). Even in unanaesthetized animals tonic convulsions are not essential for the production of retrograde amnesia with ECS. In mice, rats and chickens the current thresholds for retrograde amnesia are lower than those for tonic convulsion (1.46, 1.78, 1.88, 1.122, 1.130, 1.132, 1.133, 1.169).

Finally, since conditioned inhibition should result in a decreased speed of response, ECS subjects would be expected to respond less rapidly than controls regardless of the rewarding or punishing conditions of the learning task. Nevertheless, Herz (1.155) has demonstrated that ECS produces retrograde amnesia for both appetitive and aversive one-trial learning in the same apparatus. The animals showing amnesia respond more rapidly than controls in the aversive learning situation and more slowly than controls in the appetitive learning situation. Other investigators have demonstrated retrograde amnesia for one-trial appetitive learning (1.96, 1.125, 1.126).

Thus, although the conditioned-inhibition hypothesis has stimulated a great deal of research, the overall results do not appear to provide much support for this interpretation.

Conditioned Emotional Responses

Another interpretation of ECS-produced retention deficits is that the amnesia observed with long training-treatment intervals reflects the effects of ECS, not on memory, but on the conditioned emotional response (CER).

In the passive avoidance situation it was suggested that with FS the animal learns a nondiscriminative CER to the apparatus in general and suppresses all responses. Chorover and Schiller (1.103, 1.104) proposed that the ECS has a disinhibitive effect on the CER making the animals more active. PA and the CER would have identical behavioural consequences; either interference with consolidation or alleviation of the CER by the ECS would result in apparent forgetting. Whereas with active avoidance (AA), ECS would cause the animal to be more active and result in apparent learning. Chorover and Schiller (1.103, 1.104, 1.105) found that ECS disruption of a learned response occurred only within a few seconds

of learning and suggested that the effects of ECS on longer post-
learning intervals were on the CER. RA was seen only with very
short learning ECS intervals in an appetitively motivated situation.
It has been reported (1.188) that ECS in the one-trial PA paradigm
will alleviate the CER when given up to 24 hours after learning, but
if administered within 100 seconds of learning will produce a greater
and time-related effect indicating that RA does occur in this situation
(1.189). The ECS given after 100 seconds produces ungraded defects
in retention with time (1.190).

A single ECS given 1 hour or less before learning was less
effective than an ECS given the same time after learning (1.131), that
is, the proactive effect was less marked than the retroactive effect
of a single ECS. If ECS was alleviating a nondiscriminative CER then
equal effects would have been predicted.

According to the conditioned-inhibition hypothesis, post-
trial ECS treatments should, by inducing relaxation, facilitate
extinction. However, ECS treatments have been found to impair
extinction of both approach and avoidance responses (1.29, 1.219).

Incubation Theory

A variety of passive avoidance responses conditioned in
one-trial have been shown to change in strength or incubate over
time following learning (McGaugh, 1966; 1.91, 1.92, 1.93, 1.99, 1.190,
1.192). Incubation gradients have been demonstrated following
multiple trials in an active avoidance situation (1.82) and multitrial discriminated avoidance learning (1.192). Pinel and Cooper
(1.93) offered an explanation for the retrograde effect of ECS on
learned responses on the basis of this observation. They found that
the retrograde gradient of ECS closely paralleled the incubation
gradient of the one-trial PA response and suggested that as the
avoidance response was increasing in strength over time, the ECS was
simply halting the incubation process - producing greater defects in
retention early after learning simply because the response is weaker
at this time. Although such performance curves do sometimes parallel
the amnesic gradient, this is not always the case. In fact, in most
cases the retention curves and the amnesic gradients are not parallel
(McGaugh and Herz, 1972).

Other evidence implicates the CER in the retrograde effects
of ECS on memory, and the incubation theory. This includes McMichael's
(1966) demonstration of CER incubation gradients similar in form to
ECS-produced latency gradients in PA tasks; the demonstration that a
CER is produced in one-trial PA conditioning (1.97, 1.188); the finding
of long term ECS effects only for a PA situation in which a CER was
produced (1.104) and the finding that effects of multiple ECS's are
selective to the CER (1.8). It has been concluded by Suboski et al
(1.190, 1.191) that the temporally graded retrograde effects of ECS

at relatively long intervals are the result of an ECS produced
disruption or halting of the incubation of a CER.

A number of investigators have chosen to regard
incubation as direct evidence for memory consolidation (McGaugh,
1966; 1.99). However, Pinel (1.95, 1.96) has produced direct
evidence against this interpretation. The incubation phenomenon
results from FS-produced decreases in activity over time, but in the
one-trial passive avoidance situation in which the incubation has
most often been demonstrated, decreases in activity lead to improved
performance of the learned response and thus to the impression that
memory is improving. However, in a one-trial active avoidance
situation where decreases in activity oppose any improvements in
performance, the performance of the active avoidance response
deteriorates with time as freezing behaviour incubates (1.95). No
improvement with time is seen in one-trial learning situations such
as discriminated avoidance where decreases in activity levels do not
effect performance (1.190), or in situations where no decreases in
activity occur or in an appetitive situation where no FS is given
(1.96). Pinel et al (1971; 1971b; 1.98) report that FS or other
aversive treatments, as well as producing a tendency to freeze, have
a transient activating effect and the actual level of activity is
determined by the interaction of these two tendencies. The
incubation gradient is the result of the gradual diminuition of the
FS produced activation with the passage of time rather than any
increase in the tendency to freeze. Thus, the incubation phenomenon
seems to be of a reflexive nature and not necessarily indicative of
increases in the permanence of memory storage, improvements in memory
or the incubation of anxiety. A possible explanation of the incubation-
interruption interpretation for the relation between incubation and ECS
comes from the interaction of FS and ECS in electrocortical recordings
(1.107). Chorover and de Luca have reported that rats given ECS at
various intervals after FS do not undergo comparable seizures. The
sooner after FS is the ECS and thus the more active the animal, the
less likely is the appearance of a normal electrocorticographic
seizure. Perhaps the diminuition of the FS-produced arousal underlies
both this gradient of change in ECS produced seizures and the incubation
phenomenon. This idea is also supported by Schneider et al (1.140)
with non-contingent FS. It becomes important to have pre-ECS levels
of performance; that is, performance measured at the same time after
FS as the ECS is given to discriminate between the effects of FS and
amnesia produced by ECS (1.97).

Spevack and Suboski (1969) have suggested that the short
amnesic gradients produced when ECS is administered within the first
post-training trial minute are the only ones that represent true
amnesia, and that the longer gradients reflect incubation. However,
curves of retrograde amnesia do not directly reflect consolidation
rates. They reflect the susceptibility of memory processes to the
particular amnesic treatment administered, and as such they are

extremely sensitive to the different treatments, tasks and
experimental procedures used in various studies (Cherkin, 1969;
Dawson, 1971; McGaugh and Dawson, 1971). In particular, the amnesic
gradient obtained in any study depends on the intensity and duration
of the ECS current.

Variables operating in ECS Studies - Parameters of ECS Treatment

The present evidence seems to indicate that ECS does
interfere with the consolidation of memory. The large range of
reported consolidation times can probably be partially attributed
to experimental variables in both the ECS treatment and the learning
paradigms employed.

Site of Delivery of the ECS

The site of administration of ECS poses a number of
problems. In mice, ECS is characteristically applied via transcorneal
electrodes, whereas in rats the ECS current is administered via clips
attached to the pinnae. A number of studies have investigated these
two methods of ECS administration in both species of animals (1.45,
1.132, 1.143, 1.177, 1.196). Administration of the ECS through ear
clips or transcorneally probably causes peripheral pain which may
effect later behaviour and may lead to a conditioned fear state
(1.44, 1.196, 1.198). Nielson (1.206) has shown that simply attach-
ing earclips to rats decreases their activity in an open field, it
also increases their rate of defaecation which is often taken as a
measure of emotionality. It is probable that species differences in
thresholds and responses to ECS may be related to the differences in
treatment. With mice and rats (1.143, 1.177) a given intensity of
ECS is more effective in disrupting memory retention when delivered
across a low resistance pathway (eyes) than when administered via a
high resistance pathway (ears), even though there were no differences
in the frequency of eliciting a full tonic-extensor response or in the
duration of the convulsion once elicited. Different areas of the
brain have different thresholds for epileptic discharge, with the
hippocampus being the most susceptible (Gastaut and Fischer-Williams,
1959).

The seizure threshold of the cortex is apparently lower
anteriorly (1.122, 1.236), and it may be that this region is
critically involved in memory storage or readily elicits seizures in
other structures involved in consolidation. It might also be that
different brain structures are differently affected by the two routes
of ECS administration. Direct electrical stimulation of various
regions of brain have been employed and different effects on later
memory tests have been seen according to the precise site employed.
This technique of direct stimulation offers considerable advantages,
both in eliminating peripheral pain factors and perhaps allowing
identification of the brain regions important to the behaviour

in question. Deficits resulting from electrical stimulation of
two specific areas, the basal ganglia (principally the caudate
nucleus) and the limbic system (hippocampus and amygdala) have been
systematically investigated. Thompson (1.16) found significant
deficits in reversal learning produced by bilateral caudate
stimulation administered immediately or 17 seconds after each
response. The deficit increased with increases in voltage,
frequency, pulse duration and stimulus-train duration. Unilateral
stimulation had no effect.

Later studies (1.195, 1.207, 1.218, 1.226, 1.228) have
shown amnesia from dorsal hippocampal and amygdaloid stimulation. It
appears that to be effective such stimulation must produce afterdischarges in the amygdala; stimulation of the septum, fornix or
ventral hippocampus, which did not produce such afterdischarges
produced no interference (1.195). However, there is clear evidence
that in rats stimulation of the frontal cortex, of sufficient
intensity to produce brain seizures, produces amnesia. Zornetzer
and McGaugh (1.45) found that stimulation of the frontal cortex
produced amnesia comparable to that obtained with 50 mA ECS
administered via the pinnae. The amnesic effect was found even in
amygdalectomized rats. The amygdala is not an essential structure
for producing retrograde amnesia with seizure-inducing stimulation.

Other investigators have employed this technique of
restricted electrical stimulation to the brain. Herz et al (1.154,
1.157, 1.158, 1.159, 1.160) have used low intensity electrical
stimulation to the caudate nucleus of rats and found amnesia in a
variety of learning paradigms. No amnesia was found with comparable
stimulation of adjacent sites which appears to rule out the possibility
that the effects are due to current spread.

Criticisms of the techniques used in many of these
experiments has been made (McGaugh and Herz, 1972). In some cases
stimulation has been administered during or immediately after the
event on which the subject would have to rely in order to show
improvement on subsequent trials. Therefore any experimental
manipulation that could interfere with registration of the sensory
experience - reward, attention, set, or postural orientation - might
produce deficits that would be interpreted as amnesia. Even in the
experiments which interposed delays of several seconds between an
experience and interfering stimulation, the current intensities and
durations were often of sufficient magnitude to produce current
spread making it difficult to determine whether the target structure
or some other nearby site had been involved in production of the
deficit.

The evidence that selective brain stimulation affects
memory storage processes when it is applied immediately after learning trials, with effects diminishing with longer intervals, suggests

that minimal treatment of critical brain structures is as effective
as massive stimulation of the entire brain. ECS, although it has
greatly helped to characterize the phenomenon of memory consolidation,
has not clarified the role of various brain structures and systems
in the formation of memory.

Duration and Intensity of ECS

        Cherkin (1969) and McGaugh and Dawson (1971) have proposed
that since variations in the amnesic gradient can be produced by
varying the intensity and duration of amnesic treatments when the
task and training procedures are held constant, the degree of amnesia
may vary with the degree of disruption of neural activity produced by
the treatment. A number of workers report a graded effect of current
intensity on retention either by increasing the effective period of
ECS; or the extent of the retention deficit; or the permanence of the
RA; or the time after training at which the RA appears (1.46, 1.47,
1.48, 1.82, 1.89, 1.122, 1.130, 1.133, 1.164, 1.166, 1.169, 1.177,
1.180, 1.194, 1.209, 1.252). The threshold for convulsions changes
after the first ECS treatment which suggests that when more than one
shock is given, subsequent ones will have different potencies depending on the interval between ECS treatments (1.80, 1.197). There is
evidence that the degree of amnesia also varies with the duration of
the ECS current (1.35, 1.252). However, the evidence concerning the
effect of current duration is conflicting. Some investigators consider
the duration of the electroconvulsive current not to influence the
extent of the RA with high current intensities (1.22, 1.24, 1.157,
1.194, 1.252) or with low current intensities (1.133, 1.194). The
reason for the discrepency is not clear. Studies of the amnesic
effect of the anaesthetic flurothyl have shown that amnesia varies
with both the dosage and the duration used (Cherkin, 1969).

        There are indications that the variations in ECS intensity
and possibly duration used in different studies may account for some
of the differences in consolidation times reported.

Convulsions

        There has been considerable controversy as to whether ECS-
induced convulsions are necessary to produce amnesia. Some early
reports claim a dependence of amnesia on overt convulsions (1.31,
1.87, 1.88). Miller and Spear (1.78) claim that amnesia is positively
correlated with the severity of the convulsion despite a constant-
current ECS. Other reports indicate that overt convulsions are not
necessary for amnesia (1.68, 1.164, 1.166, 1.168, 1.195) and that
currents below the convulsion threshold may also be effective. The
convulsions seem to be all-or-none in the sense that neither the
convulsion patterns nor their time course vary systematically with
current intensity (1.166). This lack of dependence of RA on overt
convulsions is in agreement with the findings that amnesia occurs

even if the convulsion is prevented by ether anaesthesia (1.33, 1.44,
1.46, 1.47, 1.48, 1.89, 1.134, 1.217). It may be that some correlate
of the convulsion, and not simply the passage of current through the
brain, is the basis of the aversive quality of ECS (1.215). Kesner
et al (1.196) recently reported that repeated ECS treatments are not
punishing if the current is delivered through cortical electrodes
instead of ear-clip electrodes. This suggests that the rats'
pinnae may become sensitive following repeated ECS administration
via ear clips. This might account for the observation that rats
given repeated ECS treatments via ear-clip electrodes avoided the
place in a two-compartment box where the ECS was administered (1.31,
1.32).

Many of the earlier considerations of the necessity of
convulsions in producing retrograde amnesia have focused on overt
behaviour and convulsions. However, in view of the fact that amnesia
can occur in the absence of overt convulsions when the animal is
anaesthetized, it becomes necessary to look at what effect the ECS
has on neural activity in the brain. The threshold for ECS-induced
brain seizures is approximately the same as that for retrograde
amnesia (1.46, 1.47, 1.167). Following transcranial ECS in day-old
chickens it was the spike activity and not the overt convulsion or
the subsequent flattening of the EEG which was necessary for amnesia
(1.167). In mice, ether anaesthesia administered before ECS elevates
the thresholds for brain seizures and retrograde amnesia (1.44, 1.46).
Other evidence indicates that the postictal depression typically
observed after ECS is not essential for producing amnesia. In mice
anaesthetized with ether prior to ECS treatment postictal depression
is rarely seen. However, at ECS current intensities which produce
seizures, the degree of amnesia obtained is equal to, and sometimes
greater than, that produced by ECS in unanaesthetized animals (1.33,
1.46, 1.51). The degree of amnesia produced by ECS may also depend
on the period required for return of a normal EEG pattern after
treatment. The degree of amnesia produced by ECS was greater in
rats in which ECoG theta activity was absent for an extended period
following the treatment. Little or no amnesia was found in animals
in which the theta activity was present shortly after ECS treatment
(1.55, 1.56).

It appears that the passage of current through the brain
is not in itself a sufficient condition for producing amnesia.
Electroshock stimulation of sufficient intensity to produce brain
seizures is also sufficient to produce amnesia, but it is not yet
known whether the seizures are merely signs of neural disturbance
or whether they play a role in causing retrograde amnesia (McGaugh
and Herz, 1972). At ECS current levels above the brain seizure
threshold the degree of amnesia varies with current intensity. Thus
the occurrence of a seizure is not a sufficient condition for
producing maximum amnesia. The pattern of electrical activity
produced by ECS varies with current intensity. Spontaneous after

discharges occur with higher current intensities (1.45-1.48). When seizures were induced in rats by frontal cortex stimulation, the average frequency of spikes in the primary afterdischarge (PAD), the duration of the PAD and the probability of a secondary afterdischarge (SAD) varied systematically with current intensity (1.45). The secondary or spontaneous afterdischarges could be the reason for hippocampal spike activity being unrelated to the amount of RA (1.237), as spread of spontaneous afterdischarges to other cortical areas could be responsible (1.49).

ECS has been shown to impair retention when delivered as much as 24 hours after learning but was only significant up to 30 seconds (1.163). It has been suggested that this may be due to some lasting brain damage and offers another explanation for a series of ECS's being effective at long learning-ECS intervals when one is ineffective.

Physiological factors influencing retrograde amnesia

There is a problem as to whether ECS can cause physiological changes in animals. There have been reports that it can alter brain excitability, produce a loss of weight, change task performance, alter open field activity, heart rate, food motivation and cause emotionality (1.20, 1.123, 1.206, 1.239). However, other reports claim that ECS has no effect on behaviour other than interfering with memory consolidation (1.30, 1.43, 1.62, 1.75, 1.238).

The physiological state of the animal has also been reported to influence the amnesia either by extent or duration of vulnerability to ECS (1.12, 1.36, 1.37, 1.38, 1.52, 1.78, 1.134, 1.156). ECS administered to mice at night, during the peak hours of activity and metabolic rate, produces greater amnesia than treatments given during the day (1.36, 1.37, 1.38). A number of studies have shown that consolidation may be influenced by deprivation of sleep, particularly the sleep stage termed rapid-eye-movement sleep (REM). Fishbein (1.53) has shown that in mice retention is impaired if the animals are deprived of REM sleep in the interval between training and the retention test. ECS given two days after training produced amnesia in mice if they were deprived of REM sleep during this interval, and if the ECS was given shortly after they were removed from the conditions that produced REM sleep deprivation. No effect was found if ECS was delayed for an hour (1.52). Thus deprivation of REM sleep appears to act in some way to maintain the susceptibility to ECS-induced amnesia. Motivation is also an important factor (1.156, 1.231, 1.232, 1.233). The susceptibility of individual animals to ECS varies inversely as a function of body weight and it has been suggested (1.45) that with transpinnate ECS this could be due to subdermal lipid deposits as well as thickness of the skull.

A number of workers have suggested that ECS may produce state-dependent learning because of the alterations in brain

excitability (1.206, 1.230, 1.234, 1.235, 1.244, 1.245). Nielson
(1.206) found that thresholds for eliciting a learned response were
highly elevated on tests given 24 hours after an ECS treatment and
returned to levels at or near their pre-ECS values on tests given 96
hours after ECS. He also reported that over a period of 96 hours
rats recovered from the amnesic effects of an ECS treatment. These
findings led him to conclude that ECS produces brain changes which
interfere with information retrieval but not with memory-storage
processes. Nevertheless, this explanation is not supported by more
recent findings. For example, an ECS treatment affects the
performance of a previously learned response only if the animals are
tested within 2 hours after the treatment, and the impairing effects
are almost completely eliminated when the convulsions are prevented
by light anaesthesia with ether prior to the ECS treatment (1.41,
1.217). Moreover, in mice tested 24 or 96 hours after training on
a one-trial PA task retention was not affected by an ECS given 24
hours before the training (1.43). The ECS treatment given 24 hours
before training should have interfered with retention 24 hours after
training if ECS had longlasting effects (up to several days) on
retrieval processes. McGaugh and Landfield (1.50) also showed that
reinstatement of the ECS state did not enhance retention.

Place and Time of Treatment with ECS

As mentioned previously, two of the hypotheses regarding
the effects of ECS - aversive properties and competing responses -
depend on the place where the ECS treatment was given. Spevack and
Suboski (1969) concluded that when an ECS is delivered contingent on
a response, it will be aversive and produce avoidance (1.20) and
when it is delivered when an animal is not making a response it will
produce freezing behaviour (1.63, 1.64, 1.65). In contrast to the
results obtained by Lewis and Adams (1.65) it has been shown that
when an ECS was given not contingent upon a response in the apparatus,
there was no difference in the effect of ECS on the amnesia from
when it was contingent on a response (1.21, 1.61, 1.68). ECS has
been shown to be effective in producing amnesia if delivered while
an active response was being made but not if given before the response
started (1.66, 1.69). The impairment in both these reports was
attributed to fear conditioned by the ECS to the stimulus consequences
of running. But in a situation where continued responding reflects
amnesia, the ECS has been shown not to act as a negatively
reinforcing stimulus (1.59, 1.87, 1.88, 1.89, 1.117, 1.150, 1.174).

The Effect of ECS alone on Performance

A single ECS with no training is claimed to have no effect
on performance 24 hours later (1.21, 1.24, 1.59, 1.62, 1.116, 1.136,
1.140, 1.165, 1.211, Pryor et al, 1972). Repeated ECS treatments are
reported to have an aversive effect (1.18, 1.32, 1.59, 1.63, 1.67,
1.149, 1.178, 1.188, 1.197, 1.211, 1.238, 1.239, 1.249, Pryor et al,

1972). Experiments have been done using multiple ECS without
footshock to determine whether the place of treatment or the place
of recovery from the ECS were important in the development of
aversive properties. The results were contradictory, it was either
the place of treatment (1.32, 1.67) or the place of recovery (1.149,
1.249) that was involved in the development of the aversion, and
which was the determining factor in producing fear. It could be
that the extent of amnesia determines whether fear is associated
with the place of recovery or treatment with multiple ECS treatments
(1.198). However, to complicate the issue even further there have
been reports of a single ECS having an effect on activity levels
(1.141) and repeated treatments having no effect (1.120).

The Effect of ECS given before Training

A single ECS has been shown to have no effect unless given
within 1 hour before the learning or the retention trial. Even so,
the effect before training was negligible compared with ECS given 1
hour after learning (1.41, 1.127, 1.131, 1.215). In contrast
Poschel (1.18) found the proactive effects equal to the retroactive
effects, although he did use multiple trials and multiple treatments.
Darbellay and Winocur (1.239) report difficulty in training rats on
avoidance conditioning following 10 ECS treatments prior to training.
The proactive effect of ECS could be a consequence of the convulsion
because if this is prevented by anaesthesia, the proactive effect
does not occur until the ECS given 5 minutes before training (1.41,
1.215). ECS given 1 hour or less before testing with or without
convulsions does produce a deficit which is only temporary (1.215).
In all, ECS before learning in a passive avoidance task has been
found to increase latencies (1.229), decrease latencies of responding
(1.178) and to have no effect (1.140); and in an active avoidance
task to decrease latencies (1.213) or to have no effect (1.229).
Geller et al (1.147, 1.148) and Grosser et al (1.247) claim a
proactive effect of ECS, demonstrated by step-through latencies
lower on the retest than on the training trial.

It is not clear whether ECS can have proactive effects on
performance or not.

Training Variables which affect ECS-induced RA

Reinforcement Magnitude

It has been suggested that if the negative reinforcement
was increased, greater conditioning would result and this would be
reflected in a lessening of the extent of the amnesia produced by
ECS. There are a number of ways of altering the amount of
reinforcement. One way is to vary the intensity of the FS, but
various experiments have shown no conclusive evidence of this
altering the effects of ECS (1.113, 1.175, 1.187). An effect was

seen by Ray and Bivens (1.176) as a decreasing interval of ECS
effectiveness with decreased FS intensity but only after one trial.
It was suggested that insufficient intervals were investigated in
the previous studies. The duration of the FS can be altered.
Chorover and Schiller (1.103) found the avoidance and the effect of
ECS varied slightly as a direct function of FS duration.

The strength of conditioning can also be modified by
delaying FS after the step-through response (1.144, 1.147). In this
situation the disruptive effect of ECS was inversely related to the
strength of conditioning both in extent of RA and the interval
between training and ECS. A second FS produces greater conditioning
but an ECS following two FS's appeared to interfere with the retention
of the second FS only (1.139).

The amnesic gradient varies with the degree of water
deprivation in an appetitively motivated task (1.156). Under some
conditions the gradient for appetitively motivated tasks is shorter
than for aversively motivated learning (1.155).

Several studies indicate that the amnesic gradient is
influenced by the subject's familiarity with the training apparatus
prior to the training and amnesic treatment. In several instances
prior habituation was found to shorten the gradient (1.72, 1.74,
Miller and Misanin, 1969). Animals familiarized with the apparatus
without any conditioning failed to show any evidence of amnesia on
testing after one learning trial even when the ECS delay was as short
as 0.5 seconds. Whereas, if the animals were naive, they showed
amnesia with a 5 second interval. It was thought possible that
familiarization increases the aversive effects of ECS (1.74). The
extent of the familiarization, longer trials being more important
than the number, and the complexity of the task, influence the
interaction of ECS and prior familiarization (1.79).

Replications have failed to reproduce this effect (1.40,
1.115, Dawson and McGaugh, 1969c) and have indicated that under
some conditions familiarization may have no effect or may even
lengthen the amnesic gradient. It is possible that the effect of
prior familiarization varies with the task, procedures and species
used in the study as mentioned above. This leads to the general
observation that the amount of pretraining in the apparatus before
the conditioning trial (which varied in all experiments) may be an
important variable in consolidation times.

Events between Learning and ECS

Numerous recent findings show that the effectiveness of
an amnesic treatment depends on the events or conditions during the
interval between training and treatment. Detention in the apparatus

(1.110   1.137, 1.138, 1.146), socially facilitated exploratory
sessions (1.142) or a flashing light (1.76) between the learning and
the ECS increased the amnesic effects of ECS. In mice and in fish
the amnesic gradient is lengthened if the animals are retained in the
experimental apparatus after training (1.110, 1.137, 1.138, 1.146).
These results suggest that the onset of consolidation is 'triggered'
by some critical change in stimulation. Another possible interpretation is that the detention increases the animals' susceptibility
to the amnesic treatment. That is, the effect might be comparable to
that of increasing the intensity and duration of the amnesic treatment or of decreasing the time interval between training and ECS.
However, there was amnesia from detention alone which may mean that
the strength of learning was diminished. The amnesic effect of ECS
can be influenced by events occurring between the conditioning
trial and ECS and may also be influenced by procedural variables
such as handling and where the animal is kept.

Learning Task Variables

        The task used in ECS studies also introduces variability
into consolidation times. The tasks generally used are passive
avoidance including operant conditioning, active avoidance and
discriminated avoidance,all usually involving shock as the negative
reinforcer, and appetitively motivated tasks.

        Passive Avoidance - Some of the PA responses can be established
in one trial, the one-trial PA learning tasks frequently employed are
the step-down and step-through procedures with rats and mice and the
inhibition of pecking with chickens. All involve the passive
avoidance of a punishing stimulus. In the step-down procedure, the
animal is placed on a small platform a few inches above a grid floor.
The animal usually steps down from the platform within a few seconds,
where-upon it can be given a strong footshock through the grid floor.
When tested 24 hours later, the animal will be much slower to descend
than an animal not punished when it stepped down on the learning trial.

        In a stepthrough procedure, the animal is placed in a small
compartment leading through into a larger one. When the animal promptly
steps through into the second compartment it can be given a FS. One
variable here is apparently the direction the animal is facing when
it is placed in the first compartment (1.178).

        The inhibition of pecking task in chickens involves the
avoidance of pecking at a target to which it would peck before by
coating the target with an aversive chemical - methylanthranilate
(Lee-Teng et al 1.162-1.172).

        If operant conditioning of licking for water or bar
pressing in a skinner box is punished by a single shock, the learned
response is a suppression of licking or bar pressing. Operant

conditioning of a bar pressing habit has been investigated using
different schedules of reinforcement in the original acquisition of
the response. Rats have been trained on either a continuous
reinforcement schedule (CRF), a fixed ratio schedule (FR) or a
variable ratio (VR) schedule (1.70, 1.240, 1.242) and then given 1
learning trial where the rat was punished by a footshock or bar
shock for pressing the bar. ECS 10 seconds after the shock resulted
in amnesia for the habit 24 hours later only for the CRF trained
animals. Young and Day (1.243) found amnesia with both CRF and FR
schedules but the RA was only temporary, there was no amnesia 10 days
after learning. Amnesia for the extinction of a bar pressing habit
has been seen (1.150). ECS treatment between events intended for
association, between the CS and UCS, affects learning in a similar
way to ECS given after the association (1.222, 1.223, 1.224, 1.225).

In passive avoidance tasks amnesia is indicated by
continued positive responding and not by the omission of behaviour.
In these situations, if ECS halted a CER, the increase in mobility
would look like amnesia; whereas if the ECS was producing competing
responses such as freezing, it would cause an apparent increase in
learning. Similarly, the effects of FS alone would show up in the
opposite direction.

Active Avoidance - In active avoidance tasks more extensive
training is usually required to establish the response. There are
some active avoidance tasks requiring only one trial (1.31, 1.95,
1.219, 1.229). The apparatus consists of a shuttle box arrangement
of two compartments. The animal is given a FS in the compartment in
which it is placed and it either escapes into the second compartment
on receiving the FS or learns to avoid the FS by association of a
CS paired with the FS by running into the second compartment on
presentation of the CS.

In this active avoidance situation, the effect of ECS on
a CER or competing response would induce opposite effects on
performance from those seen in passive avoidance situations.
Competing responses produced by the ECS would produce apparent
amnesia, whereas any increases in activity from halting of a CER
would appear as learning.

Carew (1.219) measured passive and active avoidance
responses in the same apparatus, in both step-down and step-through
situations. In both tasks, most of the same animals which gave
evidence of RA as assessed by a PA measure gave no memory deficit
when an AA criterion was used. If discrimination, in the chosen
locus of the response is observed at the same time as latencies are
measured many animals judged amnesic by step-down or step-through
latencies actually do exhibit memory of the FS.

Discriminated Avoidance - Thus passive and active avoidance
learning situations seem to be unsuitable for testing the effects
of ECS on memory because of the confounding influence of FS, CER
and competing responses. Discriminated avoidance conditioning
techniques, where the response choice provides a relatively
unequivocal indicator of retained information, and a distinction is
made between retention and performance, are to be preferred.
Temporally ungraded effects of ECS on response choice were found
when ECS was given at relatively long intervals after learning
(1.119, 1.190) where the effect could be on the CER, however when
ECS was given at intervals less than 100 sec (1.189) or less than
30 sec (1.119) temporally graded effects were found.

Appetitive Learning - The various alternative interpretations
offered to explain the results of experiments showing retroactive
interference of ECS with learning have been primarily based on
aversive learning situations. Aversive effects, competing responses,
reduction of the fear component of CER and the incubation
explanations all apply to aversive conditioning. These problems
have led to the use of one trial appetitively motivated tasks. The
finding that ECS also interferes with performance in this situation
lends support to the idea that ECS can interfere with the
consolidation of memory.

In an experimental situation where either positive or
negative reinforcement could be given, Herz (1.155) found temporally
graded deficits in retention produced by ECS in both cases.
Quartermain et al (1.23) found a similar temporal gradient of RA
with both positive and negative reinforcement in the T-maze. It was
suggested that as the type of reinforcement here was not the major
determinant of the slope of the temporal gradient, it is likely that
the nature of the task is.

The results do not appear to be interpretable in terms of
ECS-produced fear or conditioned inhibition, both explanations would
predict that ECS would have the same effect on performance in
appetitive and aversive conditioning situations.

Multiple Trials

Further complications arise when more than one trial is
used in the original learning, with only one ECS treatment.

Multitrial experiments have shown a greater deficit in
retention after ECS when massed rather than spaced trials are given
(1.14, 1.106) and the amount of fixation occurring within a session
increases with the spacing between trials. This could be
particularly relevant to the schedules used in experiments employing
the skinner box even though only one FS is used (1.70, 1.240, 1.243).

Multitrial learning tasks involve the problem of not knowing how much consolidation occurs during training. A retention deficit has been found after an ECS 12 or 30 seconds after one trial, but no deficit when given at the same time after a second trial which followed the first (1.90, 1.105).

The number of trials also influences consolidation (1.15, 1.182). Burešová, Bureš and Gerbrandt (1.60) giving reversal training 1 hour or 24 hours after original training and ECS after reversal training only found amnesia with the long interval and a slight amnesia for the short interval. With overtraining on the original habit there was amnesia for the reversal at both intervals.

Measure of Retention

In passive avoidance tasks, the criterion of learning, that is, the maximum latency allowed during the test trial to make a response, determines to a large part the apparent training-ECS interval at which ECS ceases to be effective. The findings of Schneider et al (1.143) indicate that the gradient obtained in any study depends on the criterion used as evidence of retention. Rats were given a simple training trial on a step-down passive avoidance task, followed by an ECS treatment and a single retention test. When they were permitted a maximum of 30 seconds to respond on the retention test, the gradient was short; that is, many animals given ECS appeared to remember the punished response and did not step down. However, when the maximum latency permitted was 600 seconds, amnesia was seen even in rats given ECS 6 hours after training; that is, many of the animals responded after 30 seconds but within 600 seconds. This result helps to explain the variations in the amnesic gradient. Studies using short maximum response latencies on the retention test have typically shown short gradients (1.103), whereas studies in which long gradients were obtained have typically employed long maximum response latencies on the retention tests (1.129). Using a high cut-off latency score, ECS was found to be effective even if given 23 hours after training when tested 1 week later (1.145). Therefore, the short intervals reported for consolidation may simply result from a procedure too insensitive to demonstrate behavioural effects at longer ECS delay intervals.

Other recent data suggest that evidence of amnesia following ECS may depend on the response used as an index of retention. These studies have looked at autonomic responses. For example, if changes in heart rate are used as an index of learning, ECS may produce no amnesia (1.75, 1.123, 1.248), even when the same animals give responses indicating amnesia for inhibitory avoidance (1.26) or classically conditioned motor response (1.248). It was suggested that ECS produced amnesia for a punished response, whereas changes in heart rate indicated that the animals had learned to fear the apparatus. It may be that the consolidation rate is faster for fear

than it is for association of fear with specific cues. Or it may
be that with the procedures used (transpinneal ECS) the ECS was less
effective in disrupting activity in structures involved in retention
of nonspecific fear than in the structures involved in controlling
the overt inhibitory-avoidance response. Such an argument implies
that different aspects of learning may be mediated by different
neural structures (McGaugh and Herz, 1972). However there is
evidence of RA for heart-rate responses (1.111, 1.183, 1.246)

Task Complexity

In tasks where choices rather than latencies are reported,
task complexity seems to affect the longest ECS-delay interval which
produces retention deficits (1.79). Spatial discrimination tasks
have the shortest ECS delay intervals where ECS becomes ineffective
(1.61, 1.108, 1.120) followed by tasks involving brightness
discrimination (1.108, 1.189) and then by patterned discrimination
as the task with the longest interval (1.10). Additional evidence
linking task difficulty with retention deficits induced by post-
training ECS was reported by Thompson (1.15). Increasing the number
of trials to criterion in a multiple trial task results in more RA
(1.158). Therefore, the simpler or the shorter the task, the
shorter is the consolidation time where an ECS becomes ineffective.

Other Characteristics of Retrograde Amnesia

Permanence of RA

When ECS after training eliminates any sign of the learned
behaviour 24 hours later, it is generally considered that the memory
has been abolished permanently. This is what could be expected if
ECS disrupts or destroys the neural processes essential for the
establishment of a permanent memory trace. Conversely, if amnesic
treatments interfere with other memory processes, such as those
involved in retrieval, then the amnesia need not be permanent. It
is possible for treatments to produce temporary amnesias; this is a
common occurrence with mild concussion in human patients. However,
if all retrograde amnesia is only temporary, then it cannot be due to
interference with memory-storage processes. Thus the issue of
permanence is critical to any interpretation of experimentally
induced retrograde amnesia.

Retrograde amnesia seems to be permanent at least up to
42 days in experiments where the animals are only tested once (1.34,
1.43, 1.90, 1.102, 1.121, 1.148, 1.151, 1.153, 1.178, 1.180, 1.181,
1.209) and in some experiments with repeated testing (1.34, 1.43,
1.135, 1.139, 1.148, 1.151, 1.180, 1.185).

There have been reports of varying degrees of recovery from
RA following ECS; however most of these have involved repeated

testing of the same subjects (1.27, 1.121, 1.153, 1.193, 1.203, 1.214, 1.243). Recovery, if and when it occurs, might depend on repeated reexposure to the testing situation. However, in an adequate test for recovery animals that have been tested repeatedly must be compared with animals tested for the first time at the same interval after ECS that the repeatedly tested animals received their last test. The strength of learning also seems an important condition for recovery. Amnesia is temporary if conditioning is strong but permanent if conditioning is weak (1.90, 1.139). It may be that under some conditions ECS produced incomplete interference with memory storage, and that partial storage provides a basis for at least some recovery. This hypothesis is suggested by Pagano et al (1.209) who found that rats given low intensity ECS recovered from amnesia within 24 hours, whereas those given high intensity ECS showed no recovery even 48 hours after training and ECS treatment. Herz and Peeke (1.153) suggest that the recovery from amnesia seen after repeated testing may not be 'true' recovery but due to extinction or adaptation and habituation. With an appetitive situation, the changes in responding were in the opposite direction to that predicted by recovery. Habituation has been shown to occur in the step-through situation and ECS was effective in disrupting this as well as interfering with recall for the passive avoidance response (1.176, 1.179).

An alternative explanation for recovery from ECS-induced RA comes from the idea that if ECS only arrests trace formation rather than destroying it, the residual memory may either continue consolidating or add up. This is supported by the findings of Pagano et al (1.209) mentioned above and those of Mah et al (1.220, 1.221). Cherkin (1969) suggested that a submaximal ECS may slow but not completely stop consolidation. It has generally been assumed that retention tested 24 hours after ECS provides a measure of the consolidation achieved at the time ECS was administered. If however, some consolidation has continued to occur between ECS and the time of testing, then this will lead to an over-estimation of the amount of consolidation that occurred prior to the ECS. That there is some residual memory seems possible because there is always some interval between ECS and learning even if it is very small. So repeated testing may reinforce any residual memory. This idea is supported by the observations of Lee-Teng and Sherman (1.163) and others (1.31, 1.119, 1.120, 1.157, 1.197, 1.211) where with repeated ECS-learning treatments, the animals do eventually learn. It is suggested that there is a partial consolidation with each treatment and that these accumulate.

McGaugh and Herz (1972) conclude that it is premature to discard completely any of the theories concerning the permanence or recovery with ECS-produced amnesia or to state unequivocally that amnesic effects are due to interference with storage versus retrieval processes. Although it is likely that some instances of

recovery can be accounted for in terms of incomplete interference
with consolidation processes, we have not yet identified the
variables responsible for transience when recovery is obtained.
Even so, the numerous studies showing amnesia to be stable over
fairly long intervals do indicate that under some, if not most,
conditions the memory loss is permanent. This, of course, is all
that is required by the most general form of the consolidation
hypotheses.

Reactivation of the Memory Trace

        The permanence of ECS-induced amnesia has also been
challenged by several experiments which have shown that, by
appropriate means, memories lost after ECS can be restored. These
experiments attempt to show that arousal or 'reactivation' of the
memory trace can influence amnesia.

        There are two types of experiments; firstly, animals are
given the learning trial followed by an ECS and amnesia is seen 24
hours later. However, if a non-contingent footshock is presented
before the retention test, amnesia is not seen (1.25, 1.71, 1.94,
1.241). It was concluded that if a reminder of the learning is given
the memory can return and retrieval is possibly prevented by ECS.
A retention test prior to the reminder shock appears to be necessary
(1.25). The 'arousal' could be related to autonomic responses
produced by the reminder shock (1.26). It has been shown with two
FS-ECS treatments that although there was no memory left after the
first treatment, there was considerable retention after the second
(1.163, 1.211).

        The second type of experiment involves learning followed
by the ECS treatment 24 hours later. ECS at this time will not
produce amnesia unless arousal is reinstated by presentation of a
conditioned stimulus or non-contingent footshock (NCFS) 0.5 seconds
before the ECS (1.73, 1.83, 1.84, 1.85, 1.139). This was also the
case with ECS 30 seconds or 6 hours after learning provided the
NCFS treatment was 0.5 seconds before the ECS. NCFS 30 seconds
before the ECS was ineffective (1.139). In another experiment it
was found that a NCFS given 1 minute before training interfered
with performance (1.140). If this pretreatment was followed in
0.5 seconds by an ECS, this interference did not occur whereas it
did with ECS 30 seconds after the FS, indicating the same type of
temporal gradient as is seen in more conventional retroactive
procedures. It was suggested that ECS affects recently retrieved
memory as well as recently acquired memory (1.73, 1.83, 1.84, 1.85).

        However, these findings have not yet been confirmed in
other investigations (1.39, 1.168, 1.208, 1.220). Miller and
Springer (1.83, 1.84, 1.85) have pointed out that this recovery is

difficult to obtain and they have found it necessary to manipulate both the intensity and duration of the recovery agent in order to successfully obtain recovery of memory. However, when it does occur the reminder phenomenon is robust.

It has been suggested that the footshock given in an inhibitory avoidance task may have some effect on the amnesic qualities of ECS. There have been several attempts to account for the variation in results of ECS treatments in terms of modification of different aspects of neural activity. Chorover and DeLuca (1.107) for example, found that the pattern of brain seizures recorded from the cortex of rats is markedly influenced by a footshock administered prior to ECS treatment. They suggested that the modification in seizure pattern was due to the arousal produced by the footshock, and that it is "possible that the numerous apparent differences in the temporal characteristics of ECS-induced RA might actually reflect differences in the state of arousal at equivalent FS-ECS intervals in different experiments". (Chorover and DeLuca, 1969, p.148).

More recently Carew (1.219) has suggested that the ECS parameters used by Chorover and DeLuca (current intensity and duration) were near the threshold for producing brain seizures. At the threshold a footshock does attenuate seizures. However, as the ECS current level is increased the attenuating effect of footshock decreases, and at higher ECS intensities only normal ECoG seizure records are obtained. Thus the conclusions of Chorover and DeLuca may apply only to studies using ECS current that is near the brain-seizure threshold and in which ECS follows the footshock by a few seconds. Gold and McGaugh (1972) have found that the severity of the behavioural convulsion was attenuated by administering a footshock prior to the cortical stimulation. However, the footshock did not attenuate the cortical seizure activity.

Time of Testing and Short-Term Memory

The experimental findings reviewed so far suggest that there are at least two distinct stages in memory storage. The first stage (commonly called short-term memory) involves the formation of a template of some sort that may provide a basis for the changes involved in the permanent storage of information. It is this stage of memory that is somehow susceptible to interference produced by ECS. The long-term memory storage is invulnerable to interference by ECS .

The question arises as to how the ECS treatment is having its effect in interfering with the formation of long-term memory. If ECS is interfering or destroying the short-term memory trace, so there is nothing left for consolidation into long-term storage, it would be predicted that there would be no memory for the learning

after the ECS treatment. However, if it was just preventing the
consolidation of the short-term trace into long-term memory there
can be memory present for some short time after the treatment.

        Geller and Jarvik (1.136) found that when an ECS was
given after learning in a passive avoidance task, performance levels
were high on a retention test 1 hour after training, but gradually
deteriorated over 6 hours and there was complete amnesia at 24 hours.
Animals given ECS alone showed the effect of the treatment to be in
the opposite direction to FS alone. Geller and Jarvik suggested that
the ECS may be acting on the formation of a long term process rather
than affecting short-term memory. However, in a similar experimental
situation Ray and Barrett (1.178) report that this decrease in
retention with time following the ECS is due to the proactive effects
of ECS on responding as ECS alone induced decreasing latencies over
8 hours in their experiment. There is a procedural difference between
these two experiments - Ray and Barrett showed that Geller and Jarvik's
results could be obtained if the animal was placed in the step-through
apparatus facing toward the second compartment rather than away from
it as in their experiment. It has been shown that after ECS (1.100);
FS (1.140) or FS and ECS (1.151) that latencies are high immediately
following these treatments but approach control values over a few
hours after treatment. So the time of testing, although usually 24
hours, must be greater than 8 hours to avoid proactive effects of
ECS. Therefore there is no evidence of whether the ECS is interrupting or destroying a short-term trace or preventing its consolidation.
A study by Bovet et al (1.210) using multitrial learning with ECS
after each training session showed that analysis of the learning
curves within each session enables a distinction to be made between
the effects of ECS on short-term memory and consolidation processes
between two consecutive sessions. There was an improvement within
sessions but very little sessions with the ECS treated groups
compared with controls.

        Recently, McGaugh and Landfield (1.50) found that if the
ECS treatment was given 20 seconds after training, there was
retention of the memory 1 hour later, but amnesia subsequently
developed and there was no retention at 6 or 24 hours. Whereas, if
the treatment was closer to the learning trial (8 seconds) the
amnesia appeared earlier and there was no retention at 1 hour. These
results are difficult to interpret in terms of any non-specific
consequences of footshock and/or ECS treatments. They suggest that
a critical memory process develops within less than one minute
following training but that with ECS treatment the development of
this process (short-term memory?) is not sufficient for the
development of long-term memory. The ECS treatment was either
destroying the short-term trace or hastening its decay. This latter
idea of ECS hastening the decay of short-term memory is further
supported by the work of Miller and Springer (1.81) where the decay
of short-term retention was faster than that reported by McGaugh and

Landfield (1.50). There was retention at 15 minutes when ECS
followed immediately after the single training trial but no
retention at 30 minutes. They included a control group which
indicated that the phenomenon was not a systemic effect caused by
the interaction of footshock and ECS.

Lee-Teng (1.165, 1.170, 1.172) with ECS or SCC given
immediately after learning, has also shown retention shortly after,
which then decays. This is separable from the effects of the
aversive stimulus and the ECS. In addition, she showed that if the
shock treatment was delayed for 1 minute, there was substantial
retention at 30 minutes which increased to an asymptotic level by 1
hour. The phase 1 or short-term memory is immune or only partially
susceptible to current disruption and lasts for at least 30
minutes. Phase 2 or long-term memory storage is induced within
seconds after training, but its trace formation is a long process
involving several stages; only the beginning stage is current-
disruptable, but this phase of memory is not expressed until the
entire process is complete (1.170, 1.172).

These findings suggest that short-term memory may persist
for a short time following an amnesic treatment. This is supported
by the findings reported in the section on antibiotics. The major
question is whether such evidence indicates that the short-term
memory trace is temporary and whether it is influenced by the
amnesic agents. It has been suggested that ECS may act merely to
hasten forgetting rather than to prevent storage (Deutsch, 1969,
in McGaugh and Dawson, 1971). Such an interpretation is difficult
to accept because all animals do not reach the same level of
amnesia; in other words, the degree of forgetting eventually
attained decreased as the time between the training and the amnesic
treatment increases (McGaugh and Dawson, 1971). In addition,
Barondes and Cohen (8.51) have suggested that it is possible to
restart storage processes by giving a variety of additional treatments, but only if the treatments are given within a few hours
following training. The effect is graded - the effectiveness in
restarting storage processes decreases with time of administration
of the second treatment. It would appear to be very difficult to
interpret such effects without assuming at least two memory
processes, short-term and long-term memory.

Conclusions

After reviewing the experiments there is no doubt that
ECS given after a learning task has a retrograde amnesic effect and
no experiment contradicts this. Nothing so far makes it necessary
to reject the consolidation hypothesis of memory formation and there
is no better theory to put in its place. Experiments designed
expressly to provide evidence in support of the alternative views
have ultimately resulted in further support for the consolidation

interpretation of memory formation. However, in any particular
experiment it is not possible to account for the duration of
retrograde amnesia by the effect of ECS on the physical state of the
memory store. There is no single gradient of retrograde amnesia.
The retrograde amnesia curves are interference curves or curves of
susceptibility, not of consolidation and at best they provide only
indirect measures of memory storage processes. Behavioural or
procedural variables can be shown to have as strong or a stronger
influence on the duration of susceptibility of memories to ECS
than does the postulated time dependent change in the nature of the
memory. ECS and the events surrounding its administration have
stimulus value and learning in relation to this is as important as
learning in relation to a milder aversant stimulus such as a shock
to the feet. The nature of the acquired response to ECS whether a
CER that induces freezing or any other change in reactivity of the
animals, then interact with the behavioural test used and may show
up as an apparent increase or decrease in memory retention depending upon whether a passive or active avoidance task is used. Much
of the confounding may be eliminated by the use of a discriminated
avoidance but already the task may need more trials particularly if
an active response is required, and the time dependence between
learning and ECS becomes blurred. Not only that but the criterion
of learning has a strong effect on the apparent duration of amnesia
and this effect will depend on the difficulty of the discrimination
chosen. Absolute values of consolidation time therefore have very
little significance as to the kinetics of the consolidation process
since behavioural matters are so powerful in influencing the results.
In order to eliminate the various complications that have so far
been discovered several kinds of behavioural experiments must be
performed together using the same animal strain with the same ECS
treatment and this is apparent in the more recent papers. Ideally
a discriminated avoidance task of variable difficulty should be
responded to both actively and passively. This should be
contrasted with the effects on the same discriminations made in an
appetitive situation and then the ECS intensity should be varied
systematically for different learning-treatment intervals.

       As it becomes clearer how to design these experiments it
becomes less and less clear why they should be done. A series which
covers the behavioural and procedural variables will yield a family
of curves of retrograde amnesia each of which will be shaped by the
consolidation process and by certain of the behavioural effects of
a particular experiment. Whether, after the labour required to
produce such a family of curves, it would be possible to separate
out the curve attributable only to consolidation is by no means
certain. Yet this is the only reason for embarking on such
experiments, for there seems to be no purely psychological issue to
be solved by the use of ECS, although many points of psychological
interest have emerged from the behavioural analysis necessary for
these experiments. It would be difficult to justify continuation

of the crude ECS technique even if a true consolidation curve could be obtained since we are still ignorant of the crucial aspect of ECS necessary for amnesia. Passing large currents through the brain may act directly on biochemical brain processes required for memory formation or the action may be on the organisation of perceptual, storage, classification or search procedures occurring at a higher organizational level but still being essential for memory formation. There is much to be done to find out which of the biological consequences of ECS are directly related to the psychological consequences of memory loss.

The main benefits of the very large amount of work that has been invested in these experiments are that the consolidation hypothesis has not had to be discarded, and that the understanding of the behavioural techniques necessary for the investigation of agents that destroy memory promises to be useful in the study of other more specific amnesic treatments.

EFFECT OF VARIOUS AGENTS ON ECS-INDUCED RETROGRADE AMNESIA

Electroconvulsive shock has been variously reported to reduce RNA levels and to increase the levels of transmitters in the brain. These reports have led to several ideas as to what the ECS is doing within the CNS.

1.   A reduction in levels of RNA in the brain has been reported to follow ECS. This has been shown by direct biochemical analysis (2.2, 2.3) and by drug effects on ECS-induced retrograde amnesia. Tricyanoaminopropine (TCAP), which increases RNA levels presumably by accelerating RNA synthesis, protects against ECS-induced RA (2.2, 2.8), orotic acid, a RNA precursor, protects against ECS-induced RA presumably via some changes in the central nucleotide and/or RNA metabolism (2.16). Mg pemoline also protects against ECS-induced RA (2.14), and has also been reported to facilitate learning. It has been suggested that it increases RNA synthesis and acts as a mild stimulant.

These drugs, by producing an increase in RNA synthesis, overcome the reduction in RNA levels caused by the ECS and so prevent the occurrence of retrograde amnesia. However, there is at least one report (2.15) where TCAP did not alter either RNA levels or retrograde amnesia from ECS.

2.   ECS causes an increase in 5HT (serotonin) turnover time (2.3, 2.4, 2.5, 2.6, 2.7). Treatment with the serotonin precursor 5HTP before learning and ECS reduces the effect of the ECS in producing RA (2.3, 2.4). Likewise pretreatment with the stimulant of 5HT synthesis, pipradol also protects against ECS-induced RA (2.6).

The 5HT antagonists DBMC (2.3, 2.4) reserpine, (2.3) nialamide (2.6) amytriptyline (2.6) presumably by preventing the increase in 5HT by ECS, protect against ECS induced amnesia. p-Chlorophenylalanine, a drug shown to decrease regional brain concentrations of 5HT by 60% but having no effect on norepinephrine levels (2.17) protects against ECS-induced RA (2.4, 2.17). Treatment with nicotine also protected against ECS-induced RA (2.7).

5HT treated animals show highly impaired retention from post-training ECS, even when the shock treatment is given as long as 1 hour after training and showed an increase in whole brain 5HT concentration after ECS (2.3).

In a review of the work of his laboratory, Essman (1970) considers that 5HT plays an important role in the mediation of at least one phase of the memory consolidation process. The relationships between changes in this amine level and other events implicated in other phases of the memory consolidation process (RNA synthesis, protein synthesis and their inter-dependency) have been shown.

3.   ECS causes an increase in AChE activity and the release of bound ACh. Biochemical assay of AChE show an increase in activity after ECS (2.11). Essman (1972) determined ACh concentration at varying intervals following the administration of a single ECS to mice. There was a rapid, significant decrease in "bound" ACh within the first 10 min following ECS, contrasted with a more gradual decrease in "free" ACh. The "free" ACh reached pre-ECS base-line levels 2 hours following treatment, whereas the "bound" ACh, probably representing the labile and stable bound pools of this amine at the presynaptic nerve ending, remained decreased, even by 2 hours following a single treatment. Changes in the ACh concentration measured in a synaptosomal fraction from mouse cerebral cortex showed significant decreases in nerve ending ACh content, becoming apparent at 30 and 60 minutes following ECS, and persistent decreases were maintained for as long as 2 hours following treatment.

The anticholinergic drug scopolamine, protected against ECS induced RA when given before retention (2.11, 2.12, 3.13) and it had either no effect (2.12) or attenuated the ECS effect (2.10) when given before learning. Scopolamine given without ECS (2.12) before learning had a disruptive effect on retention.

The anticholinesterase drug eserine, when given before retention increased the ECS-induced RA (2.11) and physostigmine given before learning protected against ECS-induced RA (2.12). Physostigmine alone before retention had a disruptive effect on retention (2.12, 3.13).

Another report (2.18) claims that ECS-induced RA was not affected by physostigmine or scopolamine given at various times after learning.

Whether any of these drugs are having an effect on memory formation is extremely debatable. Considering some evidence shown in chapter 3 it seems more likely that they would have effects on the retrieval and expression of memory. There has also been consideration as to whether these drugs are producing state-dependent learning.

4.   ECS appears to provide an increase in synthesis and
utilization of norepinephrine (NE) in the brain (Essman, 1972).
An increase in NE turnover, with increased tyrosine hydroxylase
concentrations, the enzyme responsible for the rate limiting step in
NE synthesis, has been reported following ECS treatment (2.13).
Essman (2.5) found that brain NE level was not consistently altered
by electroshock, nor was the activity of brain monoamine oxidase
affected.

          Levels of other biogenic amines - dopamine and histamine
are increased following ECS (Essman, 1972).

          There is no reliable basis for assuming that multiple ECS
treatments represent a succession of the same central biochemical
changes attending a single ECS (Essman, 1972) and many biochemical
or pharmacological studies on ECS effects tends to use multiple ECS
treatments presumably in order to obtain sufficient material for
analysis.

          Multiple ECS treatments appear to be accompanied by an
increase in blood-brain barrier permeability (see Essman, 1972).
However, there is one report where a single ECS treatment which did
result in amnesia produced no alteration of blood-brain barrier
permeability (1.225). Any alteration in the permeability of the
blood-brain barrier could be due to competition for central uptake
between exogenous molecules or to selective vascular effects which
may modify ionic barriers to molecular transport. If these changes
do occur which may be undetected pharmacologically with one treatment, there would be an alteration in energy metabolism as a result
of such a change.

          Increased neuronal activity necessitates an increased
metabolic rate. Energy stores would be used up during the
convulsive activity associated with the ECS and would lead to a
decrease in ATP levels, glycogen and glucose levels in the brain.
These changes have been reported following ECS treatments and occur
also in the presence of anaesthesia preventing the overt convulsion
(Essman, 1972). In view of the variety of alterations in brain
energy metabolism resulting from ECS, it is not unexpected that
macromolecular changes and alterations in the content and metabolsim
of the brain biogenic amines may also be observed.

          As already mentioned, ECS appears to lead to a reduction
in RNA content of the brain, and as protein synthesis is intimately
linked with RNA, one would expect subsequent changes in proteins.

          The participation of brain proteins in the changes
induced by ECS has been considered in several studies. The issue of
brain proteins and their synthesis in relation to ECS probably holds
a significance for cognitive and informational processes similar to

that of nucleic acids in the brain, especially in view of the many
studies which have interrupted memory formation by the inhibition
of protein synthesis. Unfortunately, many of the studies of protein
synthesis and turnover in the brain have used multiple ECS rather
than single ECS, or titrating the effects of successive treatments.
Changes in protein synthesis in ECS in rabbits have been described
(Vesco and Giuditta, 1968). Ribosome and polysome numbers were
estimated in the cerebral cortex of rabbits immediately after the
last of six successive ECS treatments at 12-15 minute intervals.
The number of free ribosomes was increased by approximately 80%,
accompanied by a comparable decrease in the population of polysomes
as a consequence of the ECS treatment regimen. This strongly
implicates protein synthesis in the cerebral cortex as responsive
to either the direct effects of ECS or following the consequence of
such treatment on other brain substrates.

        The turnover of brain protein in rat brain was considered
following a course of ten ECS-induced seizures at two per day
(Minard and Richter, 1968). The labelling of protein and nucleic
acid fractions with glucose-^{14}C was only slightly and insignificantly
decreased. Decreases in the specific activity of protein-bound
glutamate in relation to aspartate in the total protein fraction of
ECS-treated animals suggested a rapid turnover of protein in response
to ECS. Relevant to the problem of changes in protein synthesis in
the brain with ECS is the rapidity with which changes in the
synthesis follow an electrically induced seizure. Essman (1972) has
observed that ECS induces a rapid decrease in protein.synthesis,
measured as differences in the rate of incorporation of labelled
amino acids into brain proteins between ECS and sham-treated mice.
The extent of the inhibition on whole brain incorporation produced
by ECS occurs as a function of time after ECS. A single ECS exerts
its most pronounced effects on protein synthesis within the first
30 minutes of treatment. By 1 hour after ECS there was no persisting
inhibitory effects, at least from a single seizure. From the
investigation into subcellular fractions of the mouse brain at 15
minutes post-ECS treatment, the most marked effects of ECS appear
in the cerebral cortex with the presynaptic endings (synaptosomes)
and mitochondria accounting for the greater portion of protein
synthesis and its inhibition.

        Other studies using a single ECS treatment have also shown
an inhibitory effect on incorporation of labelled amino acid into
proteins (Dunn, 1971, Dunn et al, 1971, 1.57). Cotman et al 1.57)
have reported a significant but short lasting inhibition of brain
protein synthesis and an increase in the amount of free leucine by
electroshock at intensities above the brain seizure threshold.
However they concluded that ECS induced RA was not likely to be due
to the inhibition of the protein synthesis per se but that brain
seizures and inhibition of protein synthesis are signs that the co-
ordinated function of the cells of the brain is altered by ECS to

such a degree that processes involved in memory storage are
disrupted.

In view of the multiple effects reported for ECS, whether
any of these effects are associated with the amnesia from ECS
cannot be concluded on the present evidence. In fact, even whether
these proposed changes have anything to do with the basis of memory
formation and consolidation can be debated.

TRANSMITTERS

Experiments with anticholinergic and anticholinesterase drugs led to the hypothesis that after a learning experience there is a gradual change in the level of transmitter released at a synapse during transmission. The level of ACh would be high immediately after learning during temporary storage and rapidly decline to a low point from which it would slowly increase to a new higher level underlying long-term storage (3.11, 3.13). (For a review see Deutsch, 1971).

Anticholinesterase Drugs

Di-isopropyl fluorophosphate (DFP) and physostigmine (PS) block synaptic transmission by increasing ACh levels when synaptic conductance is high. Whereas at low levels of synaptic conductance, they would facilitate transmission by preventing ACh destruction and thus aid the depolarization of the post synaptic membrane. It was shown that anticholinesterases, if administered just before the test trials, have little or no effect soon after learning but cause a deficit in relearning as the synaptic conductance improves with time (3.3, 3.8, 3.9, 3.24, 3.25,). Variations in experimental procedure were interpreted on the basis of this hypothesis. When a control animal has forgotten the task due to a lowering of synaptic conductance, anticholinesterases will produce a facilitation of relearning due to increasing the effective levels of ACh (3.5, 3.9). Altering task difficulty, the amount of training or spacing the trials will result in different amounts of learning and different synaptic conductance. The effect of DFP with undertrained habits, difficult tasks or spaced trials will be to facilitate the relearning at a time when overtraining, simple tasks or massed trials are impaired (3.4, 3.5, 3.6, 3.10). Massed trials are considered to lead to an accumulation of transmitter. The amnesic effect of DFP is only temporary, diminishing as the injection-test interval is increased, agreeing with the idea that amnesia is due to a synaptic block (3.3).

Puromycin, which is known to produce retrograde amnesia has many indirect effects on various biochemical systems. It has

been suggested that, as it effects the ACh-ChE balance in chick
embryo culture (Burkhalter, 1963) puromycin could be exerting its
effect on memory by altering the ACh-ChE balance. This idea led
to Deutsch's experiments. With puromycin in the same experimental
procedure, an increase in retention was seen at 3 days as with DFP
(3.4).

Anticholinergic Drugs

An anticholinergic drug, in reducing the amount of
transmitter that can combine with receptors, would be expected to
have most effect on retention when an anticholinesterase has no
effect - when conductance is low; and no effect when conductance
is high and an anticholinesterase produces a deficit in retention.
Scopolamine, therefore, should produce a slight retrograde amnesia
immediately after learning, complete amnesia at an intermediate
time and no deficit later when DFP and PS had no effect (3.7, 3.9,
3.21, 3.25).

Deutsch has concluded that "taken together, these results
give strong support to the notion that the physiological basis of
memory is a synaptic change" (3.9). However, these experiments are
not looking at retrograde amnesia in the classical sense but at
performance variables in the development of memories. One problem
of using drugs like these is that they are not necessarily selective
for neurones recently involved in memory and surely must have an
action on all neurones in the brain.

Weiss and Heller (1969) have criticised the experiments
of Deutsch et al on the grounds of their use of a single dose level.
The anticholinergic drugs tend to have differential effects related
to dose. However, Squire, Glick and Goldfarb (3.25) have varied the
dose of PS and of scopolamine and found a normal dose response
relationship to retention.

Levels of ACh

Slater (3.19), in order to see if the amnesic properties
of scopolamine were correlated with the reduction of brain ACh known
to occur with scopolamine (3.1) gave 3 other drugs known to reduce
ACh levels in the same situation. These did not produce amnesia,
tending to rule out the possibility that the amnesic effects of
scopolamine are due to reduced levels of brain ACh.

Performance and State-Dependent Learning

When administered before learning scopolamine has been
shown to produce state-dependent learning as well as impaired
acquisition (3.20). Although other reports claim no dissociation

of learning (3.2, 3.15, 3.16, 3.17, 3.21) two of these also report impaired acquisition (3.2, 3.17). This suggests that the drugs are having an effect on performance, which would not be unexpected. Performance effects have been seen in the rate of spontaneous alternation (Squire, 1969).

Central and Peripheral Effects

Various experiments claim that the drugs used to produce amnesia are having no peripheral effect on performance (3.2, 3.16, 3.28) judged by the administration of related compounds known to have only peripheral or peripheral and central effects. The former drugs did not produce amnesia. However, it is likely that physostigmine does have peripheral as well as central actions because it was antagonized by methscopolamine (3.25) and the drugs do affect performance (3.28).

There is some reservation about the attempt to correlate with specific memory functions, substances which have as general a distribution as the acetylcholine system. There is no doubt that these substances are somehow involved in the nature of nerve transmission, but it would be useful to distinguish this from more specific functions dealing with memory storage and retrieval. AChE activity has not yet been shown to be intimately related in a specific manner to learning. In addition, the distinction must be kept in mind between peripheral and central effects, dose-response effects, problems of tolerance and sensitization and strain and species differences, as well as various procedural problems. The side effects of drugs may interfere with the learning process.

Also, particularly with experiments on inhibition of AChE there is the problem that much of brain cholinesterase is inside neurones and probably not directly concerned with transmitter action and perhaps does not even have ACh as its main natural substrate. The role of ACh as a principal central transmitter working in a manner analogous to the skeletal neuromuscular junction is by no means accepted by neurophysiologists (Silver, 1967; 1971; Kasa, 1971).

Catecholamines and 5 hydroxytryptamine

Following the discovery of the wide cortical projection of noradrenergic neurones in the mammalian central nervous system by the fluorescence histochemistry of Falck and Hillarp, it was suggested that this system might be used in learning, either as a reinforcement mechanism or to modify neuronal metabolism in some appropriate way (Kety, 1970). This idea was backed up by the finding that compounds which had profound effects on mood in man also altered levels of biogenic amines in the brain of experimental

animals. Furthermore, agents like electroconvulsive shock which
were effective against memory increased levels of 5HT and
catecholamines in the brain. More detailed analysis of the effect
on norepinephrine metabolism showed an increase in both synthesis
and utilization of norepinephrine following ECS (Essman, 1972).

The results of early experiments on the effects of
altered biogenic amine metabolism on learning are not clear.
Chlorpromazine had no effect (3.20) on retention when given 30
minutes before testing (3.34). Amphetamine produces behavioural
excitement (e.g. 3.33) which makes learning experiments difficult,
but it has been shown to counteract the amnesic action of
scopolamine (3.1). Reserpine, which depletes catecholamine
containing neurons of their transmitters produced a loss of savings
on retest in a shuttle box when given 1 minute but not 24 hours
after learning, an effect that was counteracted by supplying excess
DOPA (3.33). DOPA alone has been found to enhance acquisition of
an avoidance response in fish. However, when Pargyline is used to
prevent the breakdown in norepinephrine, responses acquired under
the drug were not apparent on retest (3.31). Inhibition of
norepinephrine synthesis by diethyldithiocarbamate (DDC) given 30
minutes before learning (3.32) or immediately after learning (3.33)
impairs retention at 24 hours. However, in a strain of mice with
poor short term responsiveness (3.32) DDC 30 minutes before learning improved this even though retention from one to 24 hours was
reduced. DDC has large effects on reducing general activity and
if given 30 minutes before retest impairs performance (3.32). DDC
also has been reported to antagonize the amnesic effect of AXM
suggesting that AXM could act by reducing amine levels rather than
blocking protein synthesis (8.18, 8.19, 8.23). As with acetylcholine,
it is not yet clear what might be the true physiological role of
biogenic amines in the central nervous system. Recently it has
been proposed that adrenergic neurones in the cortex and
hypothalamus may innervate small arterioles, and perhaps this may
be their only function (Hartman, Zide and Udenfriend, 1972).
Compounds that interfere with amine metabolism may have their
behavioural action entirely through effects on the microcirculation
of the brain.

Note on the pharmacology of transmitter release

Even if a neuronal system using an identified transmitter
substance is uniquely involved in memory and not other functions of
the brain, it may be extremely difficult to alter such a system by
drug action. In peripheral synapses, such as the mammalian skeletal
neuromuscular junction, manoeuvres which liberate excess transmitter
are as liable to block by desensitization as to potentiate
transmission, in all but a very narrow dose range. Agents which
chronically block transmitter release soon have effects on the
sensitivity of the post synaptic membrane. Furthermore, at

peripheral adrenergic and cholinergic synapses, the release of
transmitter may affect the release of the same or different
transmitters from the same or adjacent presynaptic terminals. Thus
the release of norepinephrine may inhibit the further release from
the same terminals. (Enero, Langer, Rothlin and Stephano, 1972),
acetylcholine may facilitate or inhibit the release of
norepinephrine (Muscholl, 1970) and norepinephrine may facilitate
or inhibit the release of acetylcholine (Christ & Nishi, 1971).
Indeed, the systems of biochemical control and feedback that hedge
about the mechanisms of transmitter release seem to be too
complicated and unpredictable to be reliably manipulated by a
single pharmacological agent. Therefore, the action of such
compounds on behaviour and memory in particular is unlikely to have
a simple physiological explanation.

ANAESTHETICS, BARBITURATES, TRANQUILIZERS AND CONVULSANTS

Some of the experiments using anaesthetics or convulsants confirm that interruption of brain activity shortly after a learning experience impairs the retention of that experience.

Anaesthetics

Anaesthetics shown to be effective include ether (4.5-4.10, 4.23, 4.24, 4.27, 4.49, 4.50); carbon dioxide anaesthesia (4.3, 4.4, 4.21, 4.22, 4.28, 4.35, 4.48); halothane (4.17, 4.52, 4.55) and flurothyl anaesthesia (4.11, 4.18-4.20, 4.27). However, there have also been reports claiming that ether has no effect in producing amnesia when administered up to 5 minutes following learning (4.13, 4.14, 4.26, 4.29-4.31, 4.41, 4.49, 4.50). Part of the reason for conflicting results could be the effective dose of the anaesthetic agent, i.e. the partial pressure which is dependent on the temperature, the duration of exposure and the amount of anaesthetic (Cherkin, 1968; 4.3, 4.4, 4.18, 4.23, 4.27, 4.28). The consolidation times for the anaesthetic-sensitive mechanism appears to be of the order of 20 minutes (4.7, 4.8) whereas carbon dioxide anaesthesia gives a somewhat shorter consolidation time of about 5 minutes (4.28).

Barbiturates and Tranquilizers

The barbiturates, nembutal (4.1, 4.39) and thiopental (4.2),apparently do not produce amnesia, but pentobarbital has been reported both to impair (4.5, 4.7, 4.36) and not to impair retention (4.31, 4.51).

The tranquilizer, chlorpromazine (CPZ) has also been conflictingly reported to produce amnesia (4.16, 4.37, 4.38, 4.44-4.47) and not to produce amnesia (4.31, 4.37, 4.39). Ahmad and Achari (4.33) report that CPZ impairs learning, retrieval and consolidation, but that there was no permanent effect on the memory trace. The effect of CPZ given before learning appears to be due to an effect on acquisition, although this is not because of the state-dependent learning phenomenon (4.44-4.47). Because it was capable of producing amnesia if administered within 1 minute after learning, Johnson (4.45) concluded that CPZ impairs the consolidation of the short- to the long-term trace and also

that it impairs the short-term trace in such a way as to slow
down the extinction of learned avoidance responses.

Convulsants

The convulsant drug, pentylenetetrazol (metrazol)
likewise is controversial in its effect on retention (4.5, 4.7, 4.12,
4.32, 4.39, 4.40, 4.54) and seems to have an effect at relatively
long learning-treatment intervals (4.5, 4.7) similar to potassium
chloride in some cases.

Anaesthetics tend to give a distinctly earlier set of
temporal gradients of retrograde amnesia than do the protein
synthesis inhibitors and apparently longer than those obtained by
electro-convulsive shock. The relevant mode of action of these in
interrupting memory formation is unknown; they could be causing
spike activity perhaps like ECS preceding their anaesthetic
action, in which case a similar temporal gradient would be expected
or they could be affecting membrane structure in some way. Booth
(1970) has suggested that anaesthetics affect a non-electrical
membrane phenomenon associated with the beginning of the protein
synthesis process.

There is a considerable amount of controversy regarding
all these substances as to whether they are causing state-
dependent learning, facilitation of learning or retrograde amnesia.

With regard to the non-hydrogen bonding anaesthetics
mentioned here (carbon dioxide, halothane, diethyl ether), Porter
(1972) has offered an interpretation of their effects on memory
consolidation. This is based on their different excitant or
depressant actions in the CNS. "... for particular non-hydrogen
bonding anaesthetics, moderate retrograde excitation will enhance
memory consolidation, while either depression or severe excitation
will inhibit it. Prediction for anterograde treatment or treatment
throughout training is difficult in light of treatment effects on
input processes. This is particularly so in the case of excitation
which could conceivably interfere with or facilitate input and/or
memory processes" (Porter, 1972).

This notion could account for the conflicting reported
results for the effects of ether which shows both facilitation and
depression of memory as predicted on the basis of its dual excitant/
depressant actions. So the action of these compounds on behaviour
will in part be dependent on whether an excitant or depressant dose
is employed. Carbon dioxide, in "excitant" doses does not fit in
well with Porter's predictions but this may well be related to
carbon dioxide's multiple mechanisms of affecting CNS functions.

Porter concluded that gross CNS excitation or depression is one primary correlate of the facilitatory or inhibitory effects of _any_ agent on memory consolidation. Awareness of this general mode of action is essential to the evaluation of agents with postulated specific effects on consolidation, since many are likely to have effects on CNS activity levels (e.g. Actinomycin D (8.32), puromycin (8.43, 8.44)).

TEMPERATURE

Early reports of the effects of cooling small mammals after learning showed no retrograde amnesia for this treatment alone (5.1-5.3, 5.5, 5.6, 5.8). When cooling was combined with electroconvulsive shock given at intervals after hypothermia, consolidation time was found to be prolonged, suggesting that there had been some subliminal effect on permanent memory formation (5.3, 5.20). This has since been confirmed in experiments with fish in which greater temperature changes are possible (5.9). In both cases the absence of retrograde amnesia after simple hypothermia was probably due to the use of multitrial learning tasks which allowed a good deal of consolidation before brain cooling began.

Several more recent studies using a one-trial passive avoidance task have shown that hypothermia induced by immersion in cold water after training produces a marked performance deficit 24 hours later (5.7, 5.10-5.15, 5.18). The deficit increases with the severity of the hypothermia and decreases as the hypothermia is delayed after training. Consistent loss of memory in mice results when cooling is begun within a few minutes of learning and body temperature is taken down to about 25°C.

Other experiments have shown that dropping mice briefly into very cold or very hot water within seconds of learning also produced a performance deficit 24 hours later even when there was little change in body temperature (5.15). Suitable controls for the behavioural effects of the hypothermic treatment are therefore always necessary but when these are accounted for there undoubtedly remains a deficit in memory that is produced by cooling and that is not attributable to conditioned fear or freezing responses resulting from the stimulus of immersion into cold water (5.11), or other hypothermic treatments. In this same set of experiments isothermal water immersion or immersion into cold water that was not prolonged enough to lower body temperature were without specific amnesic effects (5.12). Neither were there any prograde effects of hypothermia (5.13).

Failure to disrupt recently acquired memories in hamsters and rats even when they were cooled to 5°C or lower within 40 minutes of learning and maintained at this temperature for up to 12 hours affirms the stability of the long term memory store (5.2, 5.8). Hypothermia, no matter how severe has only produced amnesia in mammals when the learning task is complete in one trial and cooling begins within a few minutes, preferably within seconds. The dependence of memory loss on the time delay between learning and hypothermia is similar to that found with comparable experiments using electroconvulsive shock. Therefore the effect is on short term memory and the mechanism of memory loss with hypothermia is probably through a disorganisation of neural processing by synaptic cold block rather than an effect on the metabolic reactions directly responsible for memory formation (5.2). Similar retrograde amnesia in goldfish can be produced by warming them to the point of heat narcosis (5.4) but hyperthermia in mice has not produced any deficits in the retention of a one-trial passive avoidance task (5.16, 5.17). Sudden hypothermia is an appropriate tool for investigating the time course of memory formation but because of the relatively slow fall of body temperature and the unavoidably unpleasant sensory stimuli associated with most cooling methods it is very difficult to use well. In addition cooling can produce prograde deficits in memory acquisition and retention that can be shown up with a slightly more difficult maze test even when this is delayed for 60 days after a 30 minute period of hypothermia (5.10). This suggests minor brain damage that could well impair recognition or recall. Nevertheless the results so far fit in with a two stage theory of memory storage (5.19).

ANOXIA, HYPOXIA AND HYPEROXIA

Hypoxia is a common candidate for the retrograde amnesic action of ECS, chemoconvulsants, anaesthetics and cerebral trauma. Cherkin (6.10) investigated the effects of exposure to an atmosphere of low oxygen immediately following a one-trial learning task in which ECS and halothane have been shown to produce retrograde amnesia. Memory retention was not impaired by hypoxia and hyperoxia had no significant effect on retention either.

Early reports of the effects of anoxia produced by simulated altitudes in decompression chambers, compression of the chest or hypoxia indicated an effect of retention similar to that produced by ECS (6.1-6.5), and in one experiment the effects were shown to be temporally graded (6.5). These experiments all involved more than one trial in the learning task and it was suggested that anoxia caused some brain damage (6.5).

Later reports employing shorter or even one-trial learning tasks have failed to show amnesia (6.6, 6.7, 6.9-6.11). Hypoxia used in these studies has been shown to be a non-aversive stimulus, therefore it shouldn't produce anxiety-like behaviour which could interfere with the expression of the amnesia (6.9, 6.12). The explanation may be found in the differences in animal strains and experimental conditions. It has been suggested that the failure to produce amnesia was due to the inability to produce the necessary severity of intracellular hypoxia rapidly enough for a one-trial learning task (6.9). However, Sara and Lefevre (6.13) obtained RA for a one-trial task even when hypoxia was induced gradually for 25 minutes. Lefevre and Sara (in 6.13) claimed that results showed hypoxia induces RA only within a limited, relatively narrow range of training parameters.

Temporary abolition of cortical and subcortical EEG activity was found in two experiments with anoxia produced by cerebral ischaemia (6.6, 6.7). Baldwin and Soltysik assumed that the isoelectric EEG implies the absence of unit neuronal activity and concluded because they did not obtain any amnesia that the type of recent memory involved in the delayed response task they

51

used does not require prolonged reverberatory neuronal activity but
depends on some intraneuronal change. Piracetam, a compound which
facilitates recuperation of a normal EEG-tracing after hypoxic-
hypoxia, protects memory against the amnesic action of hypoxia
produced by 96.5% nitrogen gas atmosphere (6.12, 6.13).

        Anoxia or hypoxia will deplete or reduce the available
energy supplies for the metabolic needs of the neurones and glial
cells of the brain. The function of the respiratory enzymes will
be upset, brain oxygen-tension will be decreased and there will
be a fall in brain ATP levels. Thus the energy available for the
metabolism of brain cells will drop and anaerobic formation of the
energy-rich intermediates will be insufficient for the obligatory
metabolic needs (Reichelt, 1968). One result of this lack of
energy will be on the electrical activity of the brain cells; this
will be either reduced or abolished. Most of these changes in the
respiratory enzymes' activities, glycolysis or neuro-glial ATP are
reversible provided the oxygen depression is not too pronounced or
lasts too long. If either of these occur there could be permanent
damage or death of cells.

        However, as well as a reduction in the electrical activity
in the brain, other energy requiring processes will be affected by
the reduction in available energy (e.g. protein synthesis see ch.8).
If it is conclusively established that anoxia or hypoxia can indeed
produce retrograde effects of the memory for a learning task - then
it remains to be determined (possibly by other means) at which
stage it is having its effect in the consolidation of a memory
trace.

POTASSIUM CHLORIDE

Cortical Spreading Depression

Spreading cortical depression (S.D.) has been known for
a number of years and its application to neurobehavioural research
has recently been explored.

The phenomenon was first reported by Leao (1944) who
demonstrated that chemical stimulation applied topically to the
cortex produced a slowly propagating wave of depressed electrocortical activity, which spread concentrically over the surface
of the stimulated hemisphere. That the effect of S.D. is both
reversible and limited to a single stimulated hemisphere has
provided the major reason for using S.D. in experiments on
interhemispheric transfer of memory (e.g. Bivens and Ray, 1965;
Ray and Emley, 1964; Russell and Ochs, 1963).

While the evidence is clear that S.D. produces a change
in interhemispheric transfer it certainly does not demand an
explanation solely in terms of a direct effect on neuronal function.
Schneider (1966, 1967) and Reed and Trowill (1969, 7.9) have shown
that if the response is under the control of stimuli available
during S.D., the impaired performance during retention can simply
be interpreted as due to a stimulus change, generalization
decrement or state-dependent learning.

Spreading depression has also been used to produce
retrograde amnesia in which case the criticism of the experiments
on interhemispheric transfer does not apply because S.D. is not
induced until after learning and is not present during testing.

We are only concerned here with S.D.-induced retrograde
amnesia and not with interhemispheric transfer. Several experiments
using one-trial learning tasks have shown retrograde amnesia 24
hours later when spreading depression of the cortex begins within
10 minutes after learning (7.1-7.3, 7.5). In another experiment
(7.11) amnesia was seen 24 hours later when cortical SD was
initiated at 16 minutes, but not when initiated immediately after
learning or at 256 minutes. In a multiple trial learning situation
using goldfish in shuttle box training, where ECS and antibiotics
have been shown effective in producing amnesia, KCl injected

intracranially 1 minute to 18 hours after the learning trials also
caused amnesia. 24 hours after learning the KCl had no effect.
The amnesia developed over 6 to 12 hours determined by testing at
various times after learning (7.7). In contrast to the effects
of KCl in higher vertebrates, the injection of KCl in fish
produced immediate seizures and convulsive swimming movements
which diminished in intensity over a period of 1 to 2 hours. The
convulsions caused a 20% mortality.

Hippocampal spreading depression

Puromycin has been shown to disrupt the hippocampal EEG
and also to interrupt memory formation (Barondes and Cohen, 1966;
Cohen and Barondes, 1967; Cohen, Ervin and Barondes, 1966). The
possibility that disruption of the hippocampal EEG by means other
than puromycin injections might also produce retrograde amnesia,
prompted Avis and Carlton (7.6) and Hughes (7.8) to study the
effects of hippocampal injections of KCl in retention. KCl
produced a marked attenuation of the EEG recorded at the injection
site and in addition produced subsequent amnesia for a conditioned
emotional response. However, the effect was not dependent on the
learning-treatment interval (7.8), and with these two experiments
and another (7.7) which also used multiple learning trials, KCl
was found to produce amnesia when given at relatively long periods
after learning (up to 18 hours (7.7),24 hours (7.6, 7.10) and 21
days (7.8)), intervals much greater than those reported for other
retrograde amnesia experiments with KCl, ECS etc. However, Kapp and
Schneider (7.10) found the amnesia from hippocampal S.D. 10 sec.
after learning to be permanent whereas the amnesia from S.D.
initiated at 24 hours and found at 4 days was not apparent at 21
days and the memory had apparently recovered. The effect of KCl
injected into the hippocampus is therefore more likely to be on
the ease of expression of memory at long time intervals and be
similar in nature to the hippocampal puromycin effect.

Mechanism of action of spreading depression

When overt seizures occur as a result of KCl applied to the
brain, the mechanism of memory loss could be the same as occurs
with electroconvulsive shock. The amnesia in the goldfish
experiments where there was a 20% mortality from convulsions, may
not be related at all to spreading depression.

Spreading depression is characterised by transient unit
spike activity at the edge of the wave, followed by electrical
silence and loss of excitability (Collewijn and Van Harraveld,
1966; Grafstein, 1956; Morlock, Mori and Ward, 1964). Cortical
cells are depolarized and there is a loss of K^{42} from the cortex
(Brinley, Kandel and Marshall, 1960). This could be accounted for
by an increase in ion permeability, a gain in cellular sodium and

a loss of potassium. There is also enormous swelling of nerve
cells, particularly the dendritic processes (Van Harreveld and
Malhotra, 1967). All changes it has been suggested, are due to the
release of intracellular glutamate which non-specifically affects
the permeability of adjacent cells to release their glutamate and
so on (Van Harreveld, 1971). It seems unlikely that the transient
increase in cell excitability so caused and the unit discharges at
the edge of the depressed zone is as important for the amnesic
effect as the subsequent prolonged depolarization, inexcitability,
ionic impedance and cell swelling. The passage of spreading
depression can be measured as an increase in surface negativity of
the cortex followed by a positivity (Leao, 1947) and by an increase
in cortical impedance (Leao & Ferreiva, 1971). It is most unlikely
that these indicators of the profound cellular disorganization of
S.D. are themselves direct causes of the amnesic effect as has been
suggested (Albert, 1966). Glutamate injected intravenously before
the development of the blood-brain-barrier produces changes in the
chicken forebrain which resemble spreading depression (Fifkova &
Van Harreveld, 1970) and this might be useful for the investigation
of amnesia. So far, there are no clues as to the specific
mechanism of amnesia from spreading depression.

ANTIBIOTICS AND PROTEIN SYNTHESIS

Theories of RNA and Protein Involvement in Memory Formation

During the past decade, a number of lines of evidence have suggested that macromolecular events are involved in the storage of information in the nervous system. These include demonstrations of changes in RNA and protein during learning experiences, reported transfer of memory to other animals by tissue extracts and the use of drugs to affect learning, memory storage and recall. A large number of hypotheses, based primarily on genetic and developmental principles, have been formulated dealing with the molecular basis of the memory trace. These are mainly concerned with the events which occur following electrical storage of information and lead to the permanent storage of memory traces.

Instinctive behaviour arises because of the influence of DNA and RNA on the cells of the developing nervous system. Since learning can produce long lasting patterns of behaviour as stable as instincts, it seems plausible that analagous mechanisms might be involved in both instinctive and learned behaviour.

The high turnover rates of most of the compounds in the brain suggest that the permanence of memory cannot be reasonably attributed to permanent chemical molecules. The stable representation of experience could be due to some change in configuration or substance mediated by a chemical system which, although in itself not stable, is characterised by the fact that the molecules which break down are resynthesised in a specified way, so as to maintain the essential features of the change. Such template functions are known to be served by the nucleic acids.

All RNA appears to be synthesised from a DNA template. The three RNA species involved in protein synthesis are messenger RNA, transfer RNA and ribosomal RNA. The genetic code in DNA is transmitted to mRNA in the nucleus. mRNA moves to the cytoplasm where it attaches to ribosomes which consist of ribosomal RNA and protein. Molecules of transfer RNA gather amino acids and adhere to the ribosome, and to their appropriate site on the mRNA. There

57

is at least one transfer RNA for each amino acid and these with
their associated amino acids "recognise" the appropriate site on the
RNA by complementary base pairing, and the amino acids become strung
together to form a specific polypeptide or protein. In protein
synthesis the three RNA's serve only as intermediaries between DNA
and protein. Such considerations have led workers to turn to the
possible role of RNA or proteins in the mediation of long-term
information storage.

DNA itself is stable but modifications in DNA action could
play a role (Griffith and Mahler, 1969).

A number of ways in which RNA and protein might be
involved in memory storage have been suggested.

1.   The experimental code could be recorded intracellularly in
the composition or conformation of a set of macromolecules. Thus,
if the code were known and these molecules analysed, the experience
and the adaptive behavioural response being coded would be known.
This possibility is not considered seriously by most neurobiologists
(e.g. Dingman and Sporn, 1964).

2.   The experiential code is recorded intercellularly in nerve
pathways and networks. Macromolecules serve in the process that
leads to the participation of a particular neuron in a particular
functioning network by determining whether the cell will fire in
response to input from neighbouring cells.

These theories are based on two assumptions-

1. the nervous system is pre-wired by the developmental process
    and the modification is a selection of circuits.

2. the synaptic modification associated with LTM is the consequence
    of the synthesis of new molecules.

From this there emerge two general classes of experiments
based on the new assumptions that firstly, a learning experience
should induce the synthesis of RNA and protein and the formation of
these molecules might be detected. Also the new molecule may be
capable of transferring the memory to another animal. Secondly,
drugs that interfere with the synthesis of protein or RNA might
disrupt the formation or maintenance of the memory trace. Most of
the theories of memory storage have arisen from experiments on
synthesis induced by learning, including transfer experiments.

Proteins

It has been suggested that the proteins formed from the
altered RNA function in memory storage by altering synaptic function:

1. Presynaptically, by increasing synthesis or release of
    transmitter (Barondes, 1965; Briggs and Kitto, 1962; Hyden,
    1959; 1960; Hyden and Lange, 1965; 1966; Smity, 1962) or by
    altering the release of transmitter, making it available only
    with certain characteristics of stimulation (Schmitt, 1962).

2. Changing receptor properties of the post-synaptic membrane by
    increased sensitivity or synthesis of receptor molecules,
    increased permeability to transmitter or decreased degradation
    of transmitter (Barondes, 1965).

3. By altering both pre- and post- synaptic properties by glycoproteins
    or glycolipids increasing the effective synaptic properties
    (Bogoch, 1968), or by altering the proximity of the two
    membranes with proteins (Elul, 1966).

4. Or by antibody production leading to firing of the cell (Griffith
    and Maller, 1969) or by induction of a specific memory
    "antibody" in certain neurones with an increase in synaptic
    efficacy (Szilard, 1964).

        Recently, Hyden and Lange (1970) have implicated the brain
specific protein S100 in learning.

RNA and DNA

        Some theories invoke an action of an RNA synthesised in
response to gene activation on the DNA molecule brought about by the
learning experience. Gene activation has been postulated by:-

1. Modulated frequencies of nerve impulses causes gene activation
    and the specific protein eventually synthesised will respond
    to this frequency and lead directly to an increase in
    transmitter (Hyden, 1960; Schmitt, 1962). Electrical
    impulses could alter DNA, RNA or amino acid sequences (Gaito,
    1961) or produce methylation or demethylation of a "ticket"
    on the DNA molecule leading to a synaptic change (Griffith
    and Maller, 1969). Hyden and Lange (1965; 1966) have
    suggested that DNA sites in glia and neurones are stimulated
    by environmental factors so that unique RNA is synthesised with
    a different base-ratio composition.

    Another idea was that during learning, stimulation of specific
    nerve cells causes a modification in the DNA complex such
    that DNA is activated to synthesize more RNA leading to more
    protein synthesis in synaptic regions (Gaito, 1966).

2. The neurotransmitter induces gene activation (Barondes, 1965;
    Briggs & Kitto 1962; Smith 1962).

3. Gene activation is by a substance released by the transmitter
    either by repression or derepression of genes (Barondes,
    1965; Bonner, 1966; Ungar, 1968).

4. The protein or its product inducing gene activation (8.9, 8.19).

5. Or by a foreign RNA transferred from glia to neuron and which de-
    represses neuronal DNA (Pribram, 1966).

        Other theories do not require gene activation for the
learning process. The change could be brought about by:-

1. Production of a specific RNA template by glial released RNA-
    methylation of RNA influenced by biogenic amines (Landauer,
    1964) or other RNA - (Corning and John, 1961; McConnell,
    1964a; 1964b).

2. Changes in electrical frequencies directly changing the base
    ratio of RNA (Hyden, 1959; 1960)-

3. Or nucleoprotein rearrangement (Katz and Halstead, 1950).

        Obviously with so many molecular theories of memory having
been put up, few of them can be anywhere near the truth and all of
them go further than the experimental facts allow. Of the various
experiments that gave rise to these theories those involving transfer
of behaviour between animals by the injection of brain or other
tissue extracts are not reviewed here at all. There is still much
disagreement on reproducibility although some striking effects have
been claimed. The acceleration of brain RNA or protein synthesis by
environmental stimulation and learning appears easier to replicate but
the relevance of this to memory formation is unknown.

        The present review is restricted to experiments on the
interference with memory by various drugs known to affect RNA or
protein synthesis. The first task is to try and determine whether the
behavioural effects are due to the disruption of the formation of
memory and whether this is related to the suspected metabolic action
of the drugs. If this is so then the question is whether there is
enough evidence to suggest that protein synthesis is critically
involved in memory formation or whether continuing protein synthesis
merely provides the conditions which permit the real memory reactions
to take place.

Inhibition of Memory Formation by Drugs Affecting DNA Synthesis

Cytosine arabinoside

        Cytosine arabinoside injected into the brain of goldfish
(8.33), resulting in a 95% inhibition of DNA synthesis at the time of

learning, did not produce any effect on retention. It has been
postulated that this drug acts in suppressing synthesis of DNA by
inhibiting DNA polymerase and it has no effect on protein or RNA
synthesis. This lack of interference with avoidance responding
suggests that the formation of memory does not depend on DNA
synthesis and models of memory based on this or cell replication are
not supported.

Hydroxylamine

Reinis (8.68, 8.69) has proposed that hydroxylamine may
act as a mutagen changing the transcription of activated DNA.
Hydroxylamine acts specifically on activated, derepressed DNA, leaving
behind the inactive, repressed one. Before the beginning of training,
part of the genome responsible for the production of proteins altering
the excitability of certain nerve cells during learning is repressed.
Hydroxylamine is without effect when injected before training, however
if injected intracranially from 4 hours to 3 weeks after training, it
interfered with the retention of the learned task. Reinis suggests
that training causes activation of this part of the genome and
hydroxylamine, altering the derepressed DNA, causes misreading of the
code leading to the production of a defective protein. As Reinis
mentions, biochemical proof of this hypothesis is extremely difficult
and he admits the possibility of other explanations.

Inhibition of Memory Formation by Drugs Affecting RNA Synthesis

8-Azaguanine

One of the first studies of the effects of metabolic
inhibitors on memory was done using 8-azaguanine, an inhibitor of RNA
synthesis. 8-azaguanine is incorporated in the RNA molecule thereby
producing an abnormally functioning structural analogue of RNA.

There was difficulties in interpretation of the effects of
this drug on memory. 8-azaguanine administered before learning
impaired the acquisition of a water maze habit, but had no effect on
retention when administered after training (8.1). The results may be
due to impairment of some other aspects of performance other than
interferring with memory processes. The same difficulties in
interpretation apply to the effects of 8-azaguanine on spinal fixation
time, on avoidance conditioning (8.25), on the learning of a fixed-
interval schedule (Jewett et al., 1965) and on the acquisition of a
new operant schedule (8.64). It has been suggested that 8-azaguanine
depressed motor activity as judged by lower lever-pressing rates, by
a potentiation of the effects of barbiturates (Jewett et al, 1965)
and by reduced running in an activity wheel (8.25).

It is apparent that 8-azaguanine has not been investigated
enough to warrant any conclusions as to its effect on memory.

Actinomycin D

This drug blocks the transcription by binding to guanine
nucleotides on the DNA molecule so that RNA synthesis ceases
(Goldberg et al, 1962; Reich et al, 1962). Ultimately it must have
an effect on protein synthesis but this apparently does not occur in
fish brain until several hours following the injection (8.32).

Actinomycin D differs from 8-azaguanine in that it has no
effect on acquisition in many tasks (8.40, 8.41, 8.54). However, the
toxicity produced by doses of actinomycin D large enough to cause
marked inhibition of RNA synthesis has also made the interpretation
of studies with this agent difficult.

In a number of studies actinomycin D injected before
learning in doses producing between 80 and 95% inhibition of RNA
synthesis, had no effect on acquisition or on retention up to 4 hours
after learning (8.40, 8.41). The higher doses used in the earlier
studies (8.40, 8.41) caused severe illness noticeable 10 hours after
injection and produced death within 24 hours so that retention could
not be measured at longer intervals after training. The possibility
remains that the memory seen at 4 hours was short-term memory which
may not be affected by a lack of RNA synthesis. Smaller doses had no
effect on retention at 24 hours after training (8.46, 8.60). However,
the level of inhibition of RNA synthesis achieved may have been too
low to permit the conclusion that RNA synthesis is not required for
long-term memory.

In a later study, using low doses of actinomycin D, Squire
and Barondes (8.54) found retention deficits with injection prior to
learning and also with injection 24 hours after, when tested the day
after administration of the drug. When given a week later, actinomycin
D did not produce any deficit in retention. Because the drug had had
an effect as long as 24 hours after training it was considered that
the loss of memory was not due to a lack of RNA synthesis. Recently,
Squire et al (in Cohen, 1970) using a more sensitive task, found little
retention 24 hours after a low dose of actinomycin D given prior to
training, but when given 30 minutes after training it did not affect
retention.

There are other studies which support the involvement of
RNA synthesis in memory (8.32, 8.80). However, Nakajima (8.66) has
reported that five days after very small intracerebral doses of
actinomycin D, both acquisition and retention of a spatial task were
impaired. Within five days after injection of this small dose
(1 ug), there was evidence of abnormal cerebral electrical activity
and extensive chromatolysis in the hippocampus. These effects of
actinomycin D and other evidence of cerebral abnormalities produced
by actinomycin D (Appel, 1965), support the suggestion that
behavioural effects produced by this drug may be due to actions other

than simple suppression of RNA synthesis. Perhaps both hippocampal cellular damage and the establishment of epileptogenic activity within the hippocampus contribute to behavioural impairment.

Available evidence has failed to demonstrate conclusively that RNA synthesis is necessary for memory storage. The evidence now indicates that the agents used in these experiments produce multiple effects. This fact has been a major difficulty in obtaining an adequate test of the hypothesis that RNA synthesis is involved in the formation of long-term memory.

Other Nucleic Acid Antimetabolites

Reinis (8.70) injected two antimetabolites - 2, 6-diaminopurine and 5-iodouracil, thought to interfere with RNA synthesis and producing defective proteins whose functional specificity is lost. These two drugs were found to impair retention of passive avoidance learning when given before and up to 1 hour after learning but not when given 2 hours or more after.

Inhibition of Memory Formation by Drugs Affecting Protein Synthesis

Puromycin

Puromycin is an antibiotic which acts as a powerful inhibitor of protein synthesis (Darken, 1964; Yarmolinsky and de la Haba, 1959). Puromycin structurally resembles the amino-acyl terminal of transfer RNA and the drug is presumed to act by mimicking the naturally occurring charged transfer RNA. Puromycin becomes incorporated into the carboxyl ends of the growing polypeptide chains causing their premature release from the ribosomes as peptidyl-puromycin (Allen and Zamecnik, 1962; Nathans, 1964).

The first studies employing quantifiable inhibition of protein synthesis were those of Flexner et al (8.2). Mice were given the largest dose of puromycin which could be tolerated in a single subcutaneous injection which produced 83% inhibition of cerebral protein synthesis for several hours. This had no demonstrable effect on learning or memory when injected either before or after training. However, intracerebral injections of puromycin was found to produce a complete loss of an avoidance response when injected bilaterally into temporal (hippocampal), ventricular and frontal regions or just into the temporal regions of mouse brain 24 hours after training. Frontal and/or ventricular injections had no disruptive effect. By delaying the injection time beyond 3 days it became necessary to inject into all areas to disrupt learned avoidance responses and hippocampal injections alone were ineffective. It was concluded that the hippocampal zone was the site of recent memory storage; this locus of memory storage when spread to include an extensive part of the neocortex being concerned in longer term memory storage.

The loss of memory required 12 to 20 hours to develop,
but once established it persisted for at least 3 months. Overtraining protected the response from puromycin (8.9). Puromycin
affected only recent learning, when injected after reversal
training the original learning remained intact (8.3) which meant
that the puromycin was not producing an inability to perform. The
puromycin effect was found to be dependent on the dose and hence on
the degree of protein synthesis inhibition (8.5). Studies with
substances structurally related to puromycin but without the protein
synthesis inhibiting properties were without effect. For example,
hydrolyzed puromycin and the aminonucleoside of puromycin had no
effect (8.6).

Acetoxycycloheximide (AXM), which had no effect on memory
in this situation when injected alone, protected the memory against
the puromycin induced retention deficit when they were administered
together (8.7). AXM would protect against the formation of the
abnormal puromycin peptides and mRNA would be preserved and resume
its synthesis of new protein after the drug level had fallen.
Alternatively, the retention deficit could be attributed to the
formation of the abnormal peptides.

For various reasons, it was thought that the memory
deficit in this situation was due to the formation of peptidyl
puromycin. This abnormal peptide apparently survives in the brain
for at least 8 weeks after intracerebral injection of tritiated
puromycin (8.11). The period in which the pepidyl puromycin
concentration reaches its peak coincides with the decay in responding
after injection of puromycin. In addition, puromycin in doses
effective in producing amnesia, produced swelling of the neuronal
mitochondria in the entorrhinal cortex of mice (8.13). This was not
directly related to inhibition of cerebral protein synthesis because
AXM did not produce this and in fact it substantially protected
against the swelling produced by puromycin (8.14). The extent of
the swelling was directly related to the amount of peptidyl puromycin
and it was considered that the swelling was due to the formation of
the peptide. When puromycin was neutralized with bases of certain
cations (K^+, Li^+, Ca^{++}, Mg^{++}), rather than with Na^+, it no longer had
an amnesic effect when given one day after training (8.16). It was
suggested that these cations may bind to anionic sites of neuronal
membranes and thereby protect mice from the disruptive effects of
peptidyl puromycin.

The memory deficit after injection of puromycin 24 hours
after training was found to be reversible. Intracerebral injection
of isotonic saline or water substantially reversed the retention
deficit (8.10, 8.15, 8.17, 8.52). The conclusion was drawn that
puromycin blocked the expression of the memory without substantially
altering the process that maintains the basic memory trace. However,

if puromycin was given within minutes of training or before training
with a simpler task, saline injections were not effective in
restoring memory (8.12). When puromycin is injected close to learning rather than the next day, it is likely to be preventing the
memory formation rather than just interrupting the expression by
peptidyl puromycin formation. Further studies using saline to
reverse the puromycin deficits revealed that the memory trace
appeared to be widely spread in the cortex despite the suppression
of recent memory in the hippocampus (8.15).

Under conditions where puromycin blockage of expression
can be reversed by saline injections, the puromycin is clearly not
interferring with consolidation. Flexner suggested that the abnormal
peptides are interferring with the action of normal peptides
presumably responsible for the maintenance and retrieval of the
conditioned avoidance. The saline supposedly removes the abnormal
puromycin peptides. Chorover (1969) has suggested that the action
of saline might be due to a blocking of abnormal electrical activity
induced initially by the puromycin injection and now reversed by the
saline injection permitting a return to more normal patterns of
behaviour and brain activity.

The possibility of the saline injection acting as a
reminder as in the FS reminder ECS studies is ruled out by the fact
that injections of other salts does not induce the recovery of the
memory (8.17).

The peptidyl puromycin persists for long periods in subcellular fractions of synaptosomes (nerve ending particles) from
mouse brain. This peptidyl puromycin is lost from the synaptosomes
but not from the mitochondrial fractions when the expression of
memory is restored with saline injections (8.20).

Further studies on the expression of memory and blockage
of this by puromycin have suggested the interference of adrenergic
receptors with peptidyl puromycin (8.18, 8.19, 8.22, 8.23, 8.24).

Barondes and Cohen (8.42) using a different strain of mice
to that used by Flexner, were able to train them 5 hours after
intracerebral injection of puromycin. This meant that mice could be
trained during the peak of protein synthesis inhibition and the
problem of whether protein synthesis was required for learning and
the consolidation period investigated. Mice were injected bilaterally
into the hippocampal region and trained to escape shock and choose
the correct limb of a Y-maze. Acquisition by puromycin-treated mice
was indistinguishable from that of saline-injected controls. Fifteen
minutes after training, the mice exhibited normal retention, but
after 3 hours they had total amnesia and required as many trials to
relearn the problem as naive animals. So while the mice showed
amnesia for what they had learned 3 hours before, their capacity for

learning and short term memory is retained while cerebral protein synthesis is inhibited. It was concluded that there is an initial stage of memory storage independent of protein synthesis.

Subsequent studies indicated that some of the amnesic properties of puromycin might be unrelated to inhibition of cerebral protein synthesis required for long term memory and that behavioural effects produced by puromycin might be due to general cerebral abnormality rather than to inhibition of protein synthesis, (8.43, 8.44) and that puromycin may be producing convulsive discharges in the hippocampus. It was suggested that the peptidyl-puromycin was the cause of increased susceptibility to pentylenetetrazol seizures and that the puromycin effect on memory may be due to occult seizures. AXM and cycloheximide (CXM) did not have these side effects.

In a series of experiments in Agranoff's laboratory using goldfish in a shuttle box conditioned avoidance situation, puromycin was found to produce amnesia on testing 3 days later (8.26, 8.27, 8.28, 8.29).

Varying degrees of susceptibility to the drug relative to training were found, depending upon the time of injection of puromycin and the dose used. If the inhibitor was administered either immediately before or immediately after training, memory on testing was poor. But if the injections were delayed for more than one hour after training or given 20 minutes before, no effect on memory was noted. The observation that puromycin produced no deficit in retention when injected 20 minutes before or 60 minutes after training and that it has no effect when overtraining is given (8.26), rules out non-specific actions of puromycin as the cause of lowered performance on testing.

Metrazol convulsions were potentiated by intracranial puromycin in the goldfish. AXM did not do this and in contrast to Cohen and Barondes (8.44) AXM did not prevent the puromycin potentiation of metrazol convulsions. Puromycin aminonucleoside however did potentiate the metrazol convulsions. This suggested that the convulsant activity of puromycin is not responsible for its amnesic effect in the fish. It further suggests that peptidyl puromycin is not the convulsant agent, since pretreatment with AXM which should prevent the peptidyl puromycin, did not protect against convulsions; also peptidyl puromycin is not formed with the aminonucleoside (Agranoff, 1969).

This disruptable period of consolidation appears to occur immediately after training in goldfish and apparently not during training. ECS produces memory loss in goldfish (8.27) but has a longer disruptable period than puromycin; ECS can be given up to 90 minutes after learning and still produce amnesia. This could be because maximum inhibition of protein synthesis will not occur immediately after injection. Puromycin had no effect on the rate

of learning when administered before training and produced no
postural or locomotor impairment. In an operant conditioning
situation with goldfish, puromycin immediately following a training
session did not disrupt the performance of a well-established
operant response (8.38). This suggests that the memory shown by
improvement in performance during training is not puromycin
susceptible and is short-term memory. Injection of puromycin
immediately after learning and retesting at various intervals after
showed the retention to gradually decay after 6 hours and become
completely lost over the next 2 days (8.29).

The puromycin moieties - puromycin aminonucleoside and
methyl tyrosine do not block protein synthesis or produce retention
deficits. In a further series of experiments it was shown that
consolidation could be delayed by keeping the fish in the learning
situation after training and injecting puromycin before returning
them to the home tank (8.29, 8.34, 8.35). It was postulated that
arousal or excitement evoked during training inhibits fixation and
visual stimuli in the shuttle box maintain arousal after training.
If the fish are replaced in the shuttle box for a brief period prior
to injection or puromycin, KCl or AXM, amnesia can be induced by
injection as much as 24 hours after training (8.35).

Potts and Bitterman (8.62) found that post-session
injections of puromycin produced marked retention deficits in
goldfish in a discriminative shuttle box avoidance task as well as
in a passive goal box avoidance task. However, there was a
continued improvement in the performance over weekly training sessions,
each followed immediately by an injection of puromycin. There was
some impairment but not the complete lack of retention that was
expected from the results of Agranoff's laboratory. On the basis of
their findings Potts and Bitterman (8.62) concluded that puromycin
impairs retention of consolidation of conditioned fear. According to
this hypothesis, when goldfish that have received an amnesic treatment
are tested for retention of an avoidance response, they fail to avoid
because the conditioned stimulus does not elicit fear. These studies
do not rule out the alternate possibility that puromycin interferes
with consolidation of information more generally relevant to the
instrumental behaviour. Thus in the discriminative shuttle box
avoidance, fish might have been fearful but unable to perform the
appropriate response. In a more direct measure of emotionality,
Schoel and Agranoff (8.39) used the electrocardiogram to measure
conditioned heart rate deceleration to a light-off signal paired with
a punishing electrical shock in the goldfish. Intracranial injections
of puromycin administered just before or immediately after a training
session did not appear to block formation of memory of this response.
This result is incompatible with puromycin interfering with
conditioned fear consolidation.

Huber and Longo (8.72) found that the time of injection of puromycin up to 48 hours after training or over-training did not alter the deficit in retention. They suggest that their results "question both the consolidation interference hypothesis and the idea that the retention deficit may be interference with conditioned fear". However, they did use a relatively high dose of puromycin.

Shashoua (8.63) reported that puromycin injected 90 minutes before training blocked the memory of a new swimming pattern in goldfish when tested 22 hours later. Mayor (8.65) reported retrograde amnesia with puromycin injected 5 minutes after training in the Japanese quail. However, as he did not find amnesia with AXM or with puromycin after reversal training, he put the amnesia down to peptidyl puromycin formation.

Because puromycin has multiple effects on the brain, behavioural studies with this drug appear to lead to doubt of the role of protein synthesis in memory. The experiments involving delayed injection of puromycin were originally conceived as a way of determining the role of protein synthesis in the maintenance of long-term memory storage. It now appears that the release of peptidyl puromycin into cells, and not protein synthesis inhibition itself, may be responsible for the behavioural effects of puromycin given long after training. Since these amnesic effects are reversible, these experiments do not answer this question. Unfortunately, little is currently known about this aspect of memory.

Acetoxycycloheximide

A major conclusion from the studies with puromycin is that it is not the most satisfactory drug with which to study the participation of cerebral protein synthesis in memory storage. Cycloheximide (CXM) and acetoxycycloheximide (AXM), inhibitors with even greater potency than puromycin, seem to be free from many of its defects. They produce their effect by inhibiting the transfer of amino acids from transfer RNA to polypeptide and prevent the subsequent release of the polypeptide from the polysomes without apparently damaging the ribosomes (Ennis and Lubin, 1964). Therefore there is no abortive release of abnormal peptides into the cell. When AXM is used there is no abnormal effect on neuronal cytomembranes (8.14) and AXM produces no alteration in seizure susceptibility to pentylenetetrazol (Agranoff, 1969; 8.44). For these reasons these glutarimide derivatives are advantageous for studies on memory formation.

In their first study, Flexner and Flexner (8.7) failed to find amnesia when AXM was injected 24 hours after training. They then attempted to administer AXM before training but found the mice very difficult to train (8.8). However, if reversal training was given after AXM there was retrograde amnesia. This was only a

transient amnesia, the memory persisted for a period that extended
to 3 hours, was temporally lost for up to 3 days and then returned.
This time sequence of amnesia also occurred when AXM was administered
5 minutes after training (8.8). These results supported the hypothesis
that the establishment of memory is dependent on one or more species
of mRNA which alters the rate of synthesis of one or more proteins
essential for the expression of memory, these proteins or their
products acting as inducers of their related mRNA, maintaining the
concentration of the inducer protein. In the presence of an inhibitor
of protein synthesis such as AXM, the concentration of essential
proteins could fall to levels too low for the expression of the
memory, but the apparent loss of memory would be only temporary if
the mRNA was conserved to direct protein synthesis when the inhibitor
had disappeared. According to this hypothesis, the mRNA required for
expression of memory is degraded by puromycin, but conserved in the
presence of AXM.

Serota (8.21) has found a transient amnesia in rats when
trained under the influence of AXM. Amnesia was present one day after
training but the memory returned spontaneously within 6 days. This
transient deficit in the retrieval phase was suggested to be due to
a deficiency in neurotransmitters (8.23).

Barondes and Cohen (8.46), training mice to a criterion of
9 out of 10 correct responses as did Flexner et al (8.8), also failed
to produce RA with the drug given before training. If less training
trials were given then amnesia was seen the next day if the drug was
given before training; given after training there was no or only
slight amnesia (8.46, 8.47). They suggested that deficits in retention
could be produced with AXM as long as extensive overtraining was not
given.

Doses of AXM which inhibited cerebral protein synthesis by
more than 90% were required to demonstrate this effect (8.47). The
amnesic effect found was thought not to be due to systemic illness
because subcutaneous injection of equivalent doses which inhibited
cerebral protein synthesis far less were not effective in impairing
memory. Subcutaneous administration of larger doses of AXM (8.48)
avoided the possibility of erroneous interpretation due to such
factors as increase intracranial pressure, formation of brain lesions
and scars and heterogeneous distribution of the drug. One additional
advantage found was a much more rapid onset of action of inhibiting
cerebral protein synthesis, which meant the mice could be trained
shortly after injection when they appeared completely "well" and
tested when they had completely recovered from the drug. As with
intracerebral injections before training, mice were amnesic by 6
hours and longer. The drug could be given immediately after training
to give a less marked amnesic effect but if delayed to 30 minutes,
AXM was ineffective.

The relative lack of effect of doses of AXM which inhibited
protein synthesis by nearly 90% was explained by postulating that the
residual protein synthesis was sufficient to store the information.
This was based on the idea of redundancy and the adaptive value of
the particular learning task in the natural environment. A small
amount of protein synthesizing capacity might be sufficient to mediate
memory storage if prolonged repetition rather than brief training is
given. With a more difficult task, a light-dark discrimination,
training to a criterion of 9/10 was not sufficient to overcome the
amnesic effects of AXM (8.49). Overtraining to 15/16 was necessary
to overcome the effect of AXM. AXM induced amnesia is not reversed
by saline injection (8.52).

Although the protein synthesis which appears to be required
for memory occurs during or within minutes after training, inhibition
of protein synthesis during that period is not reflected in impaired
memory until 3 or 6 hours later (8.45, 8.46, 8.47, 8.48, 8.49). This
suggested that for at least 3 hours after learning, some process other
than the synthesis of new protein is responsible for the short-term
storage of memory. Because injections of antibiotics must be given
at or near the time of training to be effective in impairing memory,
it seems as though both long and short term phases of memory begin at
the same time. Long-term memory becomes more permanent as the short-
term memory decays. Until the short-term phase which is apparently
independent of protein synthesis decays, the effects of prior
inhibition of the protein required for long-term storage cannot be
detected.

This decay of short-term memory has been confirmed by
Daniels (8.82, 8.83) injecting AXM into the hippocampus of rats
before training in a Y-maze brightness discrimination task and an
appetitive learning task. There was no amnesia for 3 hours following
training but it was apparent 4 and 6 hours after. The retrograde
amnesia observed by Daniels was not transient and was still present
7 days after treatment and training. Swanson et al (8.71) have also
observed a decay in short-term memory. In a one-trial inhibitory
avoidance task with mice, the retrograde amnesia increased as testing
was delayed from 2 hours to 2 days.

Further positive evidence that protein required for long-
term storage must be synthesized near the time of training comes
from experiments with goldfish (8.31, 8.32, 8.33, 8.36, 8.37). By
varying the time of injection of AXM before or after training and
testing 3 days later, a time-dependent difference in susceptibility
to the amnesic effects of AXM was found. Fish injected immediately
after avoidance training were amnesic when tested, whereas injections
delayed by as much as an hour after training were ineffective in
blocking memory formation. Also, in goldfish AXM administered 4
hours before training had no effect on subsequent retention.
Agranoff (8.36) found that the amnesia developed over 2 days with

injection of AXM immediately after training. He suggests that
although short-term memory appears to be converted to long-term
memory, protein synthesis is necessary for the short-term memory
to decay. Repeated injections of AXM resulted in only a partial
amnesia at a time when one injection produced complete amnesia.
Puromycin injected with AXM seems to produce more amnesia than
either drug alone (8.37) AXM therefore does not protect against
puromycin induced amnesia despite preventing the formation of
abnormal peptidyl puromycin. The amnesia from both drugs was still
evident in goldfish 7 days after training.

In all these experiments, delayed injections of AXM were
not effective in producing amnesia. Despite this evidence, a
possible requirement for continued protein synthesis for the
maintenance of long-term memories cannot be completely ruled out.
The possibility remains that protein required for maintenance of a
memory could be turned over so slowly as to be missed in these
inhibitor studies as the inhibitions usually wear off within hours
or days and cannot be maintained for any extensive period of time
without seriously affecting the behaviour of the animal.

Cycloheximide

CXM shows less sustained inhibition of cerebral protein
synthesis than AXM which allows less time for the possible development of a non-specific interference with cerebral protein which
could impair behaviour.

Amnesia from CXM, like AXM, depends on the time of injection
relative to training. The drug can be given as long as 45 minutes
before training and up to 10 minutes after (8.53, 8.77, 8.88).
Memory, presumably short-term memory, is seen following training for
between 90 minutes and 6 hours, after which time the amnesia develops
(8.50, 8.51, 8.53, 8.59, 8.73, 8.78, 8.84, 8.85). CXM has been
employed in a number of training situations and has been found to
produce amnesia at a time after the short-term has decayed. In mice
amnesia has been produced in an appetively motivated task (8.50, in
an aversively motivated T-maze (8.51) and in one trial passive
avoidance step-through task (8.53, 8.76, 8.84, 8.85) and in chickens
in a one trial passive avoidance of a lure (8.77, 8.88). Exploratory
habituation was not vulnerable to interruption by CXM (8.55).

The degree of training is an important variable in the
extent of amnesia seen; in the number of trials in the original
training (8.51, 8.56, 8.59); when footshock is delayed after the
response (8.57) or when the footshock intensity is varied (8.73) in
a one trial step through task. The number of trials also affects the
rate of decay of the short-term memory (8.59). Other psychological
variables seen to be important in studies on ECS-induced amnesia also
affect CXM induced amnesia, e.g. detention (8.29, 8.34, 8.35, 8.58)

and recovery from amnesia by using a reminder shock (8.51, 8.74, 8.76). Barondes and Cohen (8.51) using mice with inhibited cerebral protein synthesis found that manipulations that generated "arousal" could lead to the development of long-term memory provided they were introduced at a time when short-term memory still persisted and protein synthesis had recovered. If amphetamine or steriods were injected or treatment with electrical shock was given 3 hours after training in a visual discrimination task, the normal amnesic effects of a short-acting dose of CXM were not observed 7 days later. Reestablishment of the protein synthesis inhibition at the time of arousal negated the effects of the arousing agents on memory storage. It is possible that the arousal producing treatment served as a reminder of the original training. Such a state of affairs would be effective in protecting against the protein synthesis inhibitor only so long as short-term memory had not yet decayed and synthesis of protein had been reestablished. It might be expected that short-term memory remains available for manipulation affecting consolidation for the duration of the period of arousal as when goldfish are detained in the training apparatus after training, whereas under normal post-training conditions in the home tank susceptibility diminishes rapidly in an hour or so (8.29, 8.34, 8.35). Continued arousal could be holding the information in a short-term state, perhaps one of readiness of availability for the fish. For long-term storage, in addition to the information acquired during training and an intact protein synthesizing capacity, it appears that an appropriate state of arousal, which specifically directs the establishment of permanent memory may be necessary. Livingstone (1967) has speculated on the role of arousal as an order for neurons recently activated, to "print".

Squire, Geller and Jarvik (8.55) report that there is increased activity for 30 minutes following the injection of CXM, and activity is then depressed for 1 to 3 hours. Isocycloheximide which does not inhibit protein synthesis, depresses activity to the same extent as CXM, so the activity level changes may be unrelated to the amnesic effect of CXM (8.56). It was also shown that amphetamine which can antagonize the effects of CXM (8.51) did not antagonize the depression of activity (8.56). The effect of amphetamine in increasing activity in CXM treated mice was not correlated with a measurable increase in activity.

A possible mechanism for short-term memory storage has been suggested from studies using CXM and agents which inhibit the Na-K ATPase carrier system in cell membranes, known as the sodium pump. These studies have used day old chickens and a one trial passive avoidance task. Memory tested at 24 hours can be inhibited by injecting CXM 30 minutes before learning and up to 10 minutes after, whereas the sodium pump inhibitors ouabain and lithium are only effective in interferring with memory when they are injected shortly before learning, not when injected 10 minutes after. This suggested that there may be protein-independent memory processes which could only be interferred with by sodium pump inhibition very close to the time of learning. Memory tested at intervals of minutes or hours after learning is seen to decay in the presence of protein synthesis inhibition, and beyond a certain concentration of the inhibitor the memory loss cannot be increased. However, the sodium pump inhibitors can increase this rate of decay of retention when injected alone or with CXM. It is suggested that the remaining memory seen with CXM blocking protein synthesis is short-term memory and is held by membrane mechanisms dependent on the sodium pump.

Further biochemical experiments (8.79) show that inhibition of sodium transport by ouabain can also interfere with the incorporation of ^{14}C leucine into brain protein by blocking membrane transport of the amino acid. It has been suggested that accumulation of Na+ in active neurones and its subsequent extrusion by a pumping mechanism is responsible for short-term storage and is linked to long-term storage by parallel increases in the transport of amino acids as the substrate for the synthetic change needed for long-term memory.

Conclusions - Behavioural

Some of the problems found in the ECS studies with regard to training variables are apparent also in the studies using antibiotics. The amount of training and the task difficulty determines the amount of amnesia and whether or not it occurs. Reinforcement magnitude is also important. The greater the learning the less vulnerable the memory is to interference. Most of the learning tasks have required more than one trial, making clear cut decisions concerning the behavioral components susceptible to the chemical interferences difficult.

Another important factor is in the choice of dose of the inhibitor. Different experiments use different doses, although some have reported the effects of different doses in the same experimental design (Puromycin - 8.5, 8.28; AXM - 8.7, 8.46, 8.47; Actinomycin D - 8.40, 8.41). It is important to show that the dose-response relationship is a simple one, graded from zero to a maximum effect - to show that the inhibitor is interferring with only one mechanism.

The report of the reminder shock raised the question as to whether the CXM was suppressing or inhibiting the expression of an intact memory trace or whether some part of the trace was remaining intact. It is possible that the arousal idea of Barondes and Cohen is involved here. The time of injection relative to the training is another important variable. It has been assumed by many from the Flexners' work that there was interruption of memory formation when the injections were given a day or more after learning and the retrieval of this memory by saline injections cast serious doubt on

the consolidation hypothesis. However, as has been pointed out a
number of times, but not sufficiently strongly, this work is based
on the interference with the expression of memory once formed and
it has been shown by the same authors that if the injection is close
enough to the learning the memory loss is not reversible by saline
injection. These experiments are mainly not relevant to consolidation
hypothesis under review.

Conclusions - Pharmacological

To draw the conclusion, by pharmacological means, that the
synthesis of a protein or group of proteins is specifically required
for memory storage, the drugs used should specifically inhibit the
synthesis of these molecules and should not have other actions on the
brain. The drugs used so far in these studies do not satisfy this
requirement. They inhibit the synthesis of all proteins, both those
required for the normal maintenance of cell function which may
normally be degraded or have a rapid turnover and therefore need
replacement, as well as the synthesis of new proteins which may
subserve adaptive processes such as memory storage. A deletion of
constitutive proteins may result from prolonged inhibition of
cerebral protein synthesis and any behavioral deficit may be due to
this rather than to inhibition of protein synthesis specifically
required for memory formation. This problem may be lessened when
inhibition is fairly brief and when no detectable behavioral or
electrophysiological abnormalities are observed.

This raises the second problem that the drugs may have
some other action besides the one for which they are being used. It
seems that puromycin has more effects than simply blocking protein
synthesis. As already mentioned it may produce occult seizures,
indicated by the increased susceptibility to metrazol convulsions in
mice (8.43, 8.44). Puromycin has been seen to potentiate metrazol
convulsions in the goldfish. However, puromycin aminonucleoside
which does not inhibit protein synthesis nor affect memory formation
also potentiated metrazol convulsions (Agranoff, 1969; 1970a).
Puromycin also caused mitochondrial and neuronal cytomembrane
swelling (8.13, 8.14). In addition to these side effects, it
reduced the rate of respiration in guinea pig cerebral cortex (Jones
and Banks, 1969). In nerves it had an effect on conduction, reduced
the spike amplitude of electrical activity in the spinal cord of fish
(Bondeson et al, 1967) whereas the aminonucleoside did not, and
caused a reversible decrease in spike potential and positive after-
potential amplitudes of rabbit vagus nerve in vitro (Dahl, 1969),
seen also in the presence of cycloheximide. Therefore, the reduction
of nervous conduction in either case was not due to peptidyl-puromycin
formation. In the superior cervical ganglion of the rat, puromycin
and the aminonucleoside exerted a prompt and reversible depressant
effect (Paggi & Toschi, 1971). Some of the drug effects may be
secondary to the inhibition of protein synthesis e.g. the inhibition

of ganglioside synthesis by puromycin (Kanfer and Richards, 1967)
or by AXM (Barondes and Dutton, 1969). Other effects are unrelated
to protein synthesis inhibition e.g. in vitro inhibition of
cyclic AMP phosphodiesterase (Appleman and Kemp, 1966). Therefore
puromycin is not a suitable drug to use in studying the effects of
cerebral protein synthesis inhibition on memory formation. Any one
or more of these side-effects could be the cause of the amnesia.

Cycloheximide did not produce any alteration in the
susceptibility to metrazol seizures or cause any alteration in the
electrical records from mouse brain (8.43, 8.44). Acetoxycycloheximide
did not potentiate metrazol convulsions in goldfish, nor did it
prevent the puromycin potentiation of metrazol convulsions in goldfish
(Agranoff, 1969), it did not cause abnormal membrane swelling (8.14),
nor did it or Actinomycin D affect the spike potential amplitude in
vagus nerve (Dahl, 1969) nor did it effect the respiratory rate of
cortical slices (Jones and Banks, 1969). However, Antinomycin D did
produce spike discharges in the hippocampus (8.66) and caused neuronal
necrosis (Appel, 1965). Paggi and Toschi (1971) reported a depressant
effect on sympathetic ganglionic transmission with both AXM and CXM
which was slow and irreversible but the extent of the effect was much
less marked than with puromycin. CXM does have effects on activity
in mice but these appear to be dissociable from its effects on memory
(8.55, 8.56).

At the present time these two antibiotics seem preferable
to puromycin in memory studies because of their apparently more
specific action in inhibiting cerebral protein synthesis and they
produce no abnormal peptides. CXM is better than AXM in many
experiments because of its rapid onset and shorter duration of protein
synthesis inhibition.

<u>Theories</u>

The evidence to date seems to support the possibility that
synthesis of new protein at or near the time of learning is required
for long-term memory but not short-term storage of the same information.
It is not yet possible to determine whether continued synthesis of
protein is required for the maintenance of long-term memories.

If the proteins are required for memory storage, the
significance of this requirement remains unknown. There are no data
to indicate the cause and effect relationships between the
behavioral change (learning) and the chemical change (RNA and protein).
Indeed, they might be unrelated responses to separate components of
the same experience, an uncertainty that exists whenever behavioral
and chemical responses are correlated. The changes could be due to
restorational processes in the cell or to other processes not related
to encoding. For example, even if the change is tightly coupled to
learning, it may be related to the reception of sensory stimuli, to
arousal or other emotional responses. There is absolutely no
information as to what end the protein synthesis might be directed.

CONCLUSIONS

        Through susceptibility to loss by physical treatments to
the brain, and by differential sensitivity to metabolic inhibition,
memory storage can be seen to pass through a short-term stage, which
decays unless built up by the permanent storage process. This
distinction between the physiological short and long term storage
mechanisms refers only to the physical nature of the memory trace.
Short, intermediate and long term memory are also terms used by
psychologists to separate out stages in the logical processing of
information particularly in verbal learning experiments (Broadbent,
1970, Craik and Lockhart, 1972). The animal experiments reviewed
here mostly deal with time intervals longer than the decay of human
short term memory and the changing nature of the physical store is not
apparent in the threshold for the release of behaviour dependent upon
memory. Physiological short term memory probably corresponds to the
initial form of storage of information in psychological long term
memory.

        A central question in all this research has been whether
behavioural experiments can be used to determine the kinetics of the
transformation in the nature of the material storage of memory. In
the case of ECS it seems that the essential information may be
impossible to obtain because of the interferring behavioural effects
of administration of ECS. With antibiotic block of long term memory
it may be possible to come closer, because the drug can be given
before learning and not produce any obvious behavioural change
beyond the effect on memory. Nevertheless, the kind of learning
task, the difficulty of discrimination, the criteria of training and
testing all have effects on the slope of the curves of memory loss.
The use of the correct pharmacological methods particularly the
geometric variation of drug dosage and probit analysis as advocated
by Cherkin (1966) coupled with well throught out behavioural
techniques should now yield quantitative data about drug susceptibility.
It remains to be seen whether such quantitative experiments can be
interpreted in terms of a uniform rate process converting labile to
permanent memory.

77

Behavioural analysis must be given equal weight to
pharmacological methods because, as is so clear from the history
of investigations into ECS amnesia, the choice of an apparently
simple learning task does not mean that behavioural variables can
be ignored. In the end, a more complicated psychological situation
may be necessary in order to attribute behavioural change to drug
action on memory. Simple replications in different laboratories of
those experiments that have given clear cut results are needed so
that the procedural factors necessary for reliable behavioural tests
become widely known. Further behavioural analysis of agents throught
to interfere with memory formation is also necessary. Control
experiments that try to eliminate possible effects on perception or
motor control by manipulating the time relations between drug treatment and learning or recall are generally not enough. This is not
because of inadequacies of theoretical experimental design but
because, as has become clear from the use of electroconvulsive shock,
a strong and unusual experience given to an animal at any time during
the experimental period is liable to become linked to previous
experiences of the whole changing environmental complex. From out
of these links can come a host of unexpected modifications of
behaviour which are not necessarily related in any physiologically
meaningful way to the molecular action of the drugs under investigation.
State-dependent learning is one of these interactions and for some
drugs it is very strong. There must be many others, perhaps not so
strong but capable of being forced into prominence by the hazards of
experimental design.

As far as agents used to interfere with memory are concerned,
electroconvulsive shock by itself appears to have now reached a
plateau of usefulness until more is known about its physiology. It
would be a great help to know exactly which of the many cellular
consequences of ECS or other convulsants are directly responsible for
amnesia. The observation that spike discharge, as recorded by gross
electrodes, is one necessary feature is only the first step. It
should be possible to document by further neurophysiological
experiments the degree of alteration in firing pattern of neurones
produced by memory destroying ECS and then by pharmacological agents
to modify this and to test the combination for amnesic potency. A
start has been made on this by the finding that anaesthesia does not
interfere with the effect of ECS on memory but many refinements are
possible. Whether the decline of memory measured after learning in
an animal in which brain protein synthesis is inhibited corresponds
to the decline of labile memory as deduced from the ECS or other un-
specific experiments is not yet known and needs some very careful
experimentation.

The extension of behavioural techniques acquired in the
experiments on ECS, into measuring the effects of other metabolic
inhibitors of memory is now open. The need here is for inhibitors
of great specificity of action, as is apparent from the complicated

results from the use of puromycin as an inhibitor of protein synthesis. Most work has been done on inhibitors of RNA or protein synthesis but concentration of effort on this proposed stage of memory formation seems to have diverted attention from the question of how information gets from the nerve impulse code in which it enters the nervous system into a state where it becomes vulnerable to interference by inhibition of macromolecular metabolism. There are specific inhibitors of the membrane metabolic events associated with the passage of nerve impulses, the use of which may well clarify ideas about memory. Work with these substances has only just begun.

Most daunting of all is the absence of any reasonable theory of memory that can be tested with the whole animal experiments that are now possible. In spite of ingenious,difficult and detailed theorizing there is not even any conclusive evidence that memory formation involves synaptic change, let alone the very common idea that it leads to improved transmission at a synapse. Changes in the rhythmic properties of central neurones, which are known in some cases to be under direct macromolecular control (Strumwasser, 1965) could also produce the network change required for memory. Yet, the importance of patterns of synaptic connection in organised brain function leads us back to the synapse as the most probable site of plasticity. The few known naturally occurring changes in synaptic efficacy due to use of nervous pathways at critical times in development seem to depend on suppression of transmission in unused pathways rather than facilitation by use. If, as is assumed by some, learning relies on mechanisms similar to those used in the detailed patterning of synaptic connections in embryological development it would be better to look to the early stages of life history of the brain for clues as to its continuing modifiability, rather than to the sequence of molecular events needed for the manufacture of microbial enzymes (Mark, 1973).

Note on use of the tables

Each table summarises work in approximately chronological order, except that the papers by one principal investigator and his collaborators or those obviously from one laboratory are grouped together. Different groups are separated by horizontal lines.

Each entry takes the width of one double page and the comments read straight across. Full references are found listed alphabetically under first author in the reference list appropriate for the table.

Treatment and site	animals	task	trials

1.1 DUNCAN, 1945

ECS	rats	maze	no. to 3 errorless trials

1.2 DUNCAN, 1948

ECS	rats	T-maze reversal appetitive	4-7

ECS given 30 seconds or 2 hours after reversal training resulted
training when tested 30 minutes after the ECS treatment. However,
for the reversal training. It was argued that one of the effects
habits, thereby allowing older incompatible habits to regain

1.3 DUNCAN, 1949

ECS 17; 1/day transpinnate 85v.AC;200msec	rats	step-through FS AA	17; 1/day

In all groups there was no difference after first treatment.
backlegs instead of the head. The results were interpreted in
learned material undergoes a period of consolidation or perseveration.
out the effect of learning. The material rapidly becomes more
effect of cerebral electroshock was found.

1.4 HUNT AND BRADY, 1951

ECS 21;3/day	rats	skinner box FS and CS CER	no.

CS associated with FS gave rise to a CER. ECS diminishes or
treatment. (Prior to ECS treatment, on presentation of the CS

measure of retention	time of treatment	test	retention
		1/day for 30 days (with no training)	RA
response choice	30sec,2hr	30 min	RA
	30sec,2hr	24 hr	no RA

in 7 of 12 animals giving the response learned on the original
when testing was 24 hours later, there was no retention deficit
of shock may be to cause amnesia or a disorganization for recent
dominance.

no.anticipatory runs	20,40sec	every 24hr	RA
	60sec,4min 15min	every 24hr	less RA
	1,4,14hr	every 24hr	no RA

Control groups were run which consisted of shock applied to the
terms of a consolidation theory. It was suggested that newly
Early in this period a cerebral electroshock may practically wipe
resistant to such disruption; at the end of an hour no retroactive

---

bar press rates	5-6hr before training	every 24hr	

virtually eliminates the CER established prior to convulsive
there was no reduction in the bar press rates.)

Treatment and site	animals	task	trials

1.5   BRADY AND HUNT, 1951

ECS 21;3/day	rats	skinner box FS and CS CER	no.

The CER and bar pressing are incompatible. No deafness or
ECS appeared to affect the CER directly.

1.6   BRADY, 1951

ECS 21;3/day	rats	skinner box FS and CS CER	no.

There was no CER at 4 days but the CER reappeared over 90 days
response was retained throughout the experiment with no reinforce-
than controls.

1.7   BRADY, HUNT AND GELLER, 1954

ECS;21	rats	skinner box FS and CS CER	no.

1.8   GELLER, SIDMAN AND BRADY, 1955

ECS; 21	rats	skinner box FS and CS CER	no.

It was thought that the CER may be more vulnerable to ECS than the
the lever pressing habit was established. ECS treatments virtually
had no apparent effect on lever pressing in the absence of the
CER and not just to the more recently acquired learning.

---

measure of retention	time of treatment	test	retention
reaction in box, fear reactions bar press rates	5-6hr before training	4 days	

physiological incapacity were evident from the ECS treatment.

bar press rates	5-6hr before training	4 days 30 days 60 days 90 days	RA no RA no RA no RA

with presentation of the CS. In control animals (no FS) the ment, i.e. no CER. Experimental animals extinguished faster

bar press rates	every 8 or 24hr	maximum attenuation of CER
	1 every 30min	only slight attenuation of CER
	1/sec	no effect
	1 every 2 or 3 days	only slight effect

bar press rates	The CER was established prior to bar pressing habit.

lever pressing habit because it was normally conditioned after eliminated the CER acquired prior to the lever pressing, but it emotional stimulus. In this situation ECS was specific to the

Treatment and site	animals	task	trials

1.9 GERARD, 1955

ECS 1/day	hamsters	maze learning	no. 1 set/day

Cooling during the learning-ECS interval increased the consolidation hour. The temperature coefficient of 2-3 might be determined by several possible variables.

1.10   THOMPSON AND DEAN, 1955

ECS transpinnate 50mA; 500msec	rats	2 choice discriminative avoidance FS	no. to criterion

1.11   THOMPSON, 1957 (a)

ECS 1	rats	discriminative avoidance	no. to criterion
2		FS	

Two ECS treatments failed to cause a greater effect on the

1.12   THOMPSON, 1957 (b)

ECS transpinnate 50mA; 500msec	rats 30 days old	discriminative avoidance FS	no. to criterion massed
	200 days old		

There was a greater memory deficit at both ECS intervals in young

measure of retention	time of treatment	test	retention
rate of learning	5 min	every 24 hr	RA
	15 min, 1 hr	every 24 hr	slight RA
	4 hr	every 24 hr	no RA

time. ECS at 15 min produced RA equal to cooling and ECS at 1
the rate of reverberation, speed of chemical fixation or one of

---

% correct choices on relearning	10 sec, 1 hr	2 days	RA
	4 hr	2 days	no RA

% correct choices on relearning	1 min	24 hr	RA
	1 min	24 hr	same amount RA

retention deficit.

% correct choices on relearning	30sec, 15min	24 hr	RA
	30sec, 15min	24 hr	less RA

than in adult rats.

Treatment and site	animals	task	trials

1.13   THOMPSON, HARAVEY, PENNINGTON, SMITH, GANNON AND STOCKWELL,

ECS transpinnate 50mA; 500msec	rats-age: 30+40 days	two choice discriminative avoidance FS	20 massed
	50 + 60 days		
	65 day old; dark reared light reared		
ECS 2 depression of cerebral metabolic rate by hyperthyroidism		reversal of a black- white discrimination	no.
ECS and brain damage to visual cortex	65-100 days		
ECS and brain damage to anterior cortex			

There appeared to be a critical period between 40 and 50 days.
metabolic rate appeared to account for this age effect. It was
to fewer functional neurons within the brain, since brain damage
in rats is complete at about 50 days.

1.14   THOMPSON AND PENNINGTON, 1957

ECS	rats	discriminative avoidance FS	no. with inter- trial interval of
			45sec,2min 3,4 min 5,6 min

There was an optimal inter-trial interval of 3-4 minutes with

measure of retention	time of treatment	test	retention
1958			
no.errors in 20 trials on relearning	30 sec after trial 20	24 hr	RA
			less RA
			RA
			RA, no difference
no. errors	30 sec after trial 20 and 30 sec after trial 30	repeated	RA equal to controls
			little RA comparing ECS and no ECS
			RA in brain damaged compared to normals
			no effect

Neither differences in previous visual experience nor cerebral
suggested that the greater deficit in young rats may be related
increased the memory loss, and since myelination of the brain

% correct choices on relearning	30sec after last training trial	2 days	
			RA
			least RA
			RA

respect to original learning scores when ECS had least effect.

Treatment and site	animals	task	trials

1.15 THOMPSON, 1958 (a)

| ECS transpinnate 50mA; 500msec | rats | discriminative avoidance FS 45sec inter-trial interval | 10 20 30 40 |

The consolidation time increases with increasing amounts of decreases.

| | | increasing problem difficulty | 1.   3 2. 16 3. 33-40 |

Consolidation time also increases with an increase in problem

1.16 THOMPSON, 1958 (b)

| bilateral caudate ES | cats | reversal of position habit | no. |

unilateral caudate ES

ES of tegmentum

The deficit obtained with bilateral caudate stimulation was stimulus train duration.

---

measure of retention	time of treatment	test	retention
% correct choices on relearning	after last trial 30 sec 3,30 min	24 hr	RA no RA
	30sec,3min, 30 min		RA
	30sec,3min 30min		RA no RA
	30sec,3min 30min		no RA

practice (learning) up to a certain amount, from whence it

mean errors	20sec,15min		no RA
	20sec 15min		RA no RA
	20sec,15min		RA

difficulty.

errors and no. trials to relearn.	immediate	3/day	RA
	immediate		no RA
	immediate		no RA

increased with increased voltage, frequency, pulse duration and

---

Treatment and site	animals	task	trials

1.17 LEUKEL, 1957

ECS 1/trial	rats	14 unit water maze	no.

There was no difference in acquisition. The trial-ECS interval
effects on maze behaviour.

1.18 POSCHEL, 1957

ECS 10, 5/day for 2 days	rats	step-through runway. approach-avoidance	no.
proactive ECS retroactive ECS			

Proactive treatment reduced the intensity of the avoidance tendency

---

1.19 GLICKMAN, 1958

ES of ascending reticular formation	rats	extinction in conditioned avoidance	1

1.20 COONS AND MILLER, 1960

ECS 27;1/day transpinnate 50mA; 60Hz; 200msec	rats	step-through FS AA	27;1/day
pseudo ECS			

When any effects of either amnesia or conflict (as in an active
runs, learning is poorer the shorter the interval between each

measure of retention	time of treatment	test	retention
no. of errors	1 min	30 days	RA
	5 min		RA
	30 min		RA
	2 hr		no RA

determined the duration rather than the magnitude of the ECS

| running latencies | | 10 days | |

to approximately the same degree as the retroactive treatment.

| time spent at food chamber (where shocked before) | 1-2 sec | 24 hr | RA |
| | | 1 week | RA |

---

anticipatory STL (10.6sec)	20 sec	daily	RA
	60sec, 1hr		no RA
			no RA

avoidance situation) would hinder learning to make anticipatory
learning trial and ECS treatment.

Treatment and site	animals	task	trials

1.20 (Continued)

ECS 12; 1/day	rats	step-through	12;1/day
		FS (pretraining)	
		on AA) training	
		on PA, i.e.reversal	

When the effects of conflict would help and amnesia would hinder
(longer STL's) the shorter the interval between each training trial
considered greater than the aversive properties of the FS.

1.21 QUARTERMAIN, PAOLINO AND MILLER, 1965

ECS	rats	step-through	1
transpinnate		FS	
100mA; 300msec		PA	

ECS in a black bag outside the apparatus at 2.0 sec produced the
alone had no effect on retention.

1.22 PAOLINO, QUARTERMAIN AND MILLER, 1966

ECS	rats	step-through	1
transpinnate		FS	
200mA; 300msec		PA	

A 200msec ECS produced the same amount of retention deficit at 60

1.23 QUARTERMAIN, PAOLINO AND BANUAZIZI, 1968

ECS	thirsty rats	T-maze for	1
transpinnate		water	
100mA; 300msec		appetitive	
	thirsty rats	T-maze	1
		FS for	
		left choice	

Similar temporal gradients of RA can be obtained with both positive
It was suggested that as the type of reinforcement is not the major
that the nature of the task is an important determinant of the

measure of retention	time of treatment	test	retention
STL (120sec)	20 sec	daily	no RA
	60 sec		less RA
	1 hr		RA

learning to stop the avoidance response, learning is better
and the ECS treatments. The aversive properties of ECS are

measure of retention	time of treatment	test	retention
STL (180sec)	0.1-2sec	24 hr	RA
	5,7.5sec		decreasing RA
	15 sec		decreasing RA
	30 sec		little RA (20%)
	60 sec		no RA (10%)

same amount of RA as when given in the shock compartment. ECS

measure of retention	time of treatment	test	retention
STL (180sec)	60 sec	24 hr	no RA (10%)

secs as did 100mA ECS used in the previous experiment.

measure of retention	time of treatment	test	retention
no. errors	10 sec	23 hr	RA
	60 sec		RA
	1 hr		slight RA
	2 hr		slight RA
	3 hr		no RA
no. left choices on 10 trials	10 sec	23 hr	RA
	60 sec		less RA
	30 min		no RA

and negative reinforcement in a similar behavioural situation.
determinant of the slope of the temporal gradient, it is likely
length of the RA gradient.

Treatment and site	animals	task	trials

1.24 PAOLINO, QUARTERMAIN AND LEVY, 1969

ECS-transpinnate	rats	step-through	1
100mA		FS	
duration varied		PA	
200msec			
800msec			

The longer ECS duration group showed a slightly higher % stepping
(Note: the current level was much higher than 1.35). ECS alone had
group had less RA than the 800msec group, RA was still present.

1.25 QUARTERMAIN, McEWAN AND AZMITIA, 1970

ECS	rats	step-through	
transpinnate		FS	
100mA; 300msec		PA	1 test shock at T_0
			$\pm$ reminder shock (RS) outside the apparatus

As the interval between T_1 and RS increases the RS becomes
related to RS and a prior retention test in the apparatus was

In this experiment the original training was given in a different
for RS to produce long T_2 latencies – minimizing the importance of

measure of retention	time of treatment	test	retention

% stepping out
STL

	0.1 sec	24 hr	RA
	7.5–60 sec		no RA
	0.1 sec	24 hr	RA
	7.5–60 sec		no RA

out than the shorter duration group, but this was not significant.
no effect on latencies. When retested at 72 hrs - the 200msec

$$T_0 \;\overline{24\ hr}\; T_1 \;\overline{1,4\ or\ 23\ hr}\; RS \;\overline{24\ hr}\; T_2$$

STL			
	1 sec	T_1 24 hrs	RA
	1 sec	T_1; T_2 48 hr	RA
	1 sec	T_1;RS;T_2	no RA
	RS-1 hr		
	1 sec	T_1;RS;T_2	no RA
	RS-4 hr		
	1 sec	T_1;RS;T_2	RA
	RS-23 hr		

progressively less effective. The recovery was specifically

necessary for recovery from the amnesia.

	1 sec	T_1;RS;T_2	RA
	RS-4 hr		
	after T_1		

apparatus. FS had to be given in the training apparatus in order
non-specific effects of combining FS with ECS.

Treatment and site	animals	task	trials

1.26 HINE AND PAOLINO, 1970

ECS transpinnate 100mA; 500msec	rats	step-through FS PA with contingent and non- contingent FS	1 1

With FS all animals showed a drop in heart rate, whereas with ECS
On the retention test, all animals which had FS during training
or not. It was suggested that the mode of action of a reminder

1.27 QUARTERMAIN, McEWAN AND AZMITIA, 1972

ECS transpinnate 100mA; 300 msec	rats	step-through FS (1.6mA; for 2 sec) PA	1

The reminder shock (RS) was given 1 hour after T_1, T_2 was 24 hours
The RS is producing a recovery of some parts of the originally
trials. Animals not given a RS show recovery over repeated
do not show this increase in latencies with repeated tests.

1.28 MADSEN AND McGAUGH, 1961

ECS	rats	step-down FS PA	1

If ECS affects performance by inducing fear, subjects should tend
avoidance task. It was concluded therefore, as the response was

measure of retention	time of treatment	test	retention
STL (180 sec)	immediate	24 hr	RA
	60 sec		no RA
heart rate change	0-60 sec	24 hr	no RA

only and no FS-no ECS groups there was an increase in heart rate.
exhibited tachycardia - irrespective of whether they showed RA
shock could be associated with autonomic responses.

$$T_0 \text{---} 24 \text{ hr} \text{---} T_1 \text{---} 1 \text{ hr} \text{---} RS \text{---} 23 \text{ hr} \text{---} T_2 \text{---} 24 \text{ hr} \text{---} T_3 \text{-----}$$

STL (180 sec)	1 sec	T_1 (24 hr)	RA
		T_1;RS;T_2	no RA
		T_3;T_4;T_5	no RA
		T_1;noRS;T_2	RA
		T_3;T;$_4T_5$	no RA

after T_1.

learned avoidance response and this does extinguish with repeated
exposures to the training apparatus. Non-contingent FS and ECS

SDL	5 sec	24 hr	RA

not to make a response on a subsequent test in a passive
made following ECS, that ECS interferes with memory.

Treatment and site	animals	task	trials

1.29 MADSEN AND LUTTGES, 1963

ECS; 5	rats	extinction of approach response	5 daily
200msec 35mA away from maze			

No significant differences occurred until the fifth trial when the
administered in close temporal proximity to a response may cause
occurs after repeated treatments and is probably a cumulative

1.30 HUDSPETH, McGAUGH AND THOMPSON, 1964

ECS 1	rats	step-down; FS PA	1
ECS 1		no FS	1
ECS 8			8 daily

Cumulative ECS produces avoidance when administered shortly (0-20
gradually learned to avoid suggesting partial additive consolidation.

1.31 McGAUGH AND MADSEN, 1964

ECS convulsive 1	rats	discriminative place avoidance	1
9		ECS as incentive for DA	9 daily
ECS subconvulsive 1			1
9			9 daily

The latencies of subconvulsive ECS group were significantly greater
trial. ECS affects performance both by producing amnesia and by
considerably less effective than the less intensive subconvulsive

measure of retention	time of treatment	test	retention
latency of goal box entry	5 sec 1 hr	over 5 days days 1-4	no RA no RA
	5 sec 1 hr	day 5	RA no RA

immediate ECS group showed longer approach latencies. While ECS interference with or speed extinction of that response, this only process.

SDL	0-20 sec 30 min- 1 hr	24 hr	RA no RA
		24 hr	no effect on performance
	0-20 sec	24 hr	no RA

sec) after trials. The No FS groups with 8 ECS treatments

latencies and avoidance	5 sec 1 hr	24 hr	RA no RA
	5 sec-1 hr	every 24 hr	no RA
	5 sec-1 hr	24 hr	no RA
	5 sec-1 hr	every 24 hr	no RA

than those of the convulsive ECS group. The former learned in one inducing fear, but the punishing effect of these shocks is shocks and is only found with repeated treatments.

Treatment and site	animals	task	trials

1.32 DAWSON AND PRYOR,   1965

ECS 9	rats	step-through appetitive	9 1/48 hr

The places where ECS was given and where recovery occurred were
than controls or sham ECS groups. Place of recovery from ECS treat-
onset of the electro-shock.

1.33 McGAUGH AND ALPERN,   1966

ECS	mice	step-down FS	1
ECS and ether anaesthesia to prevent motor convulsion		PA	

Overt convulsions were prevented but RA still occurred; this is
shock.

1.34 LUTTGES AND McGAUGH,   1967

ECS transcorneal	mice	step-down FS PA	1

No recovery from amnesia was found with either single or repeated
task.

1.35 ALPERN AND McGAUGH,   1968

ECS Duration and intensity 200msec; 15mA	mice	step-through FS PA	1
800msec; 8mA			
400msec; 8mA			

measure of retention	time of treatment	test	retention
% time spent in compartment		24 hr after trials 7,8,9	

varied. Rats spent less time in compartment where ECS was given
ment had no effect. The aversive aspects of ECS were confined to

SDL	25 sec	24 hr	RA
	25 sec		RA

inconsistent with notions of competing responses elicited by the

SDL	15 sec	12 hr	RA
	15 sec	1 week	RA
	15 sec	1 month	RA

retention tests even though control animals had not forgotten the

SDL		24 hr	
	0 hr		RA
	1-24 hr		no RA
	0-3 hr		RA
	8-24 hr		no RA
	0-3 hr		RA
	8-24 hr		no RA

Treatment and site	animals	task	trials

1.36 STEPHENS, McGAUGH AND ALPERN, 1967

ECS (1) transcorneal
800msec; 8mA

ECS	mice	step-through	3
at 1 p.m.		FS	
		PA	
ECS			
at 9 p.m.			

ECS appears to produce greater amnesia when administered in the
rectal temperature). This could mean either that memory
that susceptibility to ECS varies directly with metabolic activity.

1.37 STEPHENS AND McGAUGH, 1968

ECS (1)	mice	step-through	1
transcorneal		PA	

ECS treatment			no. of
at 1 p.m.			massed trials
at 9 p.m.			no. of
			massed trials

At 3 minutes ECS time interval, the retention scores of 9 p.m.
At night, during crest values of the adrenal activity rhythm, the
to interact in a way which produces different results from those
trough i.e. during the day.
Therefore, the degree of RA has been shown to vary with:
1. The amount of training
2. The interval between training and ECS
3. Physiological status as indexed by the 24 hour temperature
       activity rhythm.
4. (Order of training and treatment).

1.38 STEPHENS AND McGAUGH, 1969

ECS (1)
transcorneal
800msec; 8mA

ECS	mice	step-through	3
Time of day with		FS	
3 hr phase shift		PA	
1.00 p.m. - 4 p.m.			

measure of retention	time of treatment	test	retention
STL (60sec)	5 sec	24 hr	RA
	3 min-1 hr		no RA
	5 sec,3 min		RA
	1 hr		no RA

time region of the animal's crest of activity (as measured by
consolidation rate varies inversely with metabolic activity or

STL (60sec)	5 sec,3 min	24 hr	RA
	1 hr		no RA
	5 sec,1 min	24 hr	RA
	3 min,1 hr		no RA
	1 min,3 min		RA
	5 sec,1 hr		no RA

animals were significantly poorer than those of 1 p.m. group.
training, treatment and temporal course of the experiment appear
obtained in experiments done during the animals physiological

STL (60sec)			
	5 sec,3 min	24 hr	RA
	1 hr		no RA

Treatment and site	animals	task	trials

1.38   (Continued)

9 p.m. – 12 p.m.	mice	step-through FS PA	3

At 4 p.m. the temperatures of the animals were likely to be in
to crest values at 9 p.m. These results seem to offer further
lying memory trace formation and consolidation may be quite different
rhythm, as well as during transition periods.

1.39   DAWSON AND McGAUGH,   1969(a)

ECS wound clips attached to rear of pinnae 50 mA; 500msec	rats	drinking tube FS-CS pairing PA	1

When ECS treatment was given after presentation of the stimulus
memory trace, it was totally ineffective in reducing subsequent
fear to the CS. The CS elicited fear after it was paired with FS
even though ECS did produce amnesia when administered immediately

1.40   DAWSON AND McGAUGH,   1969(b)

ECS transcorneal 20mA; 200msec	mice	step-through FS; PA FS duration determined by escape latencies	1 FAM NFAM

FAM groups were given 4 trials of prior familiarization over 4 days.

		FS duration fixed at 1 sec	FAM NFAM

The RA gradient for FAM subjects was again longer than for NFAM
did not eliminate the retrograde amnesia effects of ECS. It is
because transcorneal electrodes used here do not produce fear

measure of retention	time of treatment	test	retention
STL (60sec)	5 sec,3 min	24 hr	RA
	1 hr		no RA

transition;declining to trough values at 1 p.m. and ascending
support for the possibility that physiological processes under-
at trough and crest phases of the 24 hour temperature activity

measure of retention	time of treatment	test	retention
latency to 1st lick, 100 licks and final licks	CS;FS;ECS-immediate	24 hr	RA
	CS;FS	Day 1	
	CS;ECS-immediate	Day 2	no RA

used in the fear conditioning training i.e. reactivation of the
fear of the CS. The reactivated groups tended to exhibit more
but ECS was not effective in disrupting such re-activated fear,
after original training.

measure of retention	time of treatment	test	retention
STL escape (300 sec+ day 1 STL)	0-30 min	24 hr	RA
	60 min		no RA
	0-20 sec	24 hr	RA
	5-30 min		no RA

NFAM-FS-NECS mice had longer latencies than FAM-FS-NECS mice.

	0-20 sec	24 hr	RA
	5 min		no RA
	0 sec	24 hr	RA
	20 sec-5 min		no RA

subjects. Prior familiarization with the experimental situation
suggested that the difference from Lewis et al. 1968 (1.72) is
whereas earclips do.

Treatment and site	animals	task	trials

1.41 McGAUGH AND LONGACRE, 1969

ECS	mice	step-through	8 x 100
transcorneal		FS	(well learned)
15mA; 800msec.		AA	
ECS given on day 8			

ECS + ether
(no convulsion)

ECS with convulsion impaired retention performance only if
convulsion did not impair performance even when given immediately
proactive impairing effects of ECS on performance are due to
current. Since the impairing effects last for less than 2 hours,
amnesic effects of ECS.

1.42 DENTI, McGAUGH, LANDFIELD AND SHINKMAN, 1969

MRF-ES	rats	step-through	25
90 sec of 6 sec		FS	1 per day
on- 3 sec off;		AA	1 stim/day
0.01msec biphasic;			
300Hz			
			no stim. (implanted electrodes)
			no stim. (implanted electrodes)
			stim. 1/day

Avoidance learning is facilitated by post-trial electrical

1.43 ZORNETZER AND McGAUGH, 1969

ECS	mice	step-through	1
transcorneal		FS	
20mA; 800msec		PA	

measure of retention	time of treatment	test	retention
error scores	before training on day 8		
	2 hr	day 8 + 9	good retention
	1 hr,15 min	day 8	impaired performance
	1 hr,15 min	day 9	good retention
	1 hr,15 min+ immediate	days 8 + 9	good retention

administered 1 hour or less prior to the test. ECS without
prior to the test. These findings suggest that the brief
consequences associated with the convulsions and not to the ECS
such effects cannot readily explain the long-lasting retrograde

% correct responses	immediate- each day	0-25 days	learned faster than no shock
		26-50 days	performance did not decrease
		0-25 days	slower than controls (not implanted)
	immediate- each day	26-50 days	significant improvement

stimulation of the mesencephalic reticular formation (MRF).

STL (300 sec)	5 sec	24 hr	RA
	5 sec	48 hr	RA
	5 sec	72 hr repeat test at 1 week	RA
			RA

Treatment and site   animals   task   trials

1.43   (Continued)

Animals tested 24 hours after receiving FS + ECS showed a non-
72 hours following FS + ECS, locomotor activity was significantly
activity in animals tested 24,48 or 72 hours following ECS alone.
significantly depressed at 48 hours, but were unchanged at 24 and

In the inhibitory avoidance situation, the effects of ECS upon
time of the low response latencies (high amnesia) evidenced in

pretreatment   step-through   1
96 hr or 24 hr   FS
with NC.FS + ECS   PA

                                      FS + no ECS

Regardless of the pretreatment presumed to alter 'brain
treatment and training, all groups not given post-trial ECS
Animals given training and ECS following pretreatment all

1.44 McGAUGH AND ZORNETZER,   1970

ECS transcorneal   mice   step-through   1
                                          FS
low ECS   PA
15mA; 200msec

low ether
2.0ml for 30sec
+ low ECS

high ether
10.0ml for 30 sec
+ low ECS

high ether
+ high ECS
40mA; 800msec

Deep ether anaesthesia, but not light anaesthesia, attenuated the
current deep ether anaesthesia did not attenuate the amnesia.
indicated that the brain seizure activity produced by ECS is of
those obtained with light anaesthesia. These findings suggest that
processes which are associated with (i.e.,which result in) brain
discharge was not observed in ether protected mice. Changes in ECS
seizure activity and hence have a different effect on RA.

| measure of | time of | test | retention |
| retention | treatment | | |

significant increase in open field activity; at 48 hours and
increased. There were no significant changes in locomotor
The activity scores of animals receiving only FS were
72 hours following the treatment.

general locomotor activity cannot account for the stability over
those mice which received ECS following the learning trial.

STL (300 sec)	5 sec	24 hr	RA
		48 hr	RA
		72 hr	RA
		24 hr	good retention
		48 hr	good retention
		72 hr	good retention

excitability', and regardless of the time interval between pre-
displayed retention of the inhibitory avoidance response.
displayed RA.

STL (300 sec)			
	35 sec	24 hr	RA
	35 sec		RA
	35 sec		no RA
	35 sec		RA

amnesic effect of low current stimulation. However, with high
Electrocorticograms recorded from chronically implanted mice
shorter duration under deep ether anaesthesia in comparison with
the degree of amnesia produced by ECS depends on alteration in
seizure activity. Post-ictal depression following seizure
current intensity and duration may produce differences in brain

Treatment and site	animals	task	trials

1.45 ZORNETZER AND McGAUGH, 1970

Frontal cortex   rats
stimulation

ECS		bar press	1
transpinnate		training	
50mA; 800msec		MS	
		PA	
cortical ES			
30mA			
amygdaloid			
lesion and			
cortical ES			

After discharge following earclip ECS was shorter than with
seizure pattern with ECS. 30mA applied cortically is as effective

1.46 ZORNETZER AND McGAUGH, 1971(a)

ECS	mice		1
transcorneal			
200msec; 60Hz			
current - 1-20mA			

light ether
30 sec before ES

no ether

ES ether (E)			1
no ether (NE)		step-through	
		FS	
1-3mA E and NE		PA	
7-11mA E			
NE			
13-50mA E and NE			

measure of retention	time of treatment	test	retention

E.Co.G.activity

Seizure duration and EEG spike frequencies varied systematically with current intensity. Spontaneous secondary after discharges develop at higher stimulus intensities.

measure of retention	time of treatment	test	retention
latency to first bar press and total latency	immediate	24 hr	RA
to complete 100 presses	immediate	24 hr	RA
	immediate	24 hr	RA

cortical stimulation. The mouth shock did not alter the brain as 50mA applied via earclips.

measure of retention	time of treatment	test	retention
convulsion threshold		1-3mA	no convulsions ES appeared to be punishing
		5mA	clonic convulsion threshold
		8mA	clonic-tonic convulsion threshold
E.Co.G. primary after-discharge threshold		13.2mA	
		2.8mA	
STL (100 sec) %RA	0.5 min		
			little RA no diff-erence E and NE
			15 - 30% RA
			45 - 50% RA
			much RA no difference E and NE

Treatment and site   animals   task   trials

1.46 (Continued)

In unanaesthetized mice, the current intensities required for
for elicitation of convulsions. Light ether anaesthesia prior to
seizure and RA thresholds. The authors suggest that the results
depend on the ES current level per se, but rather on the alteration
sufficient to produce RA in ether anaesthetized mice, the P.A.D. of
postictal depression appears not to contribute to RA.

1.47 ZORNETZER AND McGAUGH,   1971(b)

ECS   mice   one-way   25 massed
transcorneal   shuttle box 10 min
200msec, plus   FS
ether   PA

5 and 12mA
15mA
20mA
20mA
30mA

The results indicate that, under some conditions, ES produces RA
activity.

1.48 ZORNETZER AND McGAUGH,   1972

The EEG spike frequency of the primary after discharge (P.A.D.)
current intensity, however, did not result in changes in the EEG

ES to frontal   rats   bar press   1
cortex   for water
                                           2mA MS
1.5mA   PA
1.5mA
2.5mA
3.5mA
6.0mA

There was no evidence of a graded effect of current intensity,
there was after discharge activity.

measure of retention	time of treatment	test	retention

eliciting brain seizures and RA were lower than that required
ES prevented the convulsions and significantly increased brain
indicate that the degree of amnesia produced by ES does not
in CNS activity produced by the ES. At ES current levels
the seizure was not followed by postictal depression.   Thus

mean avoidance responses	40 sec after last trial	24 hr	
E.Co.G. P.A.D. Primary after-discharges			
			no RA; no PAD
			some RA; no PAD
			more RA;no PAD 30%
			greater RA; PAD 70%
			RA; PAD 100%

at current levels below the threshold for E.Co.G. seizure

increased systematically with current level. Increases in
spike frequency for the spontaneous after discharge (S.A.D.).

latency to first bar press and total latency to complete 100 presses	immediate	24 hr	
			no RA; no PAD
			RA; PAD
			RA; PAD, PAD+SAD
			RA; PAD+SAD
			RA; PAD+SAD

1.5mA produced as much RA when it did as 6.0mA provided that

Treatment and site	animals	task	trials

1.48   (Continued)

Treatment and site	animals	task	trials
ES to frontal cortex	rats	bar press for water 2mA FS PA	1
1.5mA			
1.5mA			
2.5mA			
2.5mA			
3.5mA			
6.0mA			

If the motivational intensity of the learning situation is
for a bar pressing response, as current intensity was increased
magnitude of the amnesia increased. Maximal amnesia resulted when
The results suggest that the degree to which abnormal brain
determined by the motivational intensity of the learning experience.
disruptive agent and consequently the brains response in terms of
amount of frontal cortex stimulation (and concomitantly the degree
RA.

1.49 ZORNETZER, 1972

Treatment and site	animals	task	trials
midbrain ES 60 Hz for 1.0 sec	rats	bar press for water 2.0mA MS PA	1
low stimulation			

intermediate stimulation

high stimulation

The first part of this study was concerned with identification of
frontal cortex in rats previously shown to produce RA when
to be in part motor cortex. In addition to the motor projection
collateralized at the level of the substantia nigra and projected
PAD activity initiated in the midbrain and propagated to the cortex
stimulation led to the production of both a PAD and a SAD in the

1.50 McGAUGH AND LANDFIELD, 1970

Treatment and site	animals	task	trials
ECS transcorneal 15mA; 800msec	mice	step-through FS PA	1

measure of retention	time of treatment	test	retention
latency to first bar press	immediate	24 hr	
			no RA; no PAD
			some RA; PAD
			RA; PAD
			RA; PAD+SAD
			more RA; PAD+SAD
			complete RA;PAD+SAD

changed, i.e. mouth shock changed to foot shock as punishment
and as the brain's response to the current increased, the
both PAD's and SAD's occurred.
activity interferes with memory storage processes is partially
The amount of amnesia also depends on the strength of the
PAD and SAD activity. As motivational intensity increases, the
of cellular dysfunction) must also increase in order to produce

EEG and ECoG activity latency to first bar press		24 hr	
			no RA; no PAD
			no RA; PAD
			RA; PAD + SAD

the neuroanatomical projections associated with an area of
electrically stimulated. This frontal cortical region appeared
leaving this area, many fibres in the cerebral peduncle
to various regions of the limbic forebrain.
did not result in amnesia. Amnesia did result when midbrain
cortex.

STL	8 sec	1 hr	RA
	20 sec	1 hr	no RA
	20 sec	6 hr	RA
	8 sec	24 hr	RA
	20 sec	24 hr	RA

Treatment and site	animals	task	trials

1.50   (Continued)

2 ECS treatments	mice	step-through	1
ECS 1		FS	
ECS 2		PA	

The amnesia developed as short-term memory processes declined
retention. The second ECS did not produce high retention latencies
learning.

1.51 McGAUGH, DAWSON, COLEMAN AND RAWIE,   1971

ES	mice	step-through	1
transcorneal		FS	
40mA, 800msec		PA	

light ether
within 30 sec
before ES
(no convulsions)

Animals in this study at the 0.5 min ES delay interval were
less than that seen in previous studies where animals were returned

ES

ES; not restrained
ES; restrained
ES + low ether
ES + high ether

Restraining the animal has an effect comparable to that obtained by
single ES treatment could attenuate the development of a CER, the
should be shorter than that of animals given ES without ether. A
seizures and RA but no behavioural convulsions. The results were
gradient of RA produced by ECS is due to interference with the

measure of retention	time of treatment	test	retention
STL			
	20 sec 1 hr prior to testing	1 week	RA

following ECS.   Reinstatement of the ECS state did not enhance in mice given post-training ECS.   It is not state-dependent

measure of retention	time of treatment	test	retention
STL (300 sec + day 1 STL)	0.5 min	4 days	partial RA
	5 min		no RA
	10 min		partial RA
	60 min		no RA
	0.5 min	4 days	RA
	5 min		RA
	10 min		RA
	60 min		no RA

restrained by the tail before the ES.   The amount of RA seen was to the home cage during this interval.

	immediate (within 7 sec)	4 days	RA
	0.5 min		RA
	0.5 min		partial RA
	0.5 min		RA
	0.5 min		no RA

increasing the amount of punishment.   It was assumed that if a apparent RA gradient obtained with animals given ES under ether CER can be prevented by etherization; there were still brain interpreted as failing to support the hypothesis that the long incubation of a CER.

Treatment and site   animals   task   trials

1.52 FISHBEIN, McGAUGH AND SWARZ, 1971

ECS	mice	step-through	1
transcorneal		FS	
8mA; 800msec		PA	

2 days of REMD
between training
and testing
ECS

Mice were deprived of rapid eye movement sleep (REMD) for 2 days
after deprivation. Overt convulsions were avoided by giving ECS
a retention deficit. It was concluded that processes which occur
influence the storage of LTM. REM sleep deprivation may cause

1.53 FISHBEIN, 1970

partial sleep	mice	step-through	1
deprivation		FS	
REMD		PA	

Deprivation of REM sleep before training does not impair performance
consolidation of STM into LTM does not occur. It is suggested that
predominantly during the REM sleep state could be important for the

1.54 FISHBEIN, 1971

REMD	mice	step-through	1
between		FS	
training and		PA	
testing,			
tested after			
termination			
of REMD			

	T-maze	to 4/5
	discrimination	
	FS	

measure of retention	time of treatment	test	retention
STL (30 sec)	2 days + 5 min, 30 min 1,3,6,12 hr	3 days	no RA
	2 days + 5,30 min, 1hr	3 days	RA
	3,6,12 hr		no RA

immediately after training and were given ECS at various times
under light ether anaesthesia which by itself did not produce
during sleep and most predominantly during the REM sleep state,
increased neuronal excitability.

measure of retention	time of treatment	test	retention
STL (300 sec)	for 1 day before training	5sec-60min	no RA
		1-7days	no RA
	for 3 days before training	5sec-60min	no RA
		1-7days	RA

during training, nor STM for 60 minutes after, but the
endogenous processes which occur during sleep and most
conversion of memory from short-term to long-term storage.

measure of retention	time of treatment	test	retention
STL (300 sec)	for 1 day	30 min,3 hr + 24 hr	no RA
	for 3,5 or 7 days	30 min	marked RA
		3 hr	less RA
		24 hr	no RA
response choice	for 3,5 or 7 days	30 min	marked RA
		24 hr	less RA

Treatment and site	animals	task	trials

1.54   (Continued)

ECS			
transcorneal	mice	T-maze	to 4/5
8mA; 800msec		discrimination	
no REMD		FS	

REMD + ECS

1.55   LANDFIELD AND McGAUGH,   1972

ECS   rats
transpinnate
60Hz; 50mA; 1 sec

MRF-ES
50-100μA; 100 p/sec;
0.05msec pulse duration

ECS decreased the amount of theta activity. Stimulation of the
treatment enhanced the E.Co.G. theta rhythm activity. The effects
effects on memory.

1.56   LANDFIELD, McGAUGH AND TUSA,   1972(a)

ECS	rats	step-through	1
transcranial;		FS	
anterior and		PA	
posterior			
cortical screws			
15mA; 60 Hz; 1 sec			

The amount of theta activity in the E.Co.G. after training was
of the footshock whether animals had received ECS or not. ECS
that received FS-ECS, but exhibited a substantial recovery of

ECS		habituation	1
10mA; 60Hz; 1 sec		for 3 days	
		step-through	
		FS	
		PA	

measure of retention	time of treatment	test	retention
response choice			
	immediate after training	24 hr	RA
	immediate after 2 days REMD	24 hr	sig. more RA
Theta activity (4-9 Hz) on E.Co.G.			decreased theta activity
	immediate after ECS		increased theta activity

mesencephalic reticular formation (MRF) following an ECS
of these treatments on theta activity appear to parallel their

Theta rhythm of E.Co.G. STL (600 sec)	10 sec	2 days	RA - no theta
			no RA - theta

positively correlated with the degree of subsequent retention
lowered the amount of post-trial theta. Individual animals
theta after ECS, exhibited good retention 2 days later.

	5 sec	2 days	RA

Treatment and site   animals   task   trials

1.57 COTMAN, BANKER, ZORNETZER AND McGAUGH,   1971

ES transcorneal   mice   incorporation of ^{14}C-
60 Hz; 200msec
                                             leucine into brain
12mA   protein following 4 min
ether + 12mA   pulse
ether + 30mA

ether + 12mA
ether + 30mA

ether + 12mA
ether + 30mA

ether + 12mA
ether + 30mA

ether + 12mA
ether + 30mA

Electrical stimulation at 12mA produces brain seizures and RA and a
ES 12mA plus ether produces no brain seizures, no RA and has no
ES 30mA plus ether produces brain seizures, RA and a decrease in the

A significant but short-lasting inhibition of brain protein synthesis
by electroshock at intensities above the brain seizure threshold.
on brain protein synthesis. Brain seizures also correlate with RA.
protein synthesis per se. Rather, it seems likely that brain
co-ordinated function of the cells of the brain is altered to such

---

1.58 BUREŜ AND BUREŜOVÁ , 1963

ECS   rats   discriminated   to 9/10
bitemporal   avoidance
2mA; 50 Hz   FS

ECS   step-through   1
                                             FS PA

There was more RA produced by ECS than produced with spreading

measure of retention	time of treatment	test	retention
rate of protein synthesis as % of control rate			% of control rate
		0.5 min	60
		0.5 min	92
		0.5 min	74
		10 min	105
		10 min	83
		30 min	108
		30 min	115
		60 min	103
		60 min	114
		120 min	116
		120 min	104

decrease in the rate of protein synthesis.
effect on the rate of protein synthesis.
protein synthetic rate at 0.5 min and 10 min after the ES.

and an increase in the amount of free leucine were produced
At intensities below brain seizure threshold there was no effect
It is not likely that ECS-RA is due to the inhibition of
seizures and inhibition of protein synthesis are signs that the
a degree that processes involved in memory storage are disrupted.

---

response choice	1 min-2 hr	24 hr	RA
time spent in small compartment	1 min-2 hr 6 hr	24 hr	RA no RA

depression (7.3).

Treatment and site	animals	task	trials

1.59 GERBRANDT AND THOMPSON, 1964

ECS transpinnate 35mA, 75v; 200msec	rats	step-down	1/day

Performance trends during FS conditions were similar in both
last 4 trials. FS-ECS maintained a high performance in relation
the presence of either conditioned freezing or competing activity
less than 1 hour after training.

1.60 BUREŠOVÁ, BUREŠ AND GERBRANDT, 1968

ECS	rats	T-maze & 2 choice discriminative avoidance	to 9/10
		reversal of discrimination; interval between original learning and reversal short - 1 hr long - 24 hr	
		reversal with overtraining on original learning	

% correct choices provide a more sensitive measure of ECS effects
disruption of consolidation processes by ECS may always be present
and measurements appropriate to finding it.

measure of retention	time of treatment		test	retention
SDL	Phase 1 Trials 1-8	Phase 2 Trials 9-16	every 24 hr	
	FS	ECS		
	FS	ECS1 hr		
	FS	NS		
	ECS	FS		
	NS	FS		
	NS	ECS		
	NS	NS		

phase 1 and 2, also with ECS. ECS had little effect until the
to FS-ECS-1 hr and FS-NS groups. The results did not indicate
responses. An amnesic interpretation is supported when ECS was

response choice	20-30 sec	24 hr	RA
	20-30 sec		slight RA
	20-30 sec		RA
response choice	20-30 sec	24 hr	RA (poorer in retention of the reversal)

than latencies or trials to criterion. It was concluded that
in animals but experimenters have not always used situations

Treatment and site	animals	task	trials

1.61 GERBRANDT, BUREŠOVÁ AND BUREŠ, 1968

Treatment and site	animals	task	trials
ECS given outside apparatus	rats	discriminated avoidance FS	4
		reversal training	no.to 5/6

No RA was observed. Shock avoidance pre-training, or avoidance susceptible to ECS.

1.62 HERIOT AND COLEMAN, 1962

Treatment and site	animals	task	trials
ECS transpinnate 150v; 2msec pulses at 200/sec for 800msec	rats	skinner box FS	1

ECS alone had no effect on bar press rates.

1.63 ADAMS AND LEWIS, 1962(a)

Treatment and site	animals	task	trials
ECS 6	rats	step-through FS AA	6; 1/day

The ECS treatments interfered with retention of the original showed response depression. ECS given three days before training avoidance response. Adams and Lewis interpret their results to be interferes with the originally learned response. The ECS serves conditioned to stimuli evoking the original response. The response and produces apparent retrograde amnesia.

measure of retention	time of treatment	test	retention
response choice	20 sec	24 hr	no RA
	3 min	24 hr	no RA
	30 sec	24 hr	no RA

training before reversal may have made the memory trace less

bar press rate	1 min	24 hr	RA
	7 min		RA
	26 min		RA
	60 min		less RA
	180 min		no RA

avoidance responses on retraining	20 sec	3 days	RA

avoidance response. However, the no training-ECS group also
(in the shock compartment) interfered with the learning of the
due to the learning of a strong competing response which
as a UCS evoking a convulsive response, part of which becomes
conditioned convulsion competes with the originally learned

Treatment and site   animals   task   trials

1.64 ADAMS AND LEWIS, 1962(b)

ECS; 6   rats   step-through   6;1/day
transpinnate   FS
35mA; 500msec   AA

in shock compartment-
outside apparatus-

The effects of ECS are stimulus bound in the sense that a RA
the original response was learned, and the effect does not appear

ECS; 3   step-through   9;3/day
                                       FS
                                       AA

                                       extinction   5
                                       trials

                                       no extinction
                                       trials, home
                                       cage for
                                       5 days

By eliminating the CR of the apparatus for 5 days with no ECS, the
the animals were left untreated for 5 days in the home cage, they
wearing earclips was inferior to those that did not. The retrograde
animals to the place where they had received the ECS treatment but
due to the learning of strong competing responses for which ECS

1.65 LEWIS AND ADAMS, 1963

ECS; 4   rats   step-through   12; 3/day
transpinnate   FS
35mA; 300msec   AA

in shock compartment-
in safe compartment_
outside apparatus-

ECS in the shock compartment had the greatest effect on performance;
compartment and outside the apparatus there was not much effect;

measure of retention	time of treatment	test	retention
avoidance responses on retraining; jumping time	15 min	3 days after last ECS	
			RA less RA (more avoidances)

effect appears when ECS is given in the same situation in which
when ECS is given in an entirely different situation.

	5 min		
avoidance responses over 30 retraining avoidance trials		6 days after last ECS	more avoidance responses
			less avoidance responses

animals relearned the avoidance response when retrained. When
did not learn the avoidance response. The performance of animals
amnesic effects of ECS can be extinguished by returning the
where it is now not given. Retrograde amnesia was believed to be
served as an unconditioned stimulus.

avoidance responses on retraining	5 min	24 hr	
			most RA RA least RA

these animals showed little avoidance. Whereas, in the safe
these animals avoided.

Treatment and site	animals	task	trials

1.66   MISANIN AND SMITH,   1964

ECS	rats	step-through FS AA	no.
ECS		escape retraining	15

ECS significantly impaired the acquisition and retention of the
was making a running response but had virtually no effect when
response.   Impairment was attributed to fear conditioned by the

1.67   YARNELL AND ADAMS,   1964

ECS; 6	rats	jumping box FS AA	no.

Training and ECS treatments were each carried out in 3 different
ECS and the training occurred, the longer were the latencies of
The effects of ECS generalized to similar situations.

1.68   ADAMS AND PEACOCK,   1965

ECS transpinnate	rats	T-maze discriminative avoidance;	1
in goal box – in start box –		sub-convulsive transpinnate shock, 2mA in goal box	
in goal box –			
in start box –			

Response choices suggest that animals avoid the box in which both
accord with the consolidation hypothesis.

measure of retention	time of treatment	test	retention
avoidance responses on retraining	CS onset	15 min	no RA
	CS offset	15 min	RA
no.learning trials for avoidance task	CS onset	15 min	no effect
	CS offset	15 min	impaired learning

avoidance response when administered at a time when the animal
administered at a time when the animal was not making the running
ECS to the stimulus consequences of running.

latencies and % avoidances		days 9-12	RA

boxes. The more similar the stimulus situations in which the
response and the less frequent were the avoidance responses.

response latency		24 hrs	
	10sec, 1 hr		RA
	10sec, 1 hr		RA (increased latency)
running time	10 sec	24 hr	RA
	1 hr		less RA
	10 sec		RA (increased running time)
	1 hr		less RA
response choice	10 sec		no RA (13/18 chose safe box over goal box)
	1 hr		6/18 chose safe box

sub-convulsive and convulsive ECS was given, which is not in

Treatment and site	animals	task	trials

1.69 MISANIN, 1966

ECS transpinnate 300v; 500msec	rats	shuttle box AA - followed by escape training at 24 hr	50 50
ECS	rats	shuttle box, PA task inter- polated	50 50

Rats received a single ECS while performing either an escape
retraining interval of an avoidance response. ECS given during
response retraining situation; whereas ECS paired with the immobile

ECS	rats	step-through FS AA	100; 20/day
ECS	rats	step-through FS PA	100; 20/day

Animals first received training on an active avoidance response
versa. A single ECS was given after the initial training. During
responses than controls (no ECS). There was a facilitatory effect
with responses antagonistic to post-ECS training (reversal training).
interpretation of the effects of ECS.

1.70 ADAMS, PEACOCK AND HAMRICK, 1967

ECS	rats	skinner box CRF schedule FS	1
		FR5 schedule FS	1

Most suppression of bar pressing situations involve a CRF schedule
memory trace then the base line rate of responding should have no
acts as a disinhibiting stimulus, then disinhibition should be more
(But are the learning situations the same in terms of reinforcement

measure of retention	time of treatment	test	retention
mean avoidances for 15 re-training trials	following trial 50	45 min	poorer avoidance response perform-ance than no ECS
	following trial 50	45 min	RA better avoid-ance response performance than no ECS

response or an immobile response interpolated in the training-escape responding interfered with performance in the avoidance response facilitated performance.

no. passive avoidances	immediate	15 min	better learning than no ECS
no. active avoidances	immediate	15 min	better learning than no ECS

followed by training on a passive avoidance response or vice subsequent training, animals given ECS made more avoidance of ECS on training of PA and AA responses when ECS is paired These experiments claim to support a fear conditioning

bar press rates	10 sec	24 hr	RA
bar press rates	10 sec	24 hr	no RA

which produces a low rate of responding. If ECS disrupts a effect on retention of a one-trial learning. However, if ECS marked with subjects which have a low base line operant rate. and motivation?)

Treatment and site	animals	task	trials

1.71 LEWIS, MISANIN AND MILLER, 1968

Treatment and site	animals	task	trials
ECS transpinnate	rats	step-down FS	1
		strong RS- NCFS 1.6mA; 5sec	
		weak RS- NCFS 0.6mA; 5 sec	

The FS followed by ECS produces an amnesia from which partial
that at least a part of the memory remained, but that its retrieval

1.72 LEWIS, MILLER AND MISANIN, 1968

Treatment and site	animals	task	trials
ECS transpinnate 40mA; 500msec	rats	step-down FS - 5sec PA	3 FAM-no FS 1 FS trial
			no FAM trials 1 FS trial
			3,5sec NFAM trials 1 FS trial
			3,5min FAM trials 1 FS trial
			different amounts of FAM (x3)
			5 sec
			37.5 - 300sec

Familiarity with the apparatus (FAM) produced with exploratory
It was argued that prior familiarization permits a new memory (for
single ECS in a familiarized situation seems to have an effect

1.73 MISANIN, MILLER AND LEWIS, 1968

Treatment and site	animals	task	trials
ECS transpinnate 40mA; 500msec	rats	licking water tube FS-CS pairing	1
			1 + CS

24 hours after a single CS - FS pairing, brief presentation of the

measure of retention	time of treatment	test	retention
SDL	immediate	20 hr	RA
	24 hr	44 hr	partial RA
	24 hr	44 hr	RA

recovery occurs after a reminder shock (RS). The conclusion was
was prevented by the ECS.

measure of retention	time of treatment	test	retention
SDL (120sec)	immediate (contingent on offset of FS)	20 hr	no RA
	immediate	20 hr	RA
SDL (200sec)	immediate	20 hr	RA
	immediate	20 hr	no RA
	immediate	24 hr	RA
	immediate		no RA

trials with no footshock protects memory from disruption by ECS.
FS) to integrate into an existing memory system. Moreover, a
independent of its interaction with FS (i.e. it is aversive).

measure of retention	time of treatment	test	retention
licking rate	immediate	48 hr	RA
	24 hr	48 hr	no RA
	24 hr + CS	48 hr	RA

CS followed in 10 seconds by ECS will produce RA.

Treatment and site	animals	task	trials

1.74   LEWIS, MILLER AND MISANIN,   1969

ECS	rats	step-down	3 FAM-no FS
transpinnate		FS	1 FS trial
60mA; 60Hz; 500msec		PA	
		FS duration-	
immediate ECS		0.5 sec;	
with FS offset;		2.5 sec;	
delayed ECS 5sec		5.0 sec	
after FS onset			
			1 NFAM trial

In this situation 'memory consolidation' apparently occurs in less
interval approaches the conduction times of afferent neural circuits.

1.75   MENDOZA AND ADAMS,   1969

ECS	rats	conditioned	1
transpinnate		autonomic	
35mA; 500msec		response	
		FS-CS pairing	

ECS does not eliminate the conditioned fear response as indicated
or motor component. Note that ECS itself did not produce an
effect on motor performance.

1.76   MILLER, MISANIN AND LEWIS,   1969

ECS	rats	drinking tube	1
transpinnate		FS	
40mA; 500msec		CER	
flashing light for			
3 sec between FS and ECS			

The amount of RA was increased by filling the 3 sec learning-ECS
disruptive effect upon subsequent performance of the CER, it was
response mediated between learning and ECS, increasing the
itself, a primary determinant of the amnesic effects of ECS.

1.77   YARNELL,   1968

ECS	rats	hurdle cross	10; 1/day
		for social	
		contact	
		appetitive	

measure of retention	time of treatment	test	retention
SDL (300 sec)	immediate 0.5-5.0 sec from onset	20 hr	no RA
	delayed 0-4.5sec from offset	20 hr	no RA
	immediate on offset of 5 sec FS	20 hr	RA

than 0.5 seconds and is essentially instantaneous as this

| heart rate; no. boluses defecated | 12 sec | 24 hr | no RA |

by autonomic changes, even though it may eliminate the skeletal autonomic fear response. No control was done to determine the

| licking rate | 3 sec | 24 hr | partial RA |
| | 3 sec | 24 hr | complete RA |

interval with a flashing light. As the light alone had no concluded that the light stimulus and resulting orienting consequent amnesia. The time between ECS and learning is not, in

| latency of crossing | 10-15 min | 24 hr | RA |

Treatment and site	animals	task	trials

1.77   (Continued)

ECS interfered with the approach response. The results of this
of ECS. Viewed in terms of interference theory, ECS produces a
instrumental response of running. The response decrement after

1.78   MILLER AND SPEAR,   1969

Treatment and site	animals	task	trials
ECS grand mal convulsion-	rats	step-down FS PA	1
convulsion lacking the phase of hind-limb tonic extension-			

It was concluded that amnesia correlated positively with the
deprivation diet did not appear to affect the degree of amnesia in
on an ad-lib diet showed more attenuated amnesia and incomplete

1.79   MILLER,   1970

Treatment and site	animals	task	trials
ECS transpinnate 60mA; 60Hz; 500msec	rats	step-down FS-5 sec PA	1
		pretraining after 3 NFAM in; stepdown grid floor open field confinement cage	1x150 sec

All rats received 3 NFAM (5 sec) trials. Before the FS, ECS train-
of amnesia was found among the FS, ECS groups with increasing
groups showed no difference, therefore this result is not due to

Treatment and site	animals	task	trials
ECS		pretraining- massed trials distributed	1 FS trial 60 sec x 3 5 sec x 3 x 12

The time of familiarization was constant - 180 sec but distribution

Treatment and site	animals	task	trials
ECS		stepdown simple 5 sec FAM 10-150 sec FAM complex 5-20 sec FAM 37-150 sec FAM	1 FS trial 3 3 3 3

measure of retention	time of treatment	test	retention

study are consistent with the competing response or fear hypothesis crouching and freezing response or fear, which competes with the ECS would then be due to this interference.

SDL			
	immediate	24 hr	RA
	immediate	24 hr	less RA

severity of the convulsion despite the constant current ECS. A those animals exhibiting complete grand mal convulsions. Animals convulsions.

SDL (300 sec)	immediate on FS(5 sec) offset	24 hr	
			no RA
			slight RA
			more RA
			most RA

ing trial each received a pretraining trial. A decreasing degree similarity between place of FAM and training environment. FS only differential acquisition.

	immediate		no RA
			partial RA

of FAM trials was altered.

	immediate		RA
			no RA
	immediate		RA
			no RA

Treatment and site   animals   task   trials

1.79   (Continued)

3 FAM trials of different lengths 5-150 sec. There were no
due to different acquisitions.
Increasing the complexity of the learning situation increased the

ECS, NFAM   rats   step-down   1 FS trial
                                           simple &
                                           complex

FS-ECS delay in
apparatus

Detention potentiated the amnesic effect of ECS.

no ECS   FAM
                                           5,95 or 1800   3 FAM
                                           sec   1 FS trial
ECS   NFAM (5 sec)   3 FAM
                                           95 sec   1 FS trial
                                           1800 sec

Once sufficient familiarization for the FAM effect to occur has
trials is ineffectual.

                                           shuttle box   no. to
                                           AA   5 correct
                                           pretraining
                                           30 or 300 sec   3

There was no difference in acquisition with either measure between
that FAM reduces vulnerability to amnesia rather than enhancing

1.80   MISANIN,   1970

ECS 2   rats
transpinnate
300v; 500msec

Most studies use a 24 hour retention test, at which time the
excitability of the CNS which may be expressed behaviourally as
responses by which RA is evaluated.

measure of retention	time of treatment	test	retention

differences in No ECS groups, therefore the differences were not

amount of FAM needed to overcome ECS effects.

	15 sec		RA
	20 sec		no RA
	60 sec		RA

Without ECS, acquisition was unaffected by the degree of FAM

	immediate	24 hr	RA
			no RA
			no RA

taken place, further FAM (over FAM) at least up to three 1800 sec

trials to criterion or response latencies		24 hr	

FAM and NFAM. These last two studies add support to the view
acquisition.

ECS convulsion threshold	EC treatment after ECS		EC threshold
	0.09-0.38 hr		- elevated
	1.5-6 hr		- same as controls
	24 hr		- depressed
	96-384 hr		- elevated

lowered electroconvulsive threshold indicates a heightened
hyperactivity and hence as an augmentation of the active

Treatment and site	animals	task	trials

1.81 MILLER AND SPRINGER, 1971

ECS	rats	step-through	1
transpinnate		FS	
44mA; 300msec		PA	

Retention was found 15 minutes after learning and ECS but not later.

ECS	rats	step-through	
		FS	
FS and ECS		PA	
given in open field			

There was no suppression of responding by FS and ECS given outside minute retention seen with training is not due to any systemic

1.82 MISANIN, SMITH AND MILLER, 1971

ECS	rats	2 way	80
transpinnate, 60Hz;		shuttle box	
duration 1.0 and		FS	
1.5 sec		AA	
intensity- 35mA			
70mA			
140mA			

Above an ECS duration of 500msec, there was an inverted U-shaped

ECS
35mA; 50-750msec
     1.0-1.5 sec

70mA; 50msec
     200msec-1.5 sec

140mA; 50msec-1.5 sec

Altering ECS duration also had a similar inverted U-shaped function

Most ECS groups not only failed to benefit from the original learn-properties of ECS. It was suggested that the inverted U-shaped properties and amnesic properties of the ECS.

measure of retention	time of treatment	test	retention
STL (120 sec)	immediate	15 min	no RA
	immediate	30 min	RA
	immediate	60 min	RA
	immediate	120 min	RA
STL (120 sec)	immediate	15 min	no RA
	immediate	24 hr	RA
		15 min	RA

the apparatus and no training trial given. Therefore the 15
interaction of FS and ECS with performance.

no. trials to criterion on retraining	during responding		
		15 min	
			RA
			more RA
			less RA

function of ECS intensity.

	during responding	15 min	no RA
			RA
			no RA
			RA
			RA

but not significant.

ing but did worse in retraining which indicates aversive
function was due to an interaction between the aversive stimulus

Treatment and site	animals	task	trials

1.83 MILLER AND SPRINGER, 1972(a)

ECS	rats	step-through	1
transpinnate		FS	
44mA; 60Hz; 300msec		PA	

ECS +
non-contingent
RS

ECS +
NC-RS

The recovery from amnesia is partial rather than total with a non-
ECS + RS showed no suppression of STL's; the behaviour of the
recovered memory was stable over repeated test trials and a
independent of the interval between training and RS. The authors
though it is robust when it does occur. The intensity and duration
interval are all critical variables for obtaining both the reminder
were interpreted to favour a retrieval failure view of experimental

1.84 MILLER AND SPRINGER, 1972(b)

ECS	rats	step-through	1
transcorneal		FS	
50mA; 60Hz; 200msec		PA	

ECS +
NC-FS 2 hr

It was concluded that transcorneal ECS is similar to transpinnate
occur soon after acquisition.

measure of retention	time of treatment	test	retention
STL (600sec)	immediate	24 hr	RA
		+25 hr	RA
		+26 hr	RA
	immediate RS- 2 hr	24 hr	slight RA
		+25 hr	slight RA
		+26 hr	slight RA (no extinction)
	immediate RS- 2 hr	24 hr	slight RA, equal
	4 hr		at all times
	8 hr		of RS
	16 hr		
	48 hr	72 hr	
	7 days	8 days	no RA
	2 hr	5 days	no RA

contingent reminder shock. Systemic controls receiving NC-FS +
reminded animals was specific to the training situation. The
retention interval of at least 5 days. The reminder effect was
comment that recovery from amnesia is not easily obtained even
of footshock, ECS and reminder shock, as well as the FS-ECS
effect and appropriately behaved control groups. These findings
amnesia.

measure of retention	time of treatment	test	retention
STL (300sec)	8 sec	24 hr	RA
	8 sec RS 2 hr	24 hr	partial RA

ECS in that both interfere with retrieval processes that normally

Treatment and site	animals	task	trials

1.85 SPRINGER AND MILLER, 1972

ECS transpinnate 54mA ; 60Hz;300msec	rats	step-through 10 sec immersion in ice water PA	1
ECS + NC-FS as recovery agent			

The agent inducing recovery of memory need not be physically
found necessary to manipulate both the intensity and the duration
memory).

1.86 MAHUT,   1962

Thalamic ES	rats	Hebb- Williams Maze and	no.
Tegemental ES		T-maze	no.
Cortical ES			

Stimulation affected new rather than old learning and appeared to

---

1.87 WEISSMAN, 1963

ECS transpinnate intensity 17,25,35mA 50,150,450mA	rats	skinner box FS	1

Weissman claimed a dependence of RA on overt convulsions.

1.88 WEISSMAN, 1964

ECS transpinnate 150mA; 200msec	rats	skinner box FS	1

measure of retention	time of treatment	test	retention
STL (300 sec)	immediate	24 hr	RA
	RS-2 hr	24 hr	no RA

similar to the reinforcer used during training. (Note: it was
of the recovery agent in order to successfully obtain recovery of

---

	immediate		RA
	2-75 min		no RA
	immediate		no RA
	immediate		no RA

have detrimental effects on both types of learning tasks used.

---

bar press rates (5 min)			
	5 min	24 hr	no RA
	5 min		RA

| bar press rates (5 min) | 1.25-40 min | 24 hr | RA |
| | 80,160 min | 24 hr | no RA |

Treatment and site	animals	task	trials

1.89 WEISSMAN, 1965

ECS	rats	skinner box	1
intensity		FS	
15-25mA			
35-150mA			

Anti-convulsant drugs failed to protect rats against RA even

1.90 COOPER AND KOPPENAAL, 1964

ECS	rats	conditioned	1
transpinnate		drinking	
50mA;200msec		response,	
		shock PA	
			2

With two punishing shocks there was temporary suppression of an
an avoidance habit, with the animals given 2 shocks - i.e. greater
disrupt subsequent drinking at 1 and 24 hours.

1.91 PINEL AND COOPER, 1966(a)

no ECS	rats	skinner box	1
		FS	
		PA	
no ECS	rats	conditioned	1
		drinking	
		response	
		FS PA	

In both experiments there was a U-shaped retention function (Kamin
after learning but falls and then develops again over the next 8
the Kamin effect does not seem attributable to warm up factors or

1.92 PINEL AND COOPER, 1966(b)

ECS	rats	conditioned	1
transpinnate		drinking	
50mA; 300msec		response	
		FS PA	
no ECS			1

measure of retention	time of treatment	test	retention
bar press rates			
	5 min	24 hr	no or only slight RA
	5 min		more RA

though they protected against overt convulsions.

---

drinking time	within 30 sec	1 hr	RA
	30 sec	24 hr	RA
	30 sec	1 hr	RA
	30 sec	24 hr	no RA

avoidance habit. This could have been due to the development of
learning and stronger habit. ECS by itself does not seem to

bar press rates		1 min	good retention
		2 hr	poor retention
		8 hr	better retention
drinking time (forgetting)		1 min	good retention
		2 hr	poor retention
		8 hr	good retention
		25 hr	good retention

effect). Retention for an avoidance habit was high at 1 minute
hours. Because of the nature of one-trial avoidance learning,
to a temporary state of overarousal.

latency of drinking	30 sec	25 hr	RA
	2 min,4 hr		no RA
latency of drinking		10 sec	retention
		3 hr	increasing
		25 hr	over time

Treatment and site   animals   task   trials

1.92   (Continued)

Retention increased as the retest period was extended, i.e. the
over time.
Both incubation and gradient effects occur after one-trial avoidance
the gradient and incubation curves suggesting the relationship may

1.93   PINEL AND COOPER,   1966(a)

Treatment and site	animals	task	trials
ECS transpinnate 50mA; 300msec no ECS	rats	conditioned drinking response PA	1

In the one experiment where the incubation and ECS gradients were
and the ECS gradient were essentially the same. As the learned
ECS. For a consolidation hypothesis there should be an increase
be attributed to an increase in fear.

1.94   KOPPERAAL, JAGODA AND CRUCE,   1967

Treatment and site	animals	task	trials
ECS	rats	drinking tube FS PA reminder FS no reminder FS	1

A reminder FS resulted in a recovery of memory. The authors do not
ing a reminder can possibly be consonant with an interpretation
memory to form or consolidate.

1.95   PINEL,   1968

Treatment and site	animals	task	trials
no ECS	rats	step-through FS AA	1

Rather than avoiding, S's "froze" in the footshock compartment. The
It seems that ECS interrupts the incubation of the one-trial
prevalence of this freezing increased with the duration of the

measure of retention	time of treatment	test	retention

avoidance response appeared to increase in strength or incubate

training, but there were considerable differences in the shape of
be a spurious one (Note: these were separate experiments).

measure of retention	time of treatment	test	retention
latency of drinking	10sec;2 min 5 hr	25 hr	RA no RA
		10 sec 2 min 5 hr	

measured at the same time the avoidance response incubation curve
response became stronger it was less likely to be disrupted by an
in strength of storage, but not in strength of response. This may

measure of retention	time of treatment	test	retention
avoidance of drinking chamber	5 sec	24 hr + retested straight after	RA no RA RA

see how the strong avoidance exhibited by FS-ECS animals follow-
that their pre-reminder amnesia was due to any failure of the

measure of retention	time of treatment	test	retention
STL (300 sec)	5 sec 1 min 24 hr		

prevalence of this increased with duration of test-retest interval.
avoidance response rather than producing any amnesia per se. The
test-retest interval.

Treatment and site	animals	task	trials

1.96   PINEL,   1969

ECS	rats	chamber with	1
transpinnate		cul-de-sac	
60mA; 500msec		- water	
		appetitive	
no ECS			1

The no water-ECS group showed the same number of explorations as is not acting as a negative reinforcer.

ECS produced a true amnesia for one-trial appetitive training,i.e. ECS even though control S's showed no decrease in retention over within 1 min of training.

1.97   PINEL,   1970

no ECS	rats	emotional-	1
		conditioning	
		FS (CER)	
ECS 1			1
transpinnate			
50mA; 1 sec; 60Hz			

FS-reduced mobility (CER) increased in strength with time, i.e. CER producing a high rate of activity which cannot be attributed unlikely that the obtained ECS gradient is attributable to a

no ECS	rats	step-down	1
		FS PA	
ECS			1

measure of retention	time of treatment	test	retention
no. of hole explorations	10 sec, 1 min 10 min, 1 hr, 3 hr	24 hr 24 hr	RA no RA
no. of hole explorations		10 sec 1 min 10 min 1 hr 3 hr	retention remains relatively stable over a 24 hr period

the no water-pseudo ECS group, therefore it is probable that ECS

S's retained less well 24 hours after ECS than they did before the same period. To produce amnesia ECS had to be administered

activity during testing		1 min,30 min 2-24 hr	activity increased activity reduced (i.e. retention)
activity during testing	1,30 min 2-24 hr	24 hr	RA no RA

immobility increased. ECS 1 or 30 minutes after FS disrupted the to ECS being punishing or a negative reinforcer. Therefore it is gradient of ECS-induced amnesia.

activity % freezing		10 sec 3 hr	high activity reduced activity

FS produced immobility increased with time

SDL			no change

the SD latencies were not indicative of incubation.

% freezing	10 sec, 1 min 10 min, 1 hr, 3 hr	24 hr	RA no RA
SDL	10 sec, 1 min 10 min, 1 hr 3 hr		RA less RA no RA

Treatment and site	animals	task	trials

1.97   (Continued)

Measurement of latencies or % avoidance discriminates between extent before and after ECS at all training-ECS intervals. Pinel latencies produced by the ECS could be attributed to the effects on platform.

1.98   PINEL, MALSBURY AND CORCORAN,   1971 (a)

no ECS	rats	balancing on a tight rope	1

Skin resistance increased over 3 pre-FS tests. A decrease was taken as a measure of anxiety. These findings conflict with the seen in rats after a single FS is attributable to an incubation of

FS,as well as producing a relatively long-lasting tendency to which interferes with both freezing and passive avoidance. It was of this FS produced activation rather than an improvement in results in the incubation effects in rats.

1.99   IRWIN, KALSNER AND CURTIS,   1964

no ECS	rats	step-through FS PA	1

There was an initial high increase in latency due to shock stimulus, the latency increased to a maximum value after 1 hour. This process of consolidation.

1.100   IRWIN, BANUAZIZI, KALSNER AND CURTIS,   1968

ECS 12mA; 200msec	mice	hurdle cross FS PA	1 (no FS)

measure of	time of	test	retention
retention	treatment		

freezing behaviour and amnesia, since animals froze to the same
suggested that it is difficult to see how the decrease in
of ECS on freezing behaviour. NFS-ECS animals did not remain

skin	1 min		
resistance	1 hr		
	5 hr		
	24 hr		

produced by FS 1 minute and 1 hour after. Skin resistance was
hypothesis that the incubation of freezing and passive avoidance
anxiety.

freeze, has a transient activating effect on locomotor activity
argued (Pinel, 1970, 1.97) - that it is the gradual diminution
passive avoidance or an increase in the tendency to freeze which

---

STL	0 sec	good retention	
	30 sec		
	2 min	poor retention	
	15 min		
	60 min	good retention	

which fell to a relatively low level after 2 minutes, after which
gradual increase in latency was interpreted as reflecting the

hurdle cross	0-4 hr	"RA"	
latencies		increased latencies	

Treatment and site	animals	task	trials

1.100 (Continued)

ECS	mice	hurdle cross	2nd trial
		FS	with no FS
		PA	before ECS

ECS			2nd

Latencies were greatly increased immediately after a tonic-clonic
over 3-4 hours. The effect of ECS on response latencies tended to
(without FS) on a subsequent 3rd trial. Apprehension levels
correlated with subsequent hurdle-cross latencies. It was concluded
what was seen was merely an arrest of the response disposition of
formulation of the consolidation hypothesis was that registration
very early event (perhaps only seconds) followed by a relatively
phase which determines the latency or emotionality of the

1.101   LEONARD AND ZAVALA,   1964

ECS	rats	step-through	5
inside apparatus-		FS	
outside apparatus-		AA	

inside apparatus-
outside apparatus-

With ECS given either inside or outside training apparatus and
to location of ECS treatment and prior ECS had no effect. If the
ECS inside the apparatus where FS is given should decrease RA

---

measure of retention	time of treatment	test	retention
hurdle cross latencies		3 hr	no evidence for a true RA was found, the responses for pre-ECS and post-ECS trials were similar to those reported without ECS
	1-3 or 4 hr before trial		

seizure with a gradual linear decay to sham ECS control levels
be indistinguishable from the effect of a second trial alone
during first 15 seconds after placement in apparatus were highly
that a "RA" was not produced in mice by ECS or by anaesthesia;
the animals at the time the treatments were administered. A re-
and "permanent" storage of the memory trace takes place as a
labile, time-dependent integrative-elaborative-facilitative
response measured.

---

measure of retention	time of treatment	test	retention
no. errors in 10 trials	24 hr before	24 hr	no RA
			no RA same as no ECS
	after	24 hr	RA
	after		RA

either before or after training, there were no differences due
effect of ECS were due to aversiveness or competing responses,
rather than enhance it compared to outside.

Treatment and site	animals	task	trials

1.102   CHEVALIER,   1965

| ECS
transcorneal
82mA; 100Hz; 300msec | rats | circular
alley
FS | 1 |

RA was relatively permanent, without repeating testing.

1.103   CHOROVER AND SCHILLER,   1965

| ECS
transpinnate
35-50mA; 200msec | rats | step-down
FS - duration
0.5,1,2 or 4 sec
PA | 1 |

As the duration of FS increased there was a decrease in the performance.

ECS		no FS	
repeated treatments no ECS		FS	3; 1/day
ECS-3		no FS	3
ECS		FS	3
ECS		FS	3

As in previous studies, impairment in retention was inversely
earlier studies, impairment was observed only at relatively short
RA and not to aversive effects of ECS which were shown to develop

measure of retention	time of treatment	test	retention
reduction in locomotion	30 sec	1 day	RA
	30 sec	7 days	RA
	30 sec	30 days	incomplete RA

SDL (30 sec)	0.5,2,5, 10 sec	24 hr	RA
	30 sec		no RA

training-ECS interval which would result in disruption of retest

		24 hr	no increased avoidance
		4th day	no change in performance over 3 days
			avoidance increased over 3 days not yet equal to FS alone
	less than 10 sec		FS-ECS and ECS groups same
	more than 20 sec		increased avoidance over ECS alone

related to duration of the ECS-delay interval. However, unlike
(0.5-10.0 sec) ECS-delays. Impairment was attributed to brief
only after repeated ECS treatments.

Treatment and site	animals	task	trials

1.104 CHOROVER AND SCHILLER, 1966

ECS	rats	step-through	1
transpinnate		inescapable FS	
220v; 60Hz;		PA	
1 sec			

A leg shock was used to control for aversive properties of ECS.
those given ECS.

		escapable FS	
		step-down	
		1 FS	
		PA	
		1 min confinement	
		extra FS	

Confinement in the apparatus prior to ECS increased the effective-
reflect effects of ECS upon the locomotor inhibition component of
memory is limited to production of a "short-term" RA.

1.105 SCHILLER AND CHOROVER, 1967

ECS after	rats	open field	1
trial 1		maze	
35-50mA;		for food,	
60Hz; 200msec		appetitive	
ECS, after			
trial 2			2

There were only short-term amnesic effects of ECS for a positive

1.106 STEIN AND CHOROVER, 1968

hippocampal ES	rats	Hebb-	spaced trials
or		William	
caudate nucleus		Maze	massed trials
ES		appetitive	
		(well learned)	

The data suggested that memory trace consolidation could be

1.107 CHOROVER AND DeLUCA, 1969

ECS	rats	FS and ECS	1 FS
transpinnate		given in	
35-50mA; 60Hz		single	
200msec		chamber	

measure of retention	time of treatment	test	retention
STL (3 min) open field activity	1 hr	24 hr	RA

Animals given a pseudo ECS were less active in open field than

SDL (30 sec)	1 min		no RA
	2 min		no RA
	2 min		RA
	1 min		no RA

ness of the ECS. Certain passive avoidance impairments may
a CER. It is suggested that ECS-induced interference with

running time of maze	12 sec 60 sec	24 hr	RA no RA
	12 sec	24 hr	no RA

reinforcement situation.

no. errors			better retention
			disruption

facilitated or disrupted by post-trial electrical stimulation.

E.Co.G. activity	0.5,5,30 or 300 sec	continuous	

Treatment and site   animals   task   trials

1.107 (Continued)

Behavioural and E.Co.G. reactions to footshock and ECS studied under
The neural aftereffects of FS include immediate and delayed arousal
and abolition of the normal E.Co.G.(seizure) response to ECS. The
efficacy of a subsequent ECS depends more upon the severity and
se between FS and ECS. The observed variations in cortical seizure
for electrocortical activation.

1.108 CORSON, 1965

ECS   rats   spatial   no.
                                           discrimination FS
                                           brightness
                                           discrimination
                                           FS

Spatial discrimination was not affected by ECS but brightness
between experimental and control groups, therefore ECS was not

ECS   pattern D,   no.
                                           pretraining
                                           with
                                           brightness D
ECS   brightness D,   no.
                                           pretraining
                                           with
                                           pattern D

Brightness discrimination with pretraining on pattern
memory loss because other groups showed no performance disruption
with different pretraining. Therefore, task complexity is an

1.109 DAVIS, BRIGHT AND AGRANOFF, 1965

ECS   goldfish   shuttle box   20
5mA; 60Hz; 100msec   AA

Subconvulsive shock was of the same parameters as ECS,except only

measure of retention	time of treatment	test	retention

conditions comparable to those commonly used in studies of RA.
reactions which are associated, respectively, with alteration
way in which an antecedent FS affects the epileptogenic
duration of the arousal reaction than upon the time interval per
susceptibility were attributed to neural mechanisms responsible

---

response choice	30 sec	24 hr	no RA
	30 sec		RA

discrimination was. There was no response latency differences
producing fear.

	30 sec		no RA
	30 sec		RA

discrimination was disrupted by ECS. This was attributed to
with identical treatments but different habits or same habits
important variable.

---

no. trials to relearn	1-90 min	3 days	RA
	120-360 min		no RA

0.1mA. It had no significant effect.

Treatment and site	animals	task	trials

1.110 DAVIS AND HIRTZEL, 1970

ECS	goldfish	shuttle box	20
transcranial		AA	
8mA; 60Hz; 100msec			

Goldfish were returned to home tank between last trial and ECS

ITE- Fish were returned
to training or inter-trial
environment (ITE) 25 min
before ECS

ITE
ECS
ITE-ECS
ECS
ITE-ECS

Enhancement of amnesic effects of ECS occurred with exposure to
occur after 6 hours.

ITE
ECS
ITE-ECS

With ITE given 6 hours after training the RA developed at a later

The reinstatement may depend more upon evocation of specific
from a particular behavioural situation.

1.111 DAVIS AND HOLMES, 1971

ECS	Cataleptic	classically	1 session
transcranial	goldfish	conditioned	of 10
10mA; 60Hz; 2 sec		inhibition	trials
		of	
		respiration	

The retention of conditioned autonomic responses can be disrupted

measure of retention	time of treatment	test	retention
no. trials to relearn	0-1 hr	3 days	RA
	3-4 hr		partial RA
	5-24 hr		no RA

treatment.

	0 hr	1 day	partial RA
	0 hr	2 days	RA
	0 hr	4 days	RA
	4 hr	3 days	no RA
	4 hr		partial RA
	4 hr		complete RA
	6 hr		no RA
	6 hr		no RA

ITE for 25 min before ECS 4 hours after training which did not

	6 hr	7 days	no RA
	6 hr		partial RA
	6 hr		complete RA

time than ITE 4 hours after training.

emotional states than on discriminative recognition of stimuli

respiratory rate	immediate	20 min	partial RA
		1 hr	RA
		24 hr	RA
		72 hr	RA
	24 hr	72 hr	no RA

by post-session ECS in goldfish.

Treatment and site	animals	task	trials

1.112 GOLUB, CHEAL AND DAVIS, 1972

ECS	goldfish	operant	well-
transcranial		conditioning,	established
5mA; 60Hz; 1 sec		appetitive	response

Well-established patterns of operant responding were disrupted for transcranial shock following regular daily session. The ECS effect session and administration of ECS.

There are two effects of ECS neither involving a loss of memory-
1. A short term effect of the delayed ECS, attributed to an recovery period and is presumably not correlated with time
2. A long term effect produced by immediate ECS. This could be consequences which can be associated with the training

1.113 DELPRATO AND THOMPSON, 1965

ECS	rats	step-down	1
		FS 0.3mA	
		PA	
ECS		FS 2.0mA	

There were no differential effects during acquisition, but 0.3mA

1.114 THOMPSON, ENTER AND RUSSELL, 1967

ECS	rats	step-down	1
		FS	
		PA	

There was an apparent increment in the PAR at 48 hours for both FS

1.115 GALOSY AND THOMPSON, 1971

ECS	rats	step-down	1
transpinnate		FS	
40mA; 500msec		PA	
		3 FAM trials	
		of 0-37.5 sec	

FAM trials of up to 37.5 sec duration do not significantly effect than the corresponding pseudo-ECS control groups.

measure of retention	time of treatment	test	retention
rate of responding	immediate	24 hr	poor retention
	19.5 hr	24 hr	impaired performance
	immediate	48 hr	poor performance
	19.5 hr	48 hr	no effect

up to several days when the fish were convulsed by a 1 sec
varies as a function of the time elapsed between the end of a

anterograde debilitation which occurs during the post-convulsive
elapsed since the previous session.

interpreted as indicating that shock treatment has aversive
environment in a single presentation.

| SDL | 20 sec | 24 hr | no RA |
| | 20 sec | | no RA |

FS extinguished faster than pseudo-ECS or 2.0mA FS.

SDL	1 sec	24 hr	RA
	1 sec	48 hr	reduced RA
	1 sec	72 hr	RA

and FS-ECS groups, possibly due to some non-associative process.

| SDL (180 sec) | immediate | 24,48 and 72 hr | RA |

ECS-produced RA, all FAM-ECS groups having shorter latencies

    Treatment and site   animals   task   trials

1.116 KING, 1965

ECS   rats   step-through   1
transpinnate   FS PA
35mA; 60Hz; 500 msec   21 pretraining-
                                                no FS trials

FS only groups showed good retention and ECS only had no effect on

1.117 KING, 1967

ECS   rats   step-through   1
wound clips   FS
behind ears   PA
500msec; 60mA
in start box -
in goal box -

This experiment was to test conditioning explanations of amnesic
effect on latency; ECS was about equally effective as a disrupter
goal box; a gradient of decreasing effectiveness of ECS was

1.118 PFINGST AND KING, 1967

no ECS   rats   discriminative 1
                                                avoidance
                                                FS

In this experimental paradigm amnesia cannot be interpreted as

1.119 PFINGST AND KING, 1968

ECS   rats   discriminative 1
transcranial   avoidance
50-60mA; 60Hz; 500msec   FS

ECS 2   2

measure of retention	time of treatment	test	retention
STL (300 sec)	75 sec, 5 min	21-24 hr	RA
	15,60 min		no RA

performance.

STL (60 sec) on 3 test trials 15 min apart			
	5 sec		RA)
	5 sec		RA) nearly
	15 sec		RA) complete
	1 min		RA
	10 min		RA
	30 min		less RA
	60 min		less RA

effects of RA. Results did not support these. ECS alone had no
of avoidance behaviour when given in either the start box or the
obtained as the FS-ECS interval increased.

response choice		24 hr	

fear.

response choice	0-20 sec	24 hr	RA
	30-300 sec		no RA
running time	0 sec	24 hr	RA
	15-300 sec		no RA
response choice	0 sec	24 hr	
	0 sec	48 hr	no RA

Treatment and site	animals	task	trials

1.119   (Continued)

The increase in running time by some S's in every FS group
of FS in this situation, does not completely disrupt the effects of
had taken place before FS was terminated, and running time may be
choice measure.   There was an increase in retention over the day 1
FS which by itself was insufficient to produce a response choice
produce a change in response choice.

1.120   PFINGST AND KING,   1969

Treatment and site	animals	task	trials
ECS transcranial 60mA; 60Hz; 500msec	rats	discriminative avoidance FS PA	1
ECS 5 repeated FS-ECS treatments			5 1/day

ECS alone had no effect.   There was an increase in retention over
partial consolidation accumulated with repeated trials.

1.121   KING AND GLASSER,   1970

Treatment and site	animals	task	trials
ECS wound clips behind the ears 50mA; 500msec	rats	step-through FS PA	1

Animals in groups* were given repeated tests at weekly intervals
4 weeks.   For the single tests there was no recovery over 4 weeks.
avoidance responses when the ECS is of sufficient intensity and is
consolidation processes (i.e. anterior vs posterior pathway).

measure of retention	time of treatment	test	retention

suggested that ECS even if given immediately after termination
FS on later behaviour. It is possible that some consolidation
a more sensitive measure of consolidation than the response
response choice on day 3. Partial consolidation of the first
change, was added to the partial consolidation of 2nd FS to

measure of retention	time of treatment	test	retention
response choice over 10 trials	0-20 sec 30-60 sec	24 hr	RA no RA
		every 24 hr	eventually no RA

repeated testing. As ECS only had no effect, it suggests that

measure of retention	time of treatment	test	retention
STL (300 sec)	5 sec	1 day	RA
		* 2 days	RA
		3 days	RA
		* 1 week	RA
		2 weeks	RA
		* 4 weeks	RA
		6 weeks	no RA- (but controls show poor retention)

after the initial tests; in these recovery occurred over about
The authors argue that ECS produces permanent RA for passive-
effectively delivered so as to produce a complete disruption of

Treatment and site   animals   task   trials

1.122 GOLD, FARRELL AND KING, 1971

Treatment and site	animals	task	trials
ECS	rats		1
transcortical		PA	
60Hz; 500msec			
anterior placement:			
1mA			
5mA			
7.5mA			
10mA			
20mA			
posterior placement:			
1mA			
5mA			
7.5mA			
10mA			
20mA			
10mA; anterior placement			
posterior placement			

Low currents administered to anterior skull screw placements are
posterior brain structures.   Higher current values are equally
behavioural convulsion was not, in general, related to the amount
anterior and posterior ECS may be due to (a) lower thresholds for
(b) greater post-trial disruption of activity in the structures
by anterior stimulation.

1.123 ROUTTENBERG AND KAY, 1965

ECS	rats	skinner box	FS or
transpinnate		FS	no FS
20-60mA; 500msec			
		skinner box	no FS

Following one ECS significant decreases occurred in operant
descend from a platform. A non significant decrease occurred in

measure of retention	time of treatment	test	retention
STL (180 sec)	5 sec		
		24 hr	
			no RA
			RA
			RA
			RA
			complete RA
			no RA
			no RA
			no RA
			RA
			complete RA
		retest	RA
		7 days	RA

more effective in producing RA than low currents directed at
effective with both placements. It was found that the
of RA. The authors suggest that the differences between
generalized brain seizures produced by anterior stimulation; or
specifically involved in passive-avoidance learning and memory

bar press rates (30 min)	30 sec	4-6 hr	depression of responding
5 min open field activity		3 days	depression of
		4 days	activity
descent latency from platform(2 min)		4 days	shortened latency
heart rate		4 days	decreased
		9 days	decreased
bar press rates	1 hr	8 hr	depression
descent latency			shortened latency
open field activity			reduced
weight		17 days	weight loss

responding, open field activity, body weight and time taken to
heart rate.

Treatment and site   animals   task   trials

1.124   ROUTTENBERG, ZECHMEISTER AND BENTON,   1970

no ECS   rats   step-down   1
                                          FS PA
ECS
transpinnate
60Hz; 1.5 sec

Synchronized hippocampal activity was associated with FS and
hippocampal epileptiform activity was followed by behavioural and

1.125   TENEN, 1965(a)

ECS   rats   chamber   1
                                          with cul-
                                          de-sac
                                          for water,
                                          appetitive

At 3 hours there were possibly limited RA effects (but if ECS was
the number of hole explorations.)

1.126   TENEN,   1965(b)

ECS   rats   chamber   1
                                          with
                                          cul-de-sac
                                          for water,
                                          appetitive

Decreasing RA was found as the learning-ECS interval increased.

1.127   BOHDANECKY AND JARVIK,   1966

4 ECS   mice   step-through   1
                                          FS
1 ECS   PA

Effect of ECS shortly before retest was negligible compared with a
pretation that ECS given within a short time after training has an

measure of retention	time of treatment	test	retention
hippocampal activity SDL	0.5 sec	24 hr	RA

concurrent aversive responses. Tonic-clonic seizures and EEG depression.

hole	12 sec	24 hr	RA
	3 hr		slight RA

aversive one would expect the same result i.e. reduction of

hole explorations	15 sec,60 min 5 hr	24 hr	RA no RA

STL	pretreatment	24 hr	decreased latencies
	pretreatment	24 hr	no effect
	shortly before retest	24 hr	slightly decreased latencies
	12 hr before retest	24 hr	no effect

single ECS shortly after training. This supports the inter-effect in this test, in producing RA.

Treatment and site   animals   task   trials

1.128 KOPP,   1966

ECS   mice   step-through   1
                                           FS PA

The retrograde effect was temporally graded. The shorter retest
proactive, disinhibitive effect of ECS on retest performance.

1.129 KOPP, BOHDANECKY AND JARVIK, 1966

ECS   mice   step-through
transcorneal   FS PA
15mA; 200msec

FS outside the apparatus had the same effect as no punishing shock
extending to at least 1 hour for a well discriminated stimulus was

1.130 JARVIK AND KOPP, 1967

ECS   mice   step-through   1
transcorneal   FS
60Hz; 200 msec   PA
3-15mA
1mA

RA was observed at intensities of ECS too low (5mA) to elicit tonic-
necessary for producing RA.

1.131 KOPP, BOHDANECKY AND JARVIK, 1967

ECS   mice   step-through   1
transcorneal   FS
15mA; 200msec   PA

ECS   4

ECS
before retest

Only when given 1 hour before learning did ECS effect STL's 24 hr
1 hour after learning.

measure of retention	time of treatment	test	retention
STL	5 sec-1 hr 6 hr	24 hr	RA no RA

latencies observed after ECS treatment were not due to a

STL	20,80,320 sec, 5, 1 hr 6 hr	24 hr	graded RA slight RA

inside the apparatus. A temporal gradient of ECS-produced RA, demonstrated.

STL (300 sec)

	10 sec 10 sec	24 hr	RA no RA

clonic seizures. Therefore overt convulsions are not

STL (300 sec)	2-32 hr before training	24 hr	no effect
	1 hr before		increased latencies
	4 consecutive days before training	24 hr	reduced latencies
	before retest: 1-8 hr	24 hr	reduced latencies
	12-16 hr 23 hr 24 hr		no effect slight RA RA

later. ECS 1 hour before retest had less effect than ECS

Treatment and site	animals	task	trials

1.132   DORFMAN AND JARVIK,   1968(a)

20mA ECS   mice   step-through   1
60Hz; 200msec   FS   PA
transpinnate
and transcorneal
10mA ECS
transpinnate
transcorneal

5mA ECS
transpinnate and
transcorneal

At ECS current intensity of 10mA, transcorneal ECS produced more
overt convulsions at 10mA whereas transpinnate ECS was.

1.133   DORFMAN AND JARVIK,   1968(b)

ECS   mice   step-through   for 3 min
                                                PA   FS
4,5,6mA   1 or 2 FS
7,8,19mA   1 FS

4mA   less training
8-19mA

A graded decrement in retention was seen in the 6-8mA range.   The
affected by the change in training procedure.

ECS 5mA
duration: 0.1-0.6 sec
         1 - 3 sec

ECS   19mA
duration: 0.1-3 sec
           0.1 or 3 sec

A tonic extensor convulsion was not a necessary concommitant of
ECS does not flatten the temporal gradient of ECS-induced RA.
Loss of the placing response was related to the magnitude of the
even when ECS failed to effect this phenomenon. Note: that
learning that takes place in a passive avoidance situation.

measure of retention	time of treatment	test	retention
STL (300 sec)	45 sec, 1 hr	24 hr	RA
	3,6 hr		no RA
	45 sec		less RA than 20mA
	45 sec		RA
	45 sec		no RA

RA than transpinnate ECS. Transcorneal ECS was not dependent on

STL (300sec)

	0 min	24 hr	no RA
	0 min		RA
	0 min		no RA
	0 min		RA

relative amnesic efficacy of different ECS intensities was not

	0 min		no RA
	0 min		no RA
	0 min		no RA
	3-6 hr		no RA

maximal ECS-induced RA. Increasing the duration of supramaximal

retention deficit, but impaired retention could be demonstrated
supramaximal ECS does not wholly obliterate all aspects of the

Treatment and site	animals	task	trials

1. 134   ESSMAN,   1968

ECS and	mice	step-through	1
lidocaine i.p.		FS	
and saline		PA	
controls			
2,4-D and ECS			

RA occurred even though there were no overt convulsions. RA was
ECS with 2,4-D. These results were interpreted as either a drug
potentiation of the central changes produced by ECS that account

1.135   GELLER AND JARVIK, 1968(a)

ECS	mice	step-through	1
transcorneal		FS	
20mA, 200msec		PA	

Any recovery that occurs is complete within 24 hours, and no
induces only partial RA i.e. some aversive conditioning with FS
trials depending on the experimental technique.
Therefore, recovery from ECS induced amnesia did not occur with
unshocked controls and FS-ECS can be increased using a threshold

1.136   GELLER AND JARVIK, 1968(b)

ECS	mice	step-through	1
transcorneal		FS	
20mA, 200msec		PA	

There was decreased retention compared to FS controls at 1 hour,
was no significant difference from naive controls at 24 hours.
in no higher latencies than ECS following non-contingent tail
ECS affects LTM rather than STM.

measure of retention	time of treatment	test	retention
STL	immediate	24 hr	RA
	10 min		less RA
	60 min		no RA
	0-60 min		RA

not found to be a function of the interval between training and induced slowing of memory consolidation rates, or a drug induced for RA.

measure of retention	time of treatment	test	retention
STL (300 sec)	20 sec	24 hr	RA
	20 sec	24,48,72 168 hr (repeated)	RA
	20 sec	48,72, 168 hr (repeated)	RA
	20 sec	72,168 hr	RA
	20 sec	6 weeks	RA

further recovery can be demonstrated at longer intervals. ECS remains and this can be reinforced or extinguished over several

time alone or with multiple testing. The difference between FS after extinction.

measure of retention	time of treatment	test	retention
STL (300 sec)	immediate	1 hr	no RA
		2 hr	slight RA
		6 hr	slight RA
		24 hr	RA

the retention decreased over the retest intervals until there Aversive after-effects of ECS are unlikely as ECS alone results shock, which increases latencies slightly. They suggest that

Treatment and site	animals	task	trials

1.137   ROBUSTELLI AND JARVIK, 1968

ECS	mice	step-through	1
transcorneal		FS	
20mA, 200msec		PA	
home cage after FS			

detention in apparatus
after FS

30 minute detention alone with no ECS produced RA. Detention
apparatus. Detention affected performance only if given

1.138   ROBUSTELLI, GELLER AND JARVIK,   1968

ECS	mice	step-through	1
transcorneal		FS	
20mA, 200msec		PA	

no ECS plus
10 min detention
in apparatus

ECS plus detention

A similar degree of RA was found with 10 minutes detention as with
produced much more RA.

1.139   SCHNEIDER AND SHERMAN,   1968

ECS	rats	step-down	1 FS trial
transpinnate		FS	
35-50mA, 300msec		PA	

ECS given after			1 FS trial
non contingent			and NCFS
footshock (NCFS)			30 sec after
			learning

1 FS trial and
NCFS 6 hr
after learning

When rats received a brief footshock upon stepping off an elevated
afterward, amnesia was not observed 24 hours later. If a second
the electroconvulsive shock, amnesia was observed.

measure of retention	time of treatment	test	retention
STL (300 sec)			
	1 min	24 hr	RA
	5,30 min		no RA
	1,5 min	24 hr	RA
	30 min		no RA

inside the apparatus has more effect than detention outside the immediately after the training trial.

measure of retention	time of treatment	test	retention
STL (300 sec)	10 min	24 hr	slight RA
			slight RA
	10 min		more RA

ECS at 10 minutes, ECS at the end of 10 minutes detention

measure of retention	time of treatment	test	retention
SDL (30 sec)	0.5 sec	24 hr	RA
		48 hr	RA (no recovery)
	30 sec	24 hr	no RA
	6 hr		no RA
	30 sec + 0.5sec		RA
	30 sec + 30 sec		no RA
	6 hr + 0.5 sec		RA
	6 hr + 30 sec		no RA

platform, an electroconvulsive shock 30 seconds or 6 hours footshock (non contingent) was delivered 0.5 second before

Treatment and site   animals   task   trials

1.139   (Continued)

Arousal is critical to RA. It was suggested that the time-
accounted for by a single assumption; i.e. the 0.5 sec FS-ECS
retention but the 30 sec FS-ECS does not produce such after-
conditioning is strong and permanent if conditioning is weak.

1.140   SCHNEIDER,MALTER AND ADVOKAT,   1969

Treatment and site	animals	task	trials
No ECS	rats	step-down FS PA	1

SDL's increased between 1 minute and 1 hour and stabilized between

Treatment and site	animals	task	trials
ECS transpinnate 35-50mA; 300msec	rats	step-down FS	1
NCFS		PA	1
NCFS-0.5 sec ECS	rats		1
NCFS-30 sec ECS			

The pretreatment had no effect on SDL's of untrained rats.

1.141   ARON, GLICK AND JARVIK,   1969

Treatment and site	animals	task	trials
proactive ECS treatment transcorneal or transpinnate 15mA; 200msec	mice	step-through dark and light compartment	no FS

The animals behaved as though light had become more aversive to them

Treatment and site	animals	task	trials
Proactive ECS transcorneal, no light—	mice	step-through FS PA	1
light –			

measure of retention	time of treatment	test	retention

dependent data here and obtained in other studies on RA can be interval produces after-effects that interfere with subsequent effects. It was also suggested that amnesia is temporary if

measure of retention	time of treatment	test	retention
SDL (30 sec)		1 min	short latency
		1 hr	increased latency
		24 hr	same as at 1 hr

1 and 24 hours.

measure of retention	time of treatment	test	retention
SDL (30 sec)	30 min before training	1 min,1 hr or 24 hr	no effect
		1 min,1 hr or 24 hr	increased SDL
		1 min,1 hr or 24 hr	RA (decreased SDL)
		1 min,1 hr	no RA (increased SDL)
		24 hr	same as NCFS

measure of retention	time of treatment	test	retention
time spent in white compartment + or-light	24 hr before	24 hr 48 hr 1 week 4 weeks	more time spent in white compartment with no light,controls spent less time when light was on + ECS groups spent even less. The effect was not transient.

after the ECS treatment.

measure of retention	time of treatment	test	retention
STL into dark compartment	24 hr before	24 hr	both sham and ECS groups had the same latencies

ECS latencies lower than sham ECS group. Sham latencies were higher with lighted than not lighted compartment.

Treatment and site	animals	task	trials

1.141 (Continued)

Proactive ECS transcorneal 35mA; 200msec no light –	rats	skinner box	
light –			

The sham ECS treated animals made more responses on light
treatment, whereas ECS treated animals showed no preference for

Proactive ECS transcorneal 15mA; 200 msec	mice	activity box	

ECS produced increased aversion to light, which lasted a long
transpinnate ECS produced this also. Proactive effects of ECS
and bar pressing situations.

1.142 ROBUSTELLI, GELLER AND JARVIK, 1969(a)

ECS	mice	step-through FS PA	1
10 min exploratory session		step-through FS	1
ECS and 10 min exploratory session		step-through FS	1

ECS 10 minutes after training trial reduced STL's 24 hours later.
socially facilitated exploratory session for 10 minutes after
greater RA than either ECS alone or exploratory session alone.

1.143 SCHNEIDER, KAPP, ARON AND JARVIK,   1969

ECS 35–50mA; 200msec transpinnate	rats	step-through FS PA	1

transcorneal

measure of retention	time of treatment	test	retention
bar press rates + or - light onset with bar press	24 hrs before	24 hr 7 days	rate greater no difference
		24 hr 7 days	no difference no difference from sham ECS

contingent bar than on neutral bar at both intervals after either bar at both intervals.

activity in dark box	24 hr before	24 hr	increased activity

time and was not due to any peripheral visual lesion since can also influence behaviour in discriminated passive avoidance

STL		24 hr	RA
STL	10 min	24 hr	RA
STL		24 hr	RA
STL	10 min	24 hr	more RA

The PA response was partially extinguished by giving a training trial. ECS after the exploratory session produced

STL (300 and 600 sec)	10 sec - 1 hr	24 hr	RA
	6 hr		no RA
	10 sec - 6 hr		RA

Treatment and site	animals	task	trials
1.143 (Continued)			
transcorneal	mice	step-through FS PA	1
transcorneal	rats		
transpinnate			
transcorneal	mice		

The mode of delivery of ECS was shown to be more effective in rats
which ECS ceased to decrease test latencies was also shown to vary
the test trial.

1.144 ROBUSTELLI, GELLER, ARON AND JARVIK, 1969

ECS transcorneal 15mA; 200msec	mice	step-through FS PA FS delay: 0 sec	1
		FS delay: 30 sec	
		FS delay: 240 sec	

The closer the punishment to the step-through trial, the stronger
controls and ECS groups showed a decrease in latencies with an
were inversely related to the strength of the conditioned response.

1.145 ROBUSTELLI, GELLER AND JARVIK 1969(b)

ECS transcorneal 15mA; 200msec	mice	step-through FS PA	1

A typical temporal gradient was obtained and ECS was effective 23

measure of retention	time of treatment	test	retention
STL (600 sec)	10 sec - 1 hr	24 hr	RA
	6 hr		no RA
STL (30 sec)	10 sec		RA
	1 - 6 hr		no RA
	10 sec		RA
	1 - 6 hr		no RA
STL (30 and 300sec)	10 sec		RA
	1 - 6 hr		no RA

with transcorneal application. The training ECS interval at
directly with the length of cut-off criteria used to terminate

STL (600 sec)

	20 sec, 2min, 1,6 hr	24 hr	partial RA
	20 sec		complete RA
	2 min		partial RA
	1 - 6 hr		no RA
	20 sec, 2 min		
	1 hr		complete RA
	6 hr		no RA

the conditioning of the passive avoidance response. Both
increase in the delay of punishment. The amnesic effects of ECS

STL (300 sec)	10,30 min	1 week	RA
	6,23 hr		no RA
STL (1200 sec)	10,30 min		RA
	6,23 hr		less RA

hours after training with a high cut off criterion.

Treatment and site	animals	task	trials

1.146   ROBUSTELLI, GELLER AND JARVIK   1969(c)

ECS	mice	step-through	1
transcorneal		FS	
15mA; 200msec		PA	
10 min detention in apparatus. ECS and 10 min detention in apparatus.			1 1

The 10 minute detention was in the shock compartment, safe compart-
With ECS and detention the RA was greatest in the shock compartment,
complete in all of these. The amnesic effect of detention alone and

10 min detention	mice	step-through FS	1
ECS		PA	1
ECS and 10 min detention in safe compartment			1

ECS was given at various intervals after the 10 minute detention
detention in relation to ECS delay.

10 min detention			1
ECS			1
ECS and 10 min detention in safe compartment			1

There is no support to the hypothesis according to which the
altered physiological state making animals more sensitive to ECS
that the detention may weaken the retention of the original

1.147   GELLER, ROBUSTELLI AND JARVIK,   1970

ECS	mice	step-through	1
transcorneal		FS PA	
15mA; 200msec		delay of FS:	
		0 sec	
		30 sec	
		60 sec	
		120 sec	
		240 sec	

measure of retention	time of treatment	test	retention
STL (600 sec)	10 min	24 hr	RA
		24 hr	more RA
	10 min	24 hr	complete RA

ment or in a glass jar outside the apparatus.
less in the safe compartment and least outside - but virtually
ECS summed when given together.

measure of retention	time of treatment	test	retention
STL (600 sec)	10 min	24 hr	partial RA
	10,11,20 min		partial RA
	10,11,20 min		complete RA

period. There was no time-dependent decrease in the effects of

	10 min		partial RA
	10,30 min		partial RA
	6 hr		no RA
	10,30 min, 6 hr		complete RA

combined action of detention and ECS might be due to an
at the end of the detention period. It seems quite possible
response.

STL (600 sec)			
	20 sec	1 week	partial RA
	20 sec		RA
	20 sec		RA
	20 sec		RA
	20 sec		RA

Treatment and site	animals	task	trials

1.147 (Continued)

ECS had a proactive effect, demonstrated by latencies lower on the
to obtain conditioned responses of different strengths. Both
conditioned responses obtained with longer delays on punishment.

1.148 GELLER, JARVIK AND ROBUSTELLI, 1970

Treatment and site	animals	task	trials
ECS	mice	step-through	1
transcorneal		FS	
15mA; 200msec		PA	

A temporal gradient of RA was produced, with ECS still being
maintained over all retest times. There was no spontaneous recovery
when the amnesia is complete or when it is only partial.

* The step-through latencies on retest were lower than in

1.149 HARTMAN AND KIPPLE, 1966

Treatment and site	animals	task	trials
ECS treatment	rats	shuttle box	6
or recovery place		FS	
varied- inside		AA	
or outside			
apparatus			
ECS 6	rats	shuttle box	6
Treatment-		FS	
In apparatus		AA	
Outside apparatus			
Recovery-			
In apparatus			
Outside apparatus			

Allowing recovery from ECS in the test situation (in the safe
avoidance response. The place of treatment had no effect.

---

measure of retention	time of treatment	test	retention

retest than on the training trial. Delay of punishment was used
cycloheximide and ECS had a greater amnesic effect on the weaker

measure of retention	time of treatment	test	retention
STL (600 sec)	10 sec	1,2 days	RA*
		3,7 days	RA
	120 sec	1,2,3 or 7	RA
	3 hr	1,2,3 or 7	slightly less RA
	10 sec	1,3 days, 1 or 4 weeks	RA
	120 sec	1,3 days 1 or 4 weeks	RA (slightly less than 10 sec)
	3 hr	1,3 days 1 or 4 weeks	less RA

effective when given 3 hours after training. This gradient was
over a 4 week period from the amnesia produced by ECS, either

training, demonstrating a proactive effect of ECS.

---

frequency of avoidance	The place of treatment and of recovery or the effects of convulsions did not contribute to differences between experimental groups in frequency of avoidance.

STL		daily	
	10 sec		no RA
	10 sec		no RA
	10 sec		RA
	10 sec		no RA

compartment) led to decreased latencies of the conditioned

Treatment and site	animals	task	trials

1.150   GREENOUGH AND SCHWITZGEBEL,   1966

ECS	rats	skinner box	extinction
transpinnate		extinction	training for
30-35mA; 230msec			25 min

If ECS produced conditioned inhibition (Lewis and Maher, 1965)
to respond and cause ECS recipients to respond at a lower rate in
memory storage, RA for the extinction might be expected to result,
With ECS during extinction animals responded at higher rate than

1.151   GREENOUGH, SCHWITZGEBEL AND FULCHER,   1968

ECS	mice	step-through	1
transpinnate		FS	
11mA; 200msec		PA	

Independent and repeated tests over intervals of 2-72 hours
which received ECS showed increased latencies regardless of

1.152   HERZ, PEEKE AND WYERS,   1966

ECS	mice	step-through	1
		FS PA	

1.153   HERZ AND PEEKE,   1967;   PEEKE AND HERZ,   1967;   HERZ &

ECS	mice	chamber with	1
transpinnate		cul-de-sac	
18.5mA; 60 Hz; 800msec		appetitive	
		60sec drinking	
		or	
		aversive PA	
		60 sec in	
		apparatus	
		after MS	

With repeated testing the amnesia seen on day 1 had largely dis-
aversive tasks.

measure of retention	time of treatment	test	retention
no. bar presses (3 min)	30 sec	24 hr	RA

this might be expected to summate with the learned tendency not
the delayed test than non-ECS subjects. If ECS interferred with
causing ECS group to respond at a higher rate than controls.
controls.

measure of retention	time of treatment	test	retention
STL (30 sec)	5 sec	2,72 hr	RA
		2,3,24 hr	slightly less RA
		24,72 hr	RA

yielded no evidence for recovery from amnesia, although S's
training if they were tested within 3 hours after ECS.

---

measure of retention	time of treatment	test	retention
STL	immediate	22 hr	RA
PEEKE, 1968			
latency to first head poke (3 min)	75 sec	1 day	RA
	75 sec	2 day	no RA
	75 sec	3 days (repeated)	no RA
	75 sec	1 day	RA
	75 sec	3 days (separate)	RA

appeared on subsequent retention tests, on both appetitive and

Treatment and site   animals   task   trials

1.153 (Continued)

RA equal to or greater than RA in S's tested for the first time at
recovery from amnesia seen over the repeated 3 days testing may
similar in reinforced and non-reinforced control groups, possibly

1.154 WYERS, PEEKE, WILLISTON AND HERZ, 1968

caudate nucleus ES	rats	skinner box	1
or ventral hippocampal		FS	
dentate ES		PA	

180-900μA; 0.03-0.5msec   step-down   1
                               FS   PA

Electrical stimulation of caudate nucleus or ventral hippocampal
(accumbens, lateral septum, ventral thalamus, piriform cortex,
not produce RA. The RA seen with stimulation 0.1-30 seconds
not graded.

1.155 HERZ, 1969

ECS   mice   chamber with   1
transpinnate   cul-de-sac
18.5mA; 60Hz, 800msec   FS   PA

                                          appetitive

With the passive avoidance task the 15 minutes ECS did not
was not complete - suggesting a graded amnesic effect. With the
initiation of drinking) than with FS and less at 15 minutes.
The rate of memory consolidation varies as a function of the type
to be interpretable in terms of the aversive qualities of ECS nor

measure of retention	time of treatment	test	retention

day 1 was seen in S's tested for the first time on day 3. The
not have been "true" recovery since changes in behaviour were
a gradual adaption process.

bar press rates	0.1-30 sec	24 hr	RA
SDL (60 sec)	0.1 sec	24 hr	RA

dentate regions produced RA; stimulation of other regions,
substantia nigra, globus pallidus and dorsal hippocampus) did
after learning was essentially the same magnitude i.e. it was

latency to head poke, etc. (7 measures of retention)	20 sec, 15 min	24 hr	RA
	20 sec	24 hr	more RA than PA task
	15 min		less RA than PA task

produce as much RA as when given at 20 seconds, which in turn
appetitive task more RA was seen at 20 seconds (80 seconds after

of learning task. The results in the 2 experiments do not appear
in terms of conditioned inhibition.

Treatment and site	animals	task	trials

1.156 PEEKE, McCOY AND HERZ, 1969

Treatment and site	animals	task	trials
ECS transpinnate 35mA; 60Hz; 800msec water deprivation schedule 1 week prior to experiment 24 hr	mice	chamber with cul-de-sac appetitive 60 sec exposure to water	1
48 hr			
72 hr			

There was an equal amount of learning in the no ECS group. With deprivation condition ("higher drive") produced a steeper

Treatment and site	animals	task	trials
water deprivation 24 hr 48 hr 72 hr	mice	chamber with cul-de-sac appetitive	

The severe debilitation may have a direct decremental or disrupting conversion of experience into permanent memory.

1.157 WYERS AND DEADWYLER, 1971

Treatment and site	animals	task	trials
caudate nucleus ES: single square wave 500msec current level 300,600,900µA	rats	drinking from water tube MS PA	1
30 sec animals from 1st expt. retrained 24 hr later - ES			2
given 2nd treatment 24 hrs later 2 ES			3
4 ES			5

measure of retention	time of treatment	test	retention
frequency of licking			
	15 sec, 5 min	24 hr	RA
	30 min		no RA
	15 sec		RA
	5 min, 30 min		no RA
	15 sec, 5 min		RA
	30 min		no RA

the 24 hour and 48 hour deprivation schedules the higher gradient of RA.

weight loss, open field activity and frequency of head pokes	Activity, frequency of head pokes were significantly lower with the more extreme deprivation schedule.		

influence on the basic physiologic processes responsible for

measure of retention	time of treatment	test	retention
response time to 100 licks	30-300 sec	24 hr	RA temporally graded
	30 sec	24 hr	RA
	15 min		no RA
	30 sec	24 hr	RA
	120 sec		less RA
	300 sec		even less RA
	120 sec	1 each	RA
	300 sec	24 hr	RA

Treatment and site	animals	task	trials

1.157 (Continued)

There was increased retention with each trial. The rate of learn-
stimulation increased indicating that the stimulation was stopping
term memory at the time of its application. The degree of the
level.

1.158 PEEKE AND HERZ, 1971

caudate	rats	Lashley III	to a range
nucleus		maze, food	of criteria
stimulation		reinforce-	5-10 min inter-
(caudate-putamen		ment	trial
complex)			interval
single pulse			criteria:
after each trial- PTS			1/2 and 2/3
multiple pulses			
after each choice			
point - CPS			3/4 and 4/5
multiple pulses			
after each trial- MPTS			

When the criterion of the learning is an easy one, multiple
after a training trial interferes with learning, whereas a single
criterion levels, stimulation of the CPU complex whether by single
multiple stimulations are more detrimental than single pulses. It
represent a dose effect, similar to that observed with other

1.159 HERZ AND PEEKE, 1971

caudate-putamen	rats	extinction	5 min
stimulation		of over-	session
4 pulses/min		learned	
		response of	
12 pulses/min		drinking at	
		water spout	

Animals showing amnesia for learning of extinction of a response
and not more slowly as a general motor inhibition model would
single pulses were delivered.

measure of retention	time of treatment	test	retention

ing (avoidance of the tube) increased as the delay of
the encoding of the short-term associative learning into long-
deficit in the first experiment was unrelated to the current

no. trials to criterion	1,2, or 3 per day		
	PTS		no RA
	CPS		RA
	MPS		RA
	PTS		RA
	CPS		more RA
	MPS		more RA

stimulation of the caudate-putamen complex (CPU) during or
stimulation after a trial does not. At more difficult
or multiple stimulations retards the rate of learning, and
was suggested that the different stimulation conditions
amnesic agents.

time spent in contact with spout	during 1st session	1 day	
			RA
			more RA

should show this by responding at a higher rate that controls,
require. This effect was dependent on the frequency at which

Treatment and site	animals	task	trials

1.160 DEADWYLER AND WYERS, 1972

caudate nucleus stimulation single pulse	rats	habituation to light flash (LF) during drinking	6/day over 5 days
controls- light flash only ES only			
no stimulation		LF-probe trials	every 3 normal trials

Pairing caudate stimulation 100msec after each visual stimulus
no caudate stimulation, habituation proceeded at a more normal
stimulated and non-stimulated trials. The authors inferred from
with processes underlying decreased responsiveness.

1.161 HIRANO, 1966

hippocampal ES; 1/trial	cats	step-through FS AA	no. to 5/8
hippocampal es; 1/day		figural discrimination appetitive	5/day no.
hippocampal ES; 4/day		delayed reaction appetitive	no.

Delayed reaction - CS presentation was extended so that it was

---

measure of retention	time of treatment	test	retention
number of licks	100msec after	over days	took 50% more trials to habituate than controls
			habituation at normal rate

retarded habituation. During the LF-only - probe trials with
rate indicating little "transfer" of habituation between
this data a caudate effect on integration of sensory information

---

% avoidance responses	1 min	daily	no RA
response choice	1 min	daily	no RA
response choice	immediate after CS cessation	daily	RA

presented 10 seconds before UCS and response.

Treatment and site	animals	task	trials

1.162 LEE-TENG, 1966

ECS	chickens	inhibition	1
transcranial		of pecking	
28mA; 60Hz; 450msec		an aversant lure	
		by methyl-	
		anthranilate	
		PA	

ECS alone

The learning - ECS interval was measured from start of head shake.

1.163 LEE-TENG AND SHERMAN, 1966

ECS	chickens	inhibition	1
transcranial		of pecking	
28mA; 60Hz; 450msec		PA	

The learning-ECS interval was measured from the end of the 10 sec
administered at the start of the head shake. The retention seen in
had already been consolidated during the 10 sec learning trial.
retention deficit that was independent of the trial-ECS interval.

ECS 2	chickens	inhibition	2
	with trial-	of pecking	
	ECS interval,	PA	
	on 1st trial		
	of-		
	immediate		
	0 sec		
	5 sec		

The memory trace is not "all-or-none" but undergoes continuous
may be weakened by first ECS.

1.164 LEE-TENG, 1967

ECS	chickens	inhibition	1
transcranial		of pecking	
60Hz; 450msec		PA	
current intensities			
7-48mA			

There was no variation in amount of RA with changes in the
causing RA and the amount of RA did not vary with seizure pattern.

measure of retention	time of treatment	test	retention
% not pecking (10 sec)	immediate 6,11,16 sec 36 sec-24 hr	24 hrs	RA RA slight effect
			no effect
% not pecking (10 sec)	immediate 0 sec-10sec 30 sec-24 hr	24 hrs	complete RA RA (not complete) slight RA

presentation; except for the immediate group in which ECS was
the 0 sec group indicates that an appreciable amount of memory
ECS seems to have caused a smaller but constant amount of

measure of retention	time of treatment	test	retention
% not pecking	immediate	day 2	
			RA no RA no RA

strengthening during the consolidation period, even though it

measure of retention	time of treatment	test	retention
% not pecking (5 sec)	10 sec after start of head shake	24 hr	RA

intensity of ECS. Overt convulsions were not critical for

Treatment and site   animals   task   trials

1.165 LEE-TENG, 1968

Subconvulsive   chickens   inhibition   1
ES (SCC) transcranial   of pecking
12mA; 60Hz; 250msec   PA

compared with SCC-only
controls

compared with learning-
only controls

The use of sub-convulsive current (SCC) instead of a convulsive
after learning. Even though a current may prevent the formation
term memory. The possibility of the effect being due to the bad
due to the bad taste usually stopped within 30 seconds, and 2 –
5 minutes, as indexed by frequency of not head shaking after

1.166 LEE-TENG, 1969

ECS transcranial   chickens   inhibition   1
60Hz; 45msec   of pecking
current intensity   PA
0.1–7mA
8.0–120mA

ECS was given 10 sec after start of head shake. The threshold
convulsions is 12–15mA. Increasing the intensity above threshold

1.167   LEE-TENG AND GIAQUINTO, 1969

ECS transcranial   chickens
60Hz; 450msec
current intensity
5mA

10mA

15mA

Spike activities were associated with RA but the subsequent
the cause of the RA.

measure of retention	time of treatment	test	retention
% not pecking (5 sec)	SCC was given at start of head shake		
	immediate	immediate	no RA
	immediate	1-30 min	RA
	immediate	0-1 min	no RA
	immediate	2.5-30 min	RA

current enabled the animals to be tested at short intervals
of long-term memory, it does not necessarily also erase short-
taste is disfavoured because : 1 - the vigorous head shaking
the SCC seems to reduce sensitivity to the bad taste for about
pecking the lure.

% not pecking (5 sec)			
	10 sec	24 hr	no RA
	10 sec		RA

intensity for RA is 7-9mA, whereas threshold intensity for
for RA resulted in progressively more RA.

EEG recordings			
			no RA; no convulsions
			RA; no convulsions
			RA; convulsions

flattening of the trace seen at 15mA current intensity was not

Treatment and site	animals	task	trials

1.168 WEAVER AND MAGNUS, 1969

	chickens	inhibition of pecking PA	1 (metal lure)
SCC subdural above ears 12mA, 60Hz; 250 msec			1 (red lure)

SCC interval from start of head shake. A UCS (different lure with
then the chickens were given immediate subconvulsive current. No
- 1.139). Subconvulsive current without training does not decrease
effect.

1.169 LEE-TENG, 1970

ES transcranial; 60Hz; SCC-12mA; 250msec	chickens	inhibition of pecking PA	1
LECS-28mA; 450msec			
HECS-120mA; 500msec			

SCC or low ECS produced complete amnesia when given immediately
did not appreciably prolong the consolidation period, but there

There is a critical current-sensitive consolidation period of 30
intensity or duration. Within this period, the retention deficit

1.170 LEE-TENG, MAGNUS, KANNER AND HOCHMAN, 1970

SCC transcranial 12mA; 60Hz; 250msec	chickens	inhibition of pecking PA	1

Retention in the experimental group was compared with a MeA-current
return to the carton. This group indicated that pecking was
some retention at 30 minutes. Pecking was not affected by handling

SCC		inhibition of pecking PA	1

measure of retention	time of treatment	test	retention
% not pecking (5 sec)		24 hr	no RA
	immediate	4 hr	no RA
	2 min	4 hr	no RA

methyl-anthranilate) was presented 20 hours after training and "re-arousal" amnesia was seen (cf. Schneider and Sherman, 1968 the base pecking level. ECS (instead of SCC) also showed no

measure of retention	time of treatment	test	retention
% not pecking (5 sec)	0-20 sec	24 hr	RA
	30 sec-24 hr		no RA
	0-20 sec		RA
	30sec-24 hr		no RA
	0-45 sec		RA
	60sec-24 hr (measured from start of head shake)		no RA

after learning, motor convulsions are irrelevant. High ECS was a greater deficit at 45 sec than with low ECS.

seconds that cannot be prolonged by increasing the current is a function of level of current and time of delivery.

measure of retention	time of treatment	test	retention
% not pecking (5 sec)	(from head shake)		
	1 sec	1 min	no RA
	1 sec	5 min	no RA
	1 sec	30 min	RA

control group which received MeA while blinded and SCC on suppressed at 1 min and 5 min by the SCC and MeA. There was but was suppressed by SCC or MeA.

measure of retention	time of treatment	test	retention
	1 sec	5 min	no RA
	1 sec	30 min	RA
	1 sec	60,120 min	RA

Treatment and site	animals	task	trials

1.170   (Continued)

The difference was only significant at 30 min, however there is

SCC	chickens	inhibition of pecking PA	1

SCC was given 1 minute after training, there was little phase 1
Retention increased from 30 to 120 minutes. The difference between
minutes.

SCC		inhibition of pecking PA	1

The SCC was not affecting retrieval of the established memory. So

Immediate post-trial administration of transcranial current left a
hours. When current administration was delayed for 1 min after the
which increased to asymptotic level at 1 hour. These results may
Phase 1 is immune or only partially susceptible to current
Phase 2 is induced within seconds after training, but its trace
beginning stage is current-disruptable, but this phase of memory

1.171 MAGNUS AND LEE-TENG, 1971

SCC transcranial 12mA; 60Hz; 250msec	chickens	inhibition of pecking PA	1 2,1/day

1 on day 2

Experimental chickens (latent retention) were given one training
followed by a SCC when they commenced shaking their heads. On
The latent-retention controls were given a dry lure on day 1
day 2.
The results indicated that there was little latent retention
like a low dose of flurothyl (see Cherkin, 1969). The
different stages of memory consolidation.

measure of retention	time of treatment	test	retention

consistency in the direction of the differences at all times.

			(score)
1 min	5 min	no RA	.51
1 min	30 min	RA	.36
1 min	60 min	no RA	.50
1 min	120 min	no RA	.51

memory left at 30 minutes but phase 2 induction was allowed.
immediate and 1 minute SCC was significant at 30,60 and 120

5 min	24 hr	no RA	.55
30 min		no RA	.55
60 min		no RA	.55
120 min		no RA	.54

testing at these times reflects the growth of phase 2 memory.

low level of retention at 30 min which disappeared within 2
training trial, substantial retention was observed at 30 min
indicate the existence of 2 phases of measurable memory.
disruption and lasts for at least 30 min.
formation is a long process involving several stages; only the
is not expressed until the entire process is complete.

% not pecking (10 sec)	immediate	day 2	RA (92%)
	day 1- immediate day 2-5sec	day 3	RA (78%)
	SCC day 1 day 2-5 sec	day 3	RA (81%)

trial with methyl anthranilate (MeA) on the lure on day 1
day 2 they were tested for retention; followed by a second SCC.
followed by SCC and a training trial with MeA on the lure on

surviving the immediate current and the current does not act
conclusion was drawn that current and flurothyl disrupt

Treatment and site	animals	task	trials

1.172 BENOWITZ AND MAGNUS

Treatment and site	animals	task	trials
SCC 12mA; 60Hz; 280msec	chickens	inhibition of pecking PA	1

250msec

The briefer SCC allowed a larger portion of memory formation to
shorter time?) it was concluded that there is a portion of the
is passed. The current susceptible memory phase declined
depend on the duration of the SCC. The memory trace that grows
called here pre-LTM. This takes 30 min before it is behaviourally
as the memory trace is formed. The process which induces the
training. SCC doesn't speed the decline of STM but arrests one

280msec   2

250msec

The second training causes the Pre-LTM trace to continue growing
first training had been halted. The fraction amnesia from 2
sum of 2 training current intervals and do not depend on order of
physiological memory systems allow a succession of similar

measure of retention	time of treatment	test	retention
	from head shake		
% not pecking (5 sec)	immediate	24 hr	92% RA
	2 sec		79% RA
	4 sec		72% RA
	6 sec		63% RA
	10 sec		50% RA
	17 hr		no RA
	2 sec		59% RA
	8 sec		38% RA
	10 sec		37% RA

continue after passage of current (due to less current or to the
memory which does not depend on the time at which the current
exponentially. The nature of the exponential component does not
within the first 45 sec is not permanent LTM but antecedent to it,
manifest. The rate at which Pre-LTM grows decreases continously
formation of Pre-LTM remains at constant intensity following
fraction of it.

1		2			(Predicted)
2 sec	17 hr	4 sec	7 hrs	50% RA	(53)
4 sec		2 sec		60% RA	(53)
4 sec		6 sec		45% RA	(42)
6 sec		4 sec		39% RA	(42)
2 sec	6 hr	8 sec	?	20% RA	(19)
8 sec		2 sec		20% RA	(19)

exponentially from the point at which its formation after the
partial memory formations are negatively correlated with the
training. The authors suggest that under proper circumstances,
experiences.

Treatment and site	animals	task	trials

1.173 SPROTT, 1966

ECS	mice	step-down FS PA	1

No behavioural differences were seen between two typically
graded.

1.174 SPROTT AND WALLER, 1966

ECS	rats	skinner box no FS PA	no.

ECS was not acting as a reinforcing stimulus in this situation.

1.175 BIVENS AND RAY, 1967

ECS transpinnate	rats	step-down FS PA	1
ECS 10 - 1/day			10 1/day

With ECS given 1 second after training, animals will eventually
reinforcement magnitude when the intensity of the FS was varied.

1.176 RAY AND BIVENS, 1968

ECS transcorneal 50mA; 250msec	mice	step-through PA FS-0.3mA FS-1.5mA FS-2.8mA	1

As FS intensity increased, the interval during which ECS caused a
control group receiving no FS showed an increase in response
immediately after this significantly attenuated the increase in

measure of retention	time of treatment	test	retention
SDL	1-14 sec	24 hr	RA
	20-100 sec		no RA

divergent inbred strains of mice. The RA seen was temporally

bar press rates	10 sec		RA
conditioned suppression	12.5-30 sec		no RA

SDL	1 sec	24 hr	RA
	15-60 sec		no RA
	1 sec	day 1	RA
		day 10	no RA

learn but it takes longer. There was little or no effect of

STL (300 sec)	10-160 sec	24 hr	RA
	640-1600 sec		no RA
	10-160 sec		RA
	640-1600 sec		no RA
	10 sec		RA
	160-1600 sec		no RA

significant disruption of the learned response decreased. The
latency from trial 1 to trial 2 (response habituation).   ECS
latency.

Treatment and site	animals	task	trials

1.177   RAY AND BARRETT,   1969(a)

ECS 4,1/trial	mice	step-through	5
15 or 60mA; 250msec		FS 0.3 or 2.8mA	1/day
transcorneal		PA	

transpinnate

At 5 days ECS was more effective when delivered via the eyes, a
Increasing FS intensity resulted in the 60mA ECS being less
extent to which the passive avoidance response is disrupted is
delivery and intensity of the disrupting current.

ECS, 250msec	mice	step-through	1
transcorneal 5-80mA		FS PA	
same (right ear			
-right eye) 5mA-80mA			

cross (left ear
-right eye) 5-80mA
transpinnate 5-10mA
            20-80mA

The amount of disruption was inversely related to the resistance
same, cross, transpinnate).

1.178   RAY AND BARRETT   1969(b)

ECS	mice	step-through	1
transcorneal		FS	
15 or 60mA; 250msec		PA	

The No FS-ECS mice showed the same decrease in latencies over the
At retest intervals of less than 480 min following ECS-manipulation,
effects of ECS, independent of the learning situation. Thus,
only at intervals where the proactive effects of ECS had attenuated.

With pretreatment, with NCFS and/or ECS before PA trial the No FS-
groups however had latencies which decreased significantly as a

Open field activity showed the same trend. Minor procedural
in the apparatus can cause significant changes in avoidance
from 2nd compartment, latencies are inversely related to the time
compartment there is no effect of ECS on latencies in this

measure of retention	time of treatment	test	retention
STL (300 sec)	10 sec	every 24 hr	
		Day 1	no RA
		Day 5	RA
		Day 1	no RA
		Day 5	no RA

lower resistance pathway, than when delivered across the ears.
effective in disrupting retention than at the low FS level. The
in part controlled by magnitude of reinforcement, mode of

measure of retention	time of treatment	test	retention
STL (300 sec)	10 sec	24 hr	
			RA
			RA
			RA
			less RA
			RA

of the path between the two electrodes (increasing transcorneal,

measure of retention	time of treatment	test	retention
STL (300 sec)	10 sec	8-240 min	no RA
	10 sec	480 min-	
		24 hr	RA
		42 days	RA

same time period (contrary to Geller and Jarvik 1968(b) 1.136).
response latencies were largely controlled by the proactive
unconfounded measures of retention following ECS were possible

No ECS group had high latencies throughout. FS-ECS and ECS
function of time since treatment.

variations such as the direction the animal faces when placed
measures. When placed in compartment with orientation away
since ECS delivery. With orientation towards door into 2nd
experiment (Kopp, Bohdanecky and Jarvik, 1967, 1.131)

Treatment and site	animals	task	trials

1.179 BARRETT AND RAY, 1969

ECS; 1/trial transcorneal 60mA, 250msec	mice	step-through FS PA	1/day for 5 days

ECS 1/trial		step-through habituation with no FS	1/day for 5 days

Acquisition of habituation involves processes qualitatively

1.180 HUGHES, BARRETT AND RAY, 1970(a)

ECS -   40mA
transpinnate
300msec
         70mA
 	
         100mA
	rats	step-through
		FS
		PA
			1

A similar function resulted from repeated testing rather than

1.181 HUGHES, BARRETT AND RAY, 1970(b)

no ECS ECS transpinnate	rats	step-through FS PA	1 1

ECS given shortly after training produced disruption of the
training and test. A uniprocess theory was proposed.

measure of retention	time of treatment	test	retention
STL (300sec)			
	10 sec	24 hr	RA
	60 min		less RA
	10 sec	day 5	RA
	60 min		no RA
STL (300 sec)			
	10 sec	24 hr	RA
	60 min		less RA
	10 sec	day 5	RA
	60 min		less RA

similar to those controlling acquisition of a learned response.

STL	10 sec	1 day	no RA
		24 days	no RA
		42 days	RA
	10 sec	1 day	no RA
		24 days	RA
		42 days	RA
	10 sec	1 day	RA
		24 days	RA
		42 days	RA

separate testing over 42 days.

STL		42 days	good retention
	10 sec-2 min	1 day	RA
	1 hr		no RA
	10 sec-1 hr	24 days	RA
	10 sec-1 hr	42 days	RA

response suppression that increased as a function of time between

Treatment and site	animals	task	trials

1.182 BARRETT, HUGHES AND RAY, 1971

ECS	rats	discriminated	0,5
transpinnate		Y-maze	
100mA; 300msec		FS	10,15,20
			30

The RA is not due to proactive interference, punishing effects or

no ECS			15
ECS			15

Incubation of a CER occurs which asymptotes at 1 hour and then
retention. ECS and no ECS gradients were not parallel functions.
no longer confounded by the presence of a CER.

1.183 CAUL AND BARRETT, 1972

ECS	rats	conditioned	3
transpinnate		heart rate	1/day
100mA; 500msec			
		suppression	1/day
		of licking	
		responses by	
		FS	

In this study ECS was effective in attenuating both the pre-CS
bradycardia as well as the prolonged suppression of drinking as
cardiac responses with ECS raises the possibility that heart rate
on memory processes as opposed to ECS induced changes in
behavioural task.

1.184 GOLDSMITH, 1967

ECS	rats	skinner box	1
		FS	

There was no evidence of suppression of CER.

---

measure of retention	time of treatment	test	retention
errors to criterion	within 30 sec	24 hr	no RA
	within 30 sec		RA
	within 30 sec		no RA

competing responses. The amount of training was important.

		30 sec-12 hrs	
	30 sec-3 hrs	24 hrs	RA
	6-12 hrs		no RA (compared with 12 hr no ECS)

gradually dissipates such that by 12 hours it no longer affects
Therefore, ECS effects can only be assessed when performance is

heart rate	1 sec	day 2	RA
		day 3	RA
	10 sec	day 2	RA
		day 3	less RA
suppression ratios and	1 sec	over 7 days 1/day	RA
mean latency to 10 licks	10 sec		no RA

heart rate decrease and the development of the conditioned
seen in the group CS-FS. The manipulation of conditioned
may be useful to differentiate between possible effects of ECS
performance variables which are peculiar to a particular

---

latency of bar press	30 sec	24 hr	RA

Treatment and site   animals   task   trials

1.185 KINCAID, 1967

ECS   rats   step-down   1
transpinnate   FS
540v; 60Hz; 300msec   PA

Single post-trial treatment with ECS produces permanent inter-

1.186 KINCAID, 1968

ECS   rats   step-down   1
transpinnate   FS
540v; 60Hz; 300msec   PA

metrazol
convulsion

Only metrazol was capable of interferring with retention 5 minutes
convulsion. The severity of the treatment may extend the duration
rather than the extent of the convulsion.

1.187 SPEVACK, RABEDEAU AND SPEVACK, 1967

ECS   rats   step-through   1
transpinnate   FS
70mA; 200msec   PA (placed in +
in small compartment   FS in small
                                           compartment)

With confincement training rats received FS in small compartment
ing function of the FS-ECS interval.

ECS   2 or 5mA FS
transpinnate   (placed in large
50mA; 200msec   compartment and
in small compartment   shocked for
                                           entering small
                                           compartment)

The 2mA FS produced slightly higher latencies than the 5mA FS but
were shown with changes in the learning - ECS interval.

measure of retention	time of treatment	test	retention
± stepdown within 30 sec	75 sec	24 hr	RA
	75 sec	21 days	RA

ference with retention.

measure of retention	time of treatment	test	retention
± stepdown within 30 sec	90 sec	24 hr	RA
	5 min		no RA
	90 sec-5 min		RA

post-trial. The metrazol convulsion lasted longer than the ECS of the amnesic effects - severity referring to duration of action

---

measure of retention	time of treatment	test	retention
latency of entering small compartment from large	0.5-10 sec	24 hrs	RA
	5 mins		less RA
	45 mins- 2 hrs		no RA

where they were placed. With RA the latencies were a decreas-

measure of retention	time of treatment	test	retention
	0-10 sec		RA
	30 min, 2 hr, 6 hr		no RA

the difference was not significant. Temporally graded latencies

Treatment and site	animals	task	trials

1.188 SPEVACK AND SUBOSKI, 1967

ECS	rats	skinner box	1
transpinnate		contingent FS	
42mA, 500msec			
		NCFS	

Shock administered either contingent upon or between bar presses
series of seven ECS's starting 24 hours after shock raised bar
passive avoidance conditioning.

1.189 SUBOSKI, BLACK, LITNER, GREENER AND SPEVACK, 1969

ECS	rats	discriminative	1
transpinnate		avoidance	
50mA, 500msec		FS	

Rats learned to avoid retrieving a food pellet in the presence of
shock followed pellet retrieval the first time the wall was
various time intervals following shock on pellet retrieval during
found only a nongraded reduction in discriminated avoidance. At
interference with discrimination by ECS was obtained. These results
term retrograde effects attributable to possible consolidation

1.190 SUBOSKI, SPEVACK, LITNER AND BEAUMASTER, 1969

ECS	rats	discriminative	1
		avoidance	
		FS	

At long intervals between learning and ECS the RA effect occurs
latencies decreased as learning-ECS interval was lengthened from
latency gradient with increasing learning-ECS interval was
were obtained when S's were tested at the end of the shock

The conclusion was that ECS given 100 seconds to 1 hour after
with incubation of the CER.

1.191 SUBOSKI AND WEINSTEIN, 1969

ECS	rats	step-through	30
transpinnate		FS	
50mA, 500msec		PA	
no ECS			

measure of retention	time of treatment	test	retention
bar press rates	2.5–5 min	3 days	RA
	2.5–5 min	3 days	RA

reduced bar press rates. Extinction to situational cues and a
press rates, indicating that conditioned suppression occurs in

bar press rates and latency to retrieve food	0–100 sec	24 hr	graded RA
	100–3160sec		ungraded RA

an illuminated wall of the conditioning chamber when a single
illuminated. Two experiments examined the effect of ECS at
illumination. One examined long (100–3160 sec) intervals and
short (0–100 sec) intervals, however, a temporally graded
support Chorover and Schiller's (1.104) finding of only short-
disruption by ECS.

response choice	100 sec	24 hr	slight RA
	1000 sec		same–slight RA

but is not graded temporally. With a free choice the response
100 to 1000 seconds. With forced choice, a typical increasing
obtained. Latency gradients parallel to ECS-produced gradients
treatment interval rather than given ECS.

learning fails to affect memory consolidation but does interfere

20 trial test session; % avoidance	1 min	24 hr	slight RA
	1 hr		complete RA
	16 hr		no RA
		1 min	good performance
		1 hr	poor performance
		16 hr	good performance

Treatment and site	animals	task	trials

1.191 (Continued)

Rats were given a conditioning session of 30 trials in a two-way
20 trial test session or by a single ECS and a test session 24 hr
effect was obtained for percentage avoidances from the tested
from the conditioning-ECS interval, although not completely parallel
interpreted as supporting an incubation-disruption rather than a
of ECS.

1.192 BLACK AND SUBOSKI,   1971

no ECS	rats	step-through	1
		FS	
		PA	

There was no incubation gradient with response choice as the
were longest at the post-conditioning interval where discrimination
misleading measure of retention.   The bolus count was an increas-
due to generalization of fear to a greater range of stimuli.

No ECS	Rats	Y-maze	to 9/10
		discrimination	(75)
		FS	

ECS
transpinnate
50mA; 500msec

The latency changes and response choices were similar.   These
as a function of time following conditioning and that ECS disrupts

---

1.193   ZINKIN AND MILLER,   1967

ECS	rats	step-down	1
transpinnate		FS	
35mA; 200msec		PA	

The RA effect of day 1 had largely disappeared on the two subsequent
animals were tested each time and this is looking at the effect of
alone the latencies increased over the 3 days of testing.

measure of retention	time of treatment	test	retention

shuttle box followed, after either 1 min, 1 hr or 16 hrs, by a
later. The typical U-shaped intersession interval (Kamin)
groups. The groups given ECS also yielded a U-shaped function
with the intersession interval function. The results were
consolidation-disruption hypothesis for the retrograde effects

STL		10 sec- 28 hr	With STL, retention decreased from 100-3160 sec then increased to 28hrs

measure but retention was poor at 28 hours. Response latencies
was poorest. This suggests that response latency may be a
ing function of the conditioning-test interval-suggested to be

no. trials and no. of errors to criterion		1 min 2 hr	less retention more retention
	1 min 2 hr	48 hr	RA no RA

results were taken as support for freezing behaviour increasing
the incubation of freezing behaviour.

SDL (1,3 or 10 sec)	0.6 sec 0.6 sec 0.6 sec	1 day 2 days 3 days (repeated)	RA no RA no RA

trials indicating a non-permanence of RA. But the same
repeated exposure to the experimental situation of RA. With ECS

Treatment and site	animals	task	trials

1.194 MILLER, 1968

ECS	rats	step-down	1
transpinnate		FS	
35mA, 200 or 500msec		PA	
100mA; 200 or 500 msec			

ECS alone had no significant effect. ECS intensity was found to
at 48 hours ECS-only animals showed a slight increase in SDL's -
increase in latencies, whereas 3 sec group showed least increase.
35mA/200msec groups but not in the others. The decrease in RA
disruption before threshold is reached may destroy the memory
the memory only partially or temporarily.

1.195 KESNER AND DOTY, 1968

amygdala ES	cats	passive	1
		avoidance box	
		MS	

frontal cortex ES
mesencephalic reticular
formation ES

septum fornix ES
ventral hippocampus ES

1.196 KESNER, GIBSON AND LECLAIR, 1970

ECS 8; 1/trial	rats	step-down	8 1/day
transpinnate		no FS	
35mA; 60Hz; 500msec			

cranial plugs,
earclips,
xylocaine and
earclips

Xylocaine only partially reduced the ECS-induced fear state,
of the ears and not the surrounding cutaneous areas.

measure of retention	time of treatment	test	retention
SDL			
	3 sec	24 hr	RA
	30-300 sec		no RA
	3000 sec		RA

be a variable, whereas duration of ECS was not. When retested
35mA more than 100mA at 30 sec. The 3000 sec groups showed an
Absence of tonic extension was correlated with absence of RA in
found on retesting suggests a threshold in the memory process;
permanently; disruption after threshold has passed may affect

---

latency of entry	4 sec	24 hr	RA (overt convulsions not necessary)
			no RA
			no RA (overt convulsions)
			no RA
			no RA (electrical discharge)
% avoidance	immediate	day 1	no effect
		day 8	greater avoidance
	1 hr		same avoidance as controls

which could have been due to exclusive xylocaine treatment

Treatment and site	animals	task	trials

1.196 (Continued)

ECS; 10	rats	skinner box	10
earclips or		CS paired	1/day
earclips and		with ECS	
xylocaine		(CER)	

transcranial

ECS delivered via the ears induced a fear state whereas when
or prevented. The difference did not appear after the first
immediately preceding ECS treatment.

1.197 KESNER, McDONOUGH AND DOTY, 1970

ECS	cats	step-through	1
35mA; 60Hz; 5 sec		MS	
2nd MS-ECS		PA	
treatment after			
1st test			2

No amnesia was seen when a second MS-ECS treatment was given 24
no further treatment does not alter the RA from the 1st treatment
second aversive experience means a total of 8 seconds for
to create a permanent mnemonic trace. Alternatively, at time of
seizure is unable to engage all the relevant neurones to the degree

ECS	6 cats		1
ECS			1
MS-ECS			1

This was thought to be due to change in efficacy of ECS with
that some traces of the initial aversive experience have
second aversive experience.

| ECS | | | 1 |

The number of MS-ECS treatments necessary before retention is
found to decrease as the ECS interval was increased. ECS will

measure of retention	time of treatment	test	retention
suppression of response		day 10	lower suppression ratio (RA)
			less effect (no RA)

given transcranially the onset of the fear state was delayed
treatment. Fear behaviour was displayed to specific stimuli

latency over 5 trials	4 sec	24 hr	RA
	4 sec	24 hr	no RA

hours after the first and tested 24 hours later. ECS alone or
so failure was not due to fear produced by ECS,nor recovery. The
undisturbed registration of the experience and could be adequate
2nd ECS some elements are still refactory so that the second
necessary to interrupt registration.

	1 day before	24 hr	RA - in 2/6 no RA in 4/6
	8-12 days before	24 hr	RA
	15 days before	24 hr	no RA

longer delay between ECS and MS-ECS. Therefore, it was thought
survived to summate with similarly surviving traces of the

	0-15 min	24 hr	RA
	1 hr-4 hr		no RA

achieved with different MS-ECS delays was measured, and was
eventually become aversive when given without MS.

Treatment and site   animals   task   trials

1.197   (Continued)

This experiment was to test whether the shrinkage of amnesia with
regardless of MS-ECS time interval or as an interaction between MS-
It was concluded that ECS does not destroy an incipient memory trace
trace which at a later time can produce a functionally adequate

1.198   KESNER,   1971

Treatment and site	animals	task	trials
ECS	rats	step-down	no.
1/trial		no FS	
transpinnate		no FAM trials	
35mA; 60Hz; 500msec			
		200 FAM	

The larger number of pretraining trials, the earlier the
aversive and interfere with performance with a large amount of

ECS		no FS	no.

Fear is elaborated more readily in the 16-sec delay group than in
were necessary to obtain fear conditioning in the 0 sec delay group
sec delay groups primarily because of the delay of punishment. The
ECS-delay interval if ECS has only aversive properties and should
delay of punishment gradient. Fear behaviour is more readily
delaying ECS for an optimal time interval. Aversive experiences
in enhanced step-down latencies - such experiences are not recalled

Morphine		no FS	no.
injection after			
immediate ECS			

If ECS administered through the ears produces pain for an interval
an unconditioned stimulus in establishing fear behaviour. Morphine

Anterograde			
amnesic period			
- shorter		no FS	no.
- longer			

measure of retention	time of treatment	test	retention

repeated treatments occurs as a function of 2nd experience
ECS time interval and the number of experiences.
but merely arrests its development, leaving an incomplete
memory of the aversive experience.

number of treatments to SDL criterion of 30 sec	immediate	daily	RA-5.2 treatments
	immediate		no RA-1.5 treatments

conditioning of fear appears. One ECS treatment can be
prior familiarization.

no. treatments	0-10 sec	daily	decreasing RA 7-4 treatments
	16 sec		RA- 3 treatments
	30 sec		RA- 4 treatments
	60 sec		no RA-8 treatments
	300 sec		no RA-15 treatments

the 0 sec, 60 sec or 300 sec delay groups. More ECS treatments
primarily because of the ECS-induced RA and in the 60 and 300
maximum induction of fear should have occurred at the shortest
decline as the ECS-delay interval is lengthened according to a
elaborated with familiarization, multiple ECS treatments or
occurring during the post-ictal depression period do not result
(anterograde amnesia).

no.treatments	1 min	daily	RA; 7.1 treatments
	30 min		no RA-2.4 treatments

longer than the duration of the ECS, then this could serve as
significantly delayed the development of fear.

no.treatments	immediate	daily	no RA-1.9 treatments
	immediate		RA-4.3 treatments

Treatment and site   animals   task   trials

1.198   (Continued)

The anterograde amnesia could be shortened by auditory
result in registration of more intense pain and enhance the fear
but because of the RA, the ECS-induced pain is not always
animal is tested.

1.199   KESNER AND D'ANDREA,   1971

Treatment and site	animals	task	trials
ECS transcranial 35mA; 500msec	rats	skinner box bar shock	1

ECS not only blocks the storage, but also the retrieval of a new

1.200   McDONOUGH AND KESNER,   1971

Treatment and site	animals	task	trials
subseizure ES of amygdala:- bilateral ES	5 cats	passive avoidance box. MS	1
unilateral ES with contralateral amygdaloid lesion			
bilateral amygdaloid ES			
bilateral hippocampal ES			
cingulate cortex ES septum ES			

measure of retention	time of treatment	test	retention

stimulation during this period. The faster recovery should conditioning. It was concluded that ECS always produces pain, associated with the environmental situation in which the

measure of retention	time of treatment	test	retention
bar press suppression ratios	5 min	185 min	RA
	5 min	24 hr	RA
	24 hr	27 hr	RA
	24 hr	48 hr	no RA
	24 hr	27 hrs + 48 hr	RA no RA
		36 hr + 48 hr	RA no RA
		42 hr + 48 hr	RA RA
		48 hr	no RA

noxious experience.

measure of retention	time of treatment	test	retention
latency of entry into food compartment	4 sec	24 hr	
			RA
			2/5 RA (depending on placement of lesion)
	4 sec	24 hr	RA 4/4
	5 min		RA 4/4
	30 min		RA 3/4
	60 min		RA 1/2
	4 sec	24 hr	RA 4/4
	5 min		RA 4/4
	30 min		RA 2/4
	60 min		RA 1/2
	1 min	24 hr	no RA 1/1
	5 min	24 hr	no RA 1/1

Treatment and site	animals	task	trials

1.200   (Continued)

Stimulation of either the amygdala or the hippocampus will produce
stimulation can be used as a disrupting stimulus. It is suggested
spatial and temporal patterning of impulses passing through the

1.201   WILBURN AND KESNER,   1972

low frequency	4 cats	passive	1
ES of		avoidance	
non specific		box. MS	
thalamus,7 Hz			
caudate nucleus			
ES,3 Hz			
100 Hz			

Cats which received non specific thalamic stimulation consistently
ing caudate nucleus stimulation showed RA. It was suggested that
for processing aversive information into a long-term memory store.

1.202   KESNER AND CONNER,   1972

ES	rats	skinner box	1
MRF		FS contingent	
100Hz		on bar press	
		at end of 10	
		min session	
hippocampus ES			
30Hz			
MRF ES			
hippocampus ES			

It was suggested that there is a structural basis for a dual
brain reticular formation (MRF) is involved in short-term memory
rather than sequential processing of short-term and long-term must

measure of retention	time of treatment	test	retention

amnesia at the times tested. Brief, low intensity electrical
that it acts as a functional lesion by scrambling the normal
stimulated area.

measure of retention	time of treatment	test	retention
latency of entry into food compartment	4 sec	24 hr	RA 4/4
	5 min		RA 4/4
	4 sec	24 hr	no RA 4/7
	5 min		no RA 3/4
	4 sec	24 hr	RA 2/2

showed RA for mouth shock, while only half the animals receiv-
non specific thalamus, amygdala and hippocampus are all critical

measure of retention	time of treatment	test	retention
bar press suppression ratios	4 sec	64 sec	RA
	4 sec	24 hr	no RA
	4 sec	64 sec	no RA
	4 sec	24 hr	RA
	196 sec	256 sec	no RA
	196 sec	256 sec	RA- less than at 64 sec

processing of memory of aversive information, where the mid-
and the hippocampus is involved in long-term memory. Parallel
occur for aversive information.

Treatment and site	animals	task	trials

1.203   KOHLENBERG AND TRABASSO, 1968

ECS	mice	drinking chamber FS	1
ECS 2		CER	2

There was considerabte degree of forgetting in the controls after
controls 48 hours after treatment, but were markedly inferior at

---

1.204   MALDONADO,   1968

ECS	octopus	shuttle box PA	20
ECS		discriminative avoidance	30

1.205   MALDONADO,   1969

ECS	octopus	shuttle box PA	10

1.206   NIELSON,   1968

ECS transpinnate 600mA; 300msec	rats	open field activity after FS in step-down type apparatus	1

ECS produced a transient decrease in brain excitability levels
electrical stimulus, delivered to a sub-cortical area, necessary

measure of retention	time of treatment	test	retention
drinking time	10 sec	3 hr	RA
		24 hr	less RA
		48 hr	no RA
	10 sec	3 hr	RA
		24 hr	less RA
		48 hr	more RA

48 hours. Mice given ECS performed at the same levels as 24 hours and 3 hours. The shock was not response-contingent.

---

incorrect crossings	1 min	3 days	RA
number of attacks	1 min	2 days	RA
incorrect crossings and error time	1 min	3 days	RA
	6 hr		no RA

---

distance travelled; levels of activity	immediate	24 hr	increase in activity
		48 hr repeated	normal activity

lasting 4 days - determined by the increasing intensity of an to elicit a conditioned response.

Treatment and site	animals	task	trials

1.206   (Continued)

ECS; tested with :	rats	step-down	1
ear clips-			
no earclips -			
earclips-			
no ear clips -			

Recovery of the learned response occurred when ECS induced
over 24-96 hours and the recovery followed the same time course as

ECS		step-down task	1
		24 hr after	
		brain excit-	
		ability state	
		induced in a	
		T-maze	
		avoidance	
		habit	

When activity levels and brain excitability states were equalized
ance response. ECS may produce a dissociation of learning. It was
memory fixation and that memory retrieval may depend on brain

---

1.207   BARCIK,   1969

ECS	rats	step-down	1
cortical screw		FS	
electrodes		PA	
40/sec; 1.0msec			2nd with
pulse width;			FS,no ECS
30-40v; 300-900msec			
dorsal hippocampal ES			1
40/sec; 1.0msec			
pulse width			
3.0-3.6v; 10 sec			2nd with
			FS,no ECS

Amnesia can be produced by localized seizure involving the
was thought that this seizure was not as widespread as that

---

measure of retention	time of treatment	test	retention
% avoidances	immediate	24 hr	RA
	10 sec		RA
	immediate	96 hr	RA
	10 sec		RA

increases in activity levels were controlled (with ear clips) changes in brain excitability.

% avoidances	1 sec	24 hr	no RA
	4 hr		no RA
	1 sec	96 hr	no RA
	4 hr		no RA

ECS did not produce even a transient disruption of the avoid-suggested that these experiments show that ECS does not disrupt excitability states.

SDL (60 sec)	3 sec	24 hr	RA motor convulsions
		48 hr	no RA
	3 sec	24 hr	RA
	30 sec		slightly less RA
	3+30 sec	48 hrs	no RA hippocampal after discharges but no motor convulsions

hippocampus, but which does not produce motor involvement. It produced by ECS stimulation.

Treatment and site	animals	task	trials

1.208 BANKER, HUNT AND PAGANO, 1969

Treatment and site	animals	task	trials
ECS	rats	step-down	1
transpinnate		FS	2
40mA; 300msec		PA	1
ECS	rats	T-maze discrimination	1
		FS	2

A second FS several hours after training and ECS 0.5 seconds later
animals hyperactive, suggesting that this is not an appropriate
measure the animals showed no amnesia.

1.209 PAGANO, BUSH, MARTIN AND HUNT, 1969

Treatment and site	animals	task	trials
ECS	rats	step-down	1
transpinnate		FS PA	
95mA; 200msec			
55mA			

High intensity ECS produced an amnesia which lasted throughout the
only produced a temporary amnesia. Retention was depressed at 1 hr
effectiveness of ECS appears to depend not only on the time of
interference.

1.210 BOVET, BOVET-NITTI AND OLIVERIO, 1969

Treatment and site	animals	task	trials
ECS at end of each	mice	shuttle box	50 per
training session		FS PA	session
15mA, 100msec			

The analysis of the learning curves within each session enabled a
(short-term memory) and on the consolidation processes which occur

---

measure of retention	time of treatment	test	retention
SDL (30 sec)	7 hr	24 hr	no RA
	7 hr 0.5 sec		no RA
	0.5 sec		RA
response choice	0.5-30 sec	24 hr	RA
	6 hr 0.5 sec		no RA

failed to show impaired avoidance. However the second FS made
procedure in PA studies. When response choice was used as a

SDL (180 sec)	0.5 sec	1 hr	RA
		24 hr	RA
		48 hr	RA
	0.5 sec	1 hr	RA
	30 sec		no RA
	0.5 sec	24 hr	no RA
	0.5 sec	48 hr	no RA

longest retention interval tested (48 hour). Low intensity ECS
following footshock, but had returned 23 hours later. The
administration following learning, but on the intensity of the

---

% avoidances	within 2 min	every 24 hr	RA
	15 min		no RA

distinction to be made between the effects of shock on learning
in the interval between consecutive sessions (long-term memory).

Treatment and site	animals	task	trials

1.211 NACHMAN AND MEINECKE, 1969

Treatment and site	animals	task	trials
ECS	rats	skinner box	1
transpinnate		FS	
55-60mA; 200msec		PA	2 FS-ECS
			1/day
		drinking	1
		response	2 FS-ECS
		FS	1/day

The repetition of FS-training disruption treatment does not re-
on responses and the avoidance of these responses are probably a

1.212 NACHMAN, 1970

Treatment and site	animals	task	trials
ECS	rats	drinking	1 trial for
transpinnate		saccharin,	5 sec
50mA; 200msec		made sick	10 sec
		5 min later	30 sec
		with LiCl PA	

Rats which drank saccharin for 5,10, or 30 sec. and were made sick
saccharin again. An ECS given immediately after 30 sec of saccharin
ECS given immediately after 5 or 10 sec of saccharin drinking
seconds of drinking saccharin and not by 30 seconds could have been
seconds or the different ECS delay time from onset of drinking. The
gradient for ECS effects although, even at short temporal intervals,
The relatively limited effects of ECS were interpreted to be a
second experiment, ECS was found to be ineffective as a US in

1.213 PIRCH, 1969

Treatment and site	animals	task	trials
ECS; 2/day for	rats	step-through	no.
5-8 days, not		FS	
associated with		AA	
training			
transocular ECS			
150mA; 220msec			

2nd series of ECS

Studies were conducted to determine the effect of repeated ECS
performers in a two-way shuttle box. Following 14-20 training

measure of retention	time of treatment	test	retention
bar press rates	30 sec	24 hr	RA
	30 sec	daily	no RA
amount of drinking	30 sec	24 hr	RA
	30 sec	daily	no RA

produce this apparent memory impairment. FS was not contingent
result of a CER.

mean intake		72 hr	
	immediate		RA
	immediate		RA
	immediate		no RA

5 min later by an injection of LiCl learned to avoid drinking
drinking had no effect on the learned saccharin aversion while
produced some amnesic effects. The amnesia shown by 5 or 10
due to either different amounts of learning between 5 and 30
results were consistent with the idea of a brief temporal
amnesic effects occurred in only a small percentage of subjects.
result of the particularly strong type of learning used. In a
producing learned taste aversion.

% avoidances	18-24 hr	daily, 18-24 hr after final ECS 1 day 6 days	before ECS- poor avoidance after ECS- good avoidance poor avoidance same result as after one series of ECS

treatment on avoidance responding of rats which were poor
sessions, ECS was administered twice daily for 5-8 days.

Treatment and site   animals   task   trials

1.213 (Continued)

After completion of the ECS treatments, the animals underwent
follows: (1) repeated ECS treatment, without simultaneous training,
(2) the improved performance could not be explained on the basis of
performance subsided by 72-96 hours after the last ECS; (4) the
passage of time and was not dependent on relearning. This temporary
memory consolidation.

1.214 RIDDELL, 1969

ECS	rats	step-down	1
posterior		FS	
transcranial		PA	

Although there is some recovery from amnesia, as a function of time
extinguished.   It was concluded that ECS stops the memory storage
stored information.

1.215 ZERBOLIO, 1969(a)

ECS	mice	step-through	1
transcorneal		FS	
.20mA, 200msec		PA	

ether and ECS
(no convulsions)

ECS does produce a retest retention deficit when administered 1 hour
by light etherization, a retention deficit only occurs with ECS 5

ECS

ether and ECS

Animals treated with ECS with or without consulsions all show
treatment the lack of any deficits shows this effect to be only
different processes in the storage and retrieval of information.

measure of retention	time of treatment	test	retention

further behavioural testing. The results were summarized as
produced a significant improvement in avoidance responding;
spontaneous crossings in the shuttle box;(3) the improved
return to poor performance occurred spontaneously with the
effect of ECS on shuttle box performance does not involve

SDL	0.5 sec	24 hr	RA
		2-4 days	RA
		5 days	RA (slight shrinkage of latencies)

or repeated testing,this recovery is slight, labile and easily
process or it causes difficulty in the retrieval of recently

SDL (30 sec)	before learning:		
	1 hr	24 hr	deficit
	1 hr		no deficit
	30 min		no deficit
	15 min		no deficit
	5 min		deficit

before the original training. If ECS convulsions are prevented
minutes before training.

	before test:	24 hr	
	1 hr		deficit
	1 hr		deficit
	30 min		deficit
	15 min		deficit
	5 min		deficit
		48 hr retest	no deficit

comparable retention deficits on testing. 24 hours after this
temporary. Therefore, the ECS and the convulsion affect

Treatment and site	animals	task	trials

1.216 ZERBOLIO, 1969(b)

no treatment	mice	step-through	1
		FS	
		PA	

Memory storage during the first post-trial hour does not follow the biphasic character of this retention curve was interpreted as being

1.217 ZERBOLIO, 1971

ECS and etherization	mice	step-through	1
to prevent overt		FS	
convulsions		PA	
transcorneal			
20mA; 200msec			

S's show significant levels of retention on the retest trials one supporting a biphasic or multiphasic view of memory storage.

1.218 BRUNNER, ROSSI, STUTZ AND ROTH, 1970

stimulation by	rats	step-down	
subconvulsive		FS PA	
current of-			
dorsal hippocampus –			1
cortex overlying			1
hippocampus –			
septal region –			1
hippocampal lesion –			1

---

measure of retention	time of treatment	test	retention
STL (30 sec)		0-15 min	increasing
		15 min	max. retention
		15-30 min	decreasing
		30 min	min. retention
		30 min-1 hr	increasing
		1-2 hr	max retention

simple monotonic growth function indicated by the ECS work. The consistent with a multiprocess view of memory storage.

STL (30 sec)	immediate	15 min	RA
	(up to 25 sec)	30 min	less RA
		60 min	RA
		24 hr	more RA

hour or less after training. These data are interpreted as

SDL			
	immediate	24 and 48 hr	RA
	immediate		no RA
	immediate		no RA
	immediate		no RA

Treatment and site	animals	task	trials

1.219 CAREW, 1970

ECS transpinnate 45-50mA; 200msec	rats	modified step-down FS PA	1
		AA	1
ECS		modified step-through FS PA	1
		AA	

Rats were provided with cues to discriminate the place where the
down or-through onto either a black or a white surface. They could
Neither time between learning and testing nor ECS alone significantly
is observed at the same time as latencies are measured (i.e. the
amnesic by latencies actually do exhibit memory for footshock.

1.220 JAMIESON AND ALBERT, 1970

ECS transcranial 100-120mA; 500msec	rats	drinking response FS PA	1

Pairing of FS and ECS 5 hour after training did not produce amnesia.
Sherman, 1968 (1.139) cannot account for the entire retrograde
eliminating the added effect of the second FS.

measure of retention	time of treatment	test	retention
SDL	1-10 sec	24 hr	RA
	30 sec-1 hr		no RA
% alternation	1 sec		RA
	5 sec-1 hr		no RA
STL	15 sec-1 min	24 hr	RA
	5 min- 1 hr		no RA
% alternation	15 sec		RA
	30 sec-1 hr		no RA

FS was received on the floor of the apparatus, so they could step-
avoid where they were given the shock on the learning trial.
changed the alternation tendency. If another aspect of behaviour
chosen locus of step-down or step-through) many rats judged

---

latency to drink (60 sec)	0.5 sec	1 day	RA
	1 hr	1 day	no RA
		retest on day 2	extinction
	5hr NCFS+ 0.5 sec ECS	1 day	no RA
		retest on day 2	no extinction

The simple pairing of ECS and FS as suggested by Schneider and
effect of ECS. In this experiment the ECS was ineffective in

Treatment and site	animals	task	trials

1.221 MAH, ALBERT AND JAMIESON, 1972

Treatment and site	animals	task	trials
ECS transcranial 25mA; 400msec	rats	drinking response FS	1
2ECS		PA	
2ECS			
2ECS			
2ECS			

The disruptiveness of the second ECS is time dependent. The
disinhibitory effects of the ECS's. These findings were
continue after ECS.

1.222 KRAL, 1970

Treatment and site	animals	task	trials
ECS transpinnate 40mA; 500msec	rats	taste aversion with toxic drug illness	1

Rats were allowed to drink sour water for 10 minutes and 30 minutes
taste-illness interval, 2 or 25 minutes after tasting. The ECS
that the memory is kept in a labile form during the CS-US interval

1.223 KRAL, 1971(a)

Treatment and site	animals	task	trials
ECS transpinnate 60mA; 700msec	rats	drinking sweet or sour water	1
		taste aversion to sweet water by illness induced by LiCl 4 hrs after tasting	1

measure of retention	time of treatment	test	retention
approach latency (60 sec)	5 min	2 days	v. slight RA
	1 hr		no RA
	5 min + 1 hr		RA
	5 min + 24 hr		v. slight RA
	24 hr + 25 hr	3 days	no RA
	5 min + 2 hr	2 days	RA
	+ 3 hr		v. slight RA
	+ 6 hr		no RA

retention deficit does not appear to be due to punishing or
interpreted as indicating that memory consolidation can

---

sour water intake		5 extinction trials over 15 days	
	-2 or -25 min	trials 1,2,	RA
	-2 or -25 min	trials 3,4	no RA

later were injected with a toxic drug. ECS was given in the
retarded learning but could not prevent it. It was assumed
and that ECS disrupts this.

sweet & sour water intake	within 30 sec of tasting	3 days	no effect i.e. no RA for CS
sweet water intake	after CS:		
	0 hr	3 days	RA
	2 hr		RA
	4 hr		RA
			(all equal)

Treatment and site   animals   task   trials

1.223   (Continued)

A interpolation of ECS during the interval between a taste (CS) and
of a taste aversion (Kral, 1970, 1.222). Possible interpretations
Experiments to test these produced negative results. It was
dissociation of taste - illness events, the individual events

1.224   KRAL,   1971(b)

Treatment and site	animals	task	trials

ECS- posterior
transcranial
60mA; duration:-
  0.4 sec
  0.8 sec
  1.6 sec
  3.2 sec
	rats	taste aversion
		to sour water
		by LiCl injection
		30 min after
		tasting
			1

1.0 sec;current:
  12mA
  60mA
	same rats
	as above after
	extinction to
	sour water
	aversion
		taste aversion
		to sweet water
			1

The results suggest that ECS treatment between events intended
relationships similar to those obtained with post-association-ECS

1.225   ST. OMER AND KRAL,   1971

Treatment and site	animals	task	trials
ECS posterior transcranial 60mA; 600msec. pretreatment with supravital dye-trypan blue before ECS	rats	taste aversion to sweet water induced by LiCl illness 30 min after tasting	1

Trypan blue mitigates the dysrhythmic effects of ECS on brain EEG
of the blood brain barrier which is reported to occur with ECS.
avoidance learning, suggesting that increased permeability of the
induced decrement in taste avoidance learning.

measure of retention	time of treatment	test	retention

an induced illness (US) has been shown to impede the learning were - RA for the CS or proactive interference of ECS with US. suggested that there was a third possible interpretation - remaining independently in memory.

measure of retention	time of treatment	test	retention
sour water intake	15 min after CS	3 days	
			RA
			increased RA
			increased RA
			complete RA
sweet water intake	15 min after CS	3 days	
			v.slight RA
			RA

for association affects learning according to parametric paradigms.

measure of retention	time of treatment	test	retention
sweet water intake	15 min after CS	3 days	RA
			RA

and was thought to do so by preventing increased permeability This dye did not prevent the disruptive effect of ECS on blood brain barrier may not be the mechanism of an ECS-

Treatment and site	animals	task	trials

1.226 LIDSKY AND SLOTNICK, 1970

Transcorneal	mice	chamber	1
ECS		with shock	
		bars	
hippocampal ES		FS	
cortical ES		PA	

These three modes of stimulation had no effect on retest behaviour,
account for the typical effects of ECS on memory consolidation.

1.227 LIDSKY AND SLOTNICK, 1971

bilateral ES:	mice	step-through	1
thalamus		FS	
cortex		PA	
amygdala			
hippocampus			
ECS-transcorneal			
hippocampus			
unilateral stimulation			
hippocampus			
ECS			

With ECS or hippocampal stimulation, the extent of retention
treatment, with no deficits at a 7 hour delay.

1.228 McINTYRE, 1970

Bilateral	rats	skinner box	no.
convulsions elicited		FS	
by unilateral		CER	
amygdaloid stimulation			
unilateral			
amygdaloid stimulation			
with no convulsions			
bilateral convulsion-			
anterior limbic field			

measure of retention	time of treatment	test	retention
latency, exploratory activity, freezing	40 sec	24 hr	RA
	40 sec		RA
	40 sec		no RA

Interference with hippocampal activity may be sufficient to

STL (300 sec) exploratory activity	immediate	24 hr	
	7-33 sec		no RA
	mdn 15 sec		no RA
			moderate RA
			severe RA
			severe RA
			less RA than bilateral stim.
	0 hr	24 hr	severe RA
	2.5 hr		partial RA
	7 hr		no RA
	0 hr	24 hr	severe RA
	2.5 hr		partial RA
	7 hr		no RA

disruption varied inversely with the interval between FS and

---

suppression ratio		up to 6 weeks	RA
			no RA
			no RA

Treatment and site	animals	task	trials

1.228 (Continued)

Bilateral convulsions elicited by unilateral amygdaloid stimulation
response in rats. The amnesic effect was primarily retrograde in
was stable for at least six weeks. Unilateral amygdaloid stimul-
convulsions and did not disrupt CER acquisition, nor did bilateral
ictal period of depression, which follows an amygdaloid convulsion,

---

1.229   POSLUNS AND VANDERWOLF,   1970

Treatment and site	animals	task	trials
Proactive ECS transpinnate 300msec	rats	step-through FS AA	to 9/10
ECS 300msec–2sec			25
Proactive ECS	rats	jump escape task FS AA	1
ECS			1
		jump escape FS AA	1
		drinking tube FS PA	1
		drinking tube MS PA	1
		step-down FS PA	1

In attempting to explain why the longest ECS delay interval which
experimental reports, Chorover and Schiller (1965, 1.103) suggested
of a specific discrimination of cues". Therefore a fundamental
discriminative learning. In this experiment for testing 24 hours
beside the platform or for training they were placed in the
This group was tested in the normal way. There was no significant
tended to freeze where ever they were placed.

measure of retention	time of treatment	test	retention

were demonstrated to induce amnesia for a conditioned emotional
nature with additional prograde influence in some animals, and
ation in previously unstimulated animals did not cause
convulsions elicited from the anterior limbic field. The post-
was shown to interfere with CER acquisition.

---

measure of retention	time of treatment	test	retention
no.escape responses in trials to criterion	24 hr before	24 hr after ECS	improved acquisition
	after first avoidance session	24 or 50 hr	no effect
latency to jump	24 hr before	24 hr after ECS	no effect on performance
latency to jump	1 or 30 sec	24 hr	no RA
latency to jump	1 sec	24 hr	no RA
latency	30 sec	24 hr	RA
drinking latencies (30 sec)	1,30,60 sec 300 sec	24 hr	RA no RA
SDL (30 sec)	1,10 sec 30,60 sec	24 hr	RA no RA

produced retention deficits varied so greatly among
that ECS induced RA only in tasks which"depend upon retention
assumption is that the step-down task requires specific
after PA training the animals were placed on the grid floor
apparatus with the platform removed and 1 sec later given FS.
difference in test latencies and in all situations rats

Treatment and site	animals	task	trials

1.229   (Continued)

| 5 proactive
ECS treatments
over 4 days | rats | jump
escape FS
AA | 1 |
| | | step-down
FS PA | 1 |

The ECS 1 sec after learning in a one-trial escape task, or 30 sec
deficits. One ECS had no anterograde effect upon escape but
sec after passive-avoidance training in a situation similar to the
passive-avoidance tasks, ECS produced temporally graded retention
before training increased retention deficits produced by one post-
task. Perhaps ECS concomitantly induces a slight memory impair-
effects combine synergistically to produce retention deficits in

1.230   WISHAW AND DEATHERAGE,   1971

| Hippocampal
electrographic
seizures | rats | one-way
jump
avoidance | daily for
5 days
until 5
correct
successively |

The avoidance response does not transfer from the preictal to
an animal has learned in the postictal phase, the response is
induced from other hippocampal loci. When trained in the postictal
normal condition.

| | | 2 choice
brightness
discrimination | daily
to 9/10 |
| | | 2 choice
pattern
discrimination | |

It was suggested that seizures disrupt normal hippocampal function
"state-dependent" effects occur on tasks in which the primary

measure of retention	time of treatment	test	retention
latencies	1 sec	24 hr	no RA
SDL	12,20 sec	24 hr	RA

after active avoidance acquisition, induced no retention
facilitated avoidance acquisition 24 hours later. The ECS 30
escape task produced retention deficits and, in two other
deficits (up to 10 and 60 sec, respectively). Five ECS's
training ECS in a passive avoidance task but not in the escape
ment and a slight impairment of movement inhibition, and these
passive-avoidance tasks.

reponse latency to jump (60 sec)	24 hr after final training	after treatment 10 sec-1 hr	severely disrupted performance
		24 hr	normal performance

postictal stage but can be learned in the postictal stage. Once
transferable to the postictal phase of electrographic seizures
conditions they could learn but this did <u>not</u> transfer to the

response choice	24 hr after 10 trials	postictal	normal performance
	24 hr after 10 trials	postictal	normal performance

in the control of movement and that disruption and hence
measure of performance involves movement.

| Treatment and site | animals | task | trials |

1.231 ROBBINS AND MEYER, 1970

ECS transpinnate 35mA; 500msec	rats	2 choice discriminative avoidance or approach FS-S appetitive -F	to 11/12 on each of 3 tasks
Order of tasks- $F_1S_2F_3$			
$F_1S_2F_3$			
$S_1F_2S_3$			
$S_1F_2S_3$			

Rats were taught 3 tasks and given ECS after the third. Retention both cases, the older habit was impaired because it had the same of the type of incentive used to establish the habit.

1.232 HOWARD AND MEYER, 1971

ECS transpinnate 35mA; 500msec order of tasks- $F_1S_2F_3$	rats	2 choice discriminative avoidance or approach FS-S appetitive F	to 11/12 on each of 3 tasks
$F_1S_2F_3$			
$S_1F_2S_3$			
$S_1F_2S_3$			

This was a replication of 1.231 with sham-ECS used as a control. given, showed no impairment of retention under any conditions. Is at on post-treatment trials with positive reinforcement (S,F,S-F and groups. So interference between tasks is not sufficient in

1.233 GLENDENNING AND MEYER, 1971

ECS transpinnate 35mA ; 500msec ECS sham ECS	rats	two 2-choice discriminations order of tasks - S_1S_2	to 11/12
ECS sham ECS		S_1F_2	

measure of retention	time of treatment	test	retention
mean trials to relearn	immediately after-	tested 24 hr after on	
	F_3	F_1	RA
	F_3	S_2	no RA
	S_3	S_1	RA
	S_3	F_2	no RA

of the first or second task was measured 24 hours later. In
motivation as that task after which ECS was given, regardless

mean trials to relearn	immediately after-	tested 24 hr after 3rd task on	
	F_3	F_1	RA
	F_3	S_2	no RA
	S_3	S_1	RA
	S_3	F_2	no RA

The sham-ECS groups, which had earclips attached but no ECS was
ECS serving as a punishing stimulus? Running times were looked
F,S,F,-F). There was no difference between ECS and sham-ECS
itself to produce the impairments.

mean trials to relearn	immediately after S_2 or F_2	tested 24 hr after on	
		S_1	RA "RA"
		S_1	no RA "no RA"

Treatment and site	animals	task	trials

1.233 (Continued)

The amount of interaction between two successively learned
habits were acquired under similar or different conditions of
ECS effects, but motivationally related retroactive interference
obtained with three-habit training paradigms.

1.234 THOMPSON AND NEELY, 1970

ECS	rats	step-down	1
transpinnate		FS	
50mA; 250msec		PA	

ECS

ECS itself had minimal effect on performance. Retention was best

ECS

Retention was best when ECS-training and ECS-retention intervals

ECS 2

ECS 1

It was concluded that ECS is able to produce a state in which learn-

1.235 THOMPSON AND GROSSMAN, 1972

ECS	rats	three	to 11/12
transpinnate		2 choice	on each
50mA; 300msec		discriminations	task
		S_1 and S_3 (shock)	
		F_2 (food)	

measure of retention	time of treatment	test	retention

discriminations was a marked function of whether or not the
incentive/motivation. There were no motivational - specific
was found which was much larger than has previously been

---

measure of retention	time of treatment	test	retention
SDL	25 min before training and test	24 or 48 hr	no RA
	25 min before training		RA
	25 min before test		RA

when training and retention conditions were identical.

	25 min before training	35,45, 15,55 min	RA
		25 min	no RA

were identical.

	(1)immediately after training (2) 20 min before test	24 sor 48 hr	less RA
	immediately after training		RA

.ing is dissociated from the normal state.

mean trials to relearn S_1	immediately after S_3	24 hr after S_3	RA
F_2			no RA

Treatment and site	animals	task	trials

1.235   (Continued)

| 2nd ECS 15 min before retest | rats | three 2 choice discriminations | |

A state-dependent hypothesis was proposed to explain these data.
of a second ECS creates conditions favourable to the recall of

---

1.236   VARDARIS AND GEHRES,   1970

| Posterior cortex ES | rats | step-through FS PA | 1 |
| no ECS | | | 1 |

4 rats had anomalous avoidance scores and also had abnormal brain
The brain seizure pattern was related to retention of passive

1.237   VARDARIS AND SCHWARTZ,   1971

| dorsal hippocampal ES | rats | step-through FS PA | 1 |
| no ECS | | | 1 |

There was no consistent relation between duration of spike activity
that RA results from propagation of the after-discharges and not
hippocampal seizure activity but two showed no retention deficit.

---

measure of retention	time of treatment	test	retention
mean trials to relearn	immediately after S_3	24 hr after S_3	
S_1			no RA
F_2			RA

ECS produces retrograde dissociative effects. The administration dissociated information.

STL (600 sec)	3 sec	24 hr	RA
	1 hr		no RA
EEG	3 sec-1 hr	48 hr retest	no RA

seizure records in response to brain stimulation. avoidance tendency.

| STL (600 sec) | 3 sec | 24 hr | RA |
| EEG | 3 sec | 48 hr retest | no RA |

or depression and the step-through latencies. It was suggested from seizures in hippocampus per se because all rats exhibited

---

Treatment and site	animals	task	trials

1.238 WINOCUR AND MILLS, 1970

ECS 1/day	rats	skinner box	no.
transpinnate		CRF schedule	
45mA; 250msec		FS	
CS-ECS contingent		no FS	
CS-FS			
CS-ECS non contingent			
CS only			

Fear produced by ECS contingent on bar pressing was as effective
that ECS interferes with normal functioning by inducing conditioned
ECS are more closely related to the convulsive response itself than
seizure. CS was on for 3 minutes before FS or ECS, so RA for CS

1.239 DARBELLAY AND WINOCUR, 1971

ECS	rats	2 choice	15/day
transpinnate		avoidance	
45mA; 250msec		conditioning	
10 treatments		to 9/10	
paired with CS (light)		to CS of light	
		(LCS)	
		or tone (TCS)	
10 treatments		or no specific	
not paired (with CS)		CS (NCS)	

Over the 10 treatment days the ECS groups failed to show normal
defecation. After this treatment these Ss required a greater
effect which was not related to specific CS pairings. It was
and disruptive enough to restrict new learning in an aversive

---

1.240 YOUNG AND GALLUSCIO, 1970

ECS	rats	skinner box	1
transpinnate		FS	
50mA;500msec		CRF schedule	
		FR schedule	1

measure of retention	time of treatment	test	retention

suppression
of bar
pressing

	over 20 days		no RA,suppression
			suppression
			RA,no suppression
			no suppression

as FS-induced fear in establishing a CER. There was no evidence
inhibition or increased motor activity. Traumatic effects of
to any noxious after-effects occurring during recovery from the
would be unlikely.

no. trials to criterion	ending 3 days before training	over days	mean no.trials 55.8 LCS 57.1 TCS 40.6 NCS
			33.9 LCS 30.1 TCS 22.1 NCS

weight gain, while exhibiting greater amounts of urination and
number of trials to reach criterion on the avoidance problem, an
concluded that the stressful effects of ECS were persistent
situation.

---

no. bar presses during extinction and rate of responding	immediate	24 hr	RA
	immediate		no RA

Treatment and site   animals   task   trials

1.240   (Continued)

The amount of training and FS-ECS interval were made constant.
for FS only on the continuous reinforcement schedule and not on the
eliminate suppression of responding in FR group due to the effect
response rate which a partial reinforcement schedule generates.

1.241 GALLUSCIO,   1971

ECS	rats	skinner box	1
transpinnate		FS	
50mA; 500msec			
		reminder FS	1
		4 hr after ECS	

1.242 YOUNG AND DAY, 1971

ECS	rats	skinner box	
transpinnate		bar press	
50mA; 500msec		CRF, FS	1
		VR, FS	1

The variable ratio-ECS (VR-ECS) group did not show the partial
ECS group. There was a non-significant difference between the
the effect of ECS is independent of the acquisition response rate.

1.243 YOUNG AND GALLUSCIO, 1971

Pretraining on	rats	skinner box	1
CRF + FR schedules		FS	
ECS			
transpinnate			
50mA; 500msec			

Suppression of the lever press response due to FS was reduced by
10 days after there was apparent spontaneous recovery of the CER
There was a declined rate of responding of ECS groups, greater for

---

1.244 DeVIETTI AND LARSON, 1971

ECS	rats	drinking	1
transpinnate		chamber	
92mA; 60Hz; 200msec		MS	
NCFS 24 hr after		PA	
training			

measure of retention	time of treatment	test	retention

Offset of FS initiated onset of the ECS. ECS produced amnesia
fixed ratio schedule. It was not clear whether ECS failed to
of the partial reinforcement schedule itself or due to the higher

mean no. lever presses	immediate	24 hr	RA
			partial RA

mean no. lever presses	immediate on offset of FS	24 hr	
			RA
			no RA

reinforcement effect during extinction when compared to the CRF-
number of responses made by both groups. The results suggest that

mean no. lever presses	immediate	24 hr	RA
	immediate	10 days	no RA

the ECS regardless of the acquisition reinforcement schedule.
since there were no differences between FS only and FS-ECS groups.
FR than for CRF schedules.

---

licking latency	0.5 sec	24 hr after treatment	"RA"
		96 hr	no RA

Treatment and site	animals	task	trials

1.244   (Continued)

| NCFS-ECS
24 hr before | rats | extinction
training | 3 |

Results of both experiments indicated that the combination of FS
suggest these data indicate that experiments that have used
demonstrate the disruption of memory formation as a consequence of

1.245   MAYSE AND DeVIETTI,   1971

| ECS
transpinnate
92mA; 60Hz, 200msec | rats | water
T-maze
FS | to 4
successive
correct
trials |

FS-ECS
delivered 24 hr
before retraining -
before training -

before retraining and
training

water
T-maze
FS

ECS alone was not effective in either treatment order. FS-ECS
dependency but not when given only 24 hours before retraining.
the task was looked at, here the FS-ECS produced state-dependency
notion that amnesia observed 24 hours after a training trial FS
effect rather than a failure of memory fixation.

1.246   DeVIETTI AND KALLIOINEN,   1972

| ECS
transpinnate
92mA; 60Hz; 200msec | rats | fear
conditioned
to tone FS | 1 |

These results show that ECS can produce retrograde amnesia when an

measure of retention	time of treatment	test	retention
licking latency	24 hr before	96 hr	RA

and ECS can produce state-dependent learning. The authors
procedures involving footshock followed closely by ECS to
ECS are also subject to a state-dependent interpretation.

| trials to criterion on retraining | | 3 days | |

Training	Retraining		
no FS-ECS	FS-ECS		no RA
FS-ECS	no FS-ECS		"RA"-(state dependency)
FS-ECS	FS-ECS		no RA

reversal
of choice

Training	Retraining		
no FS-ECS	FS-ECS		"RA"
FS-ECS	no FS-ECS		"RA"
FS-ECS	FS-ECS		no RA

administered 24 hour prior to training produced state
Because state dependency effects are task dependent reversal of
in both treatment orders. The second experiment supports the
followed 0.5 sec later by ECS may be due to a state dependency

| heart rate deceleration | 0.5 sec | 24 hr | RA |

autonomic index of retention is employed.

Treatment and site	animals	task	trials

1.247 GROSSER, PERCY AND PIERCE, 1971

ECS	mice	step-through	
transpinnate		FS PA	
10mA; 200msec		1sec	
		duration	
		FS	

The 2-sec and 4-sec groups showed test latencies lower than their
the other ECS times but not with these two groups. A proactive
authors than one involving memory consolidation.

1.248 NAITOH, 1971

ECS-multiple	ewes	pavlovian	2/day for
cortical		conditioning	12 days
100mA; 60Hz; 1 sec			
		CS-MHS condit-	
		ioning of -	
		motor CR	
		EEG CR	
		heart rate	
		BP responses	

The CS-clicks were followed in 12 sec by mild head shock (MHS).
response (CR) or other CR's, such as conditional EEG, heart rate and
significantly attenuated the motor CR, but did not interfere with
responses.

1.249 OLSEN AND HAGSTROM, 1971

ECS 7	rats	step-down	7
place of recovery:		no FS	
shock compartment-		PA of ECS	
dissimilar place-			

Over 7 days, ECS in the same compartment led to greater avoidance
compartment. The SDLs increased in both groups but this difference
conclusion that part of the aversive effect developed as a function

---

measure of retention	time of treatment	test	retention
STL (180 sec)	0 sec	24 hr	RA
	1 sec		RA
	2 sec		max.RA
	4 sec		max.RA
	8 sec		no RA

training STL's. There was considerable variation in STL's with
effect of ECS interpretation seems more acceptable to the

---

		over 12 days	
leg flexion	1 min		attenuated (RA)
EEG			no effect
heart rate			no effect
blood pressure			no effect

CS-ECS was ineffectual in establishing a motor conditioned
blood pressure responses. ECS given after each CS-MHS pairing
acquisition of conditioned EEG, heart rate and blood pressure

---

SDL	daily	over 7 days	greater avoidance
			less avoidance

of that compartment than when ECS was given in a different
was not apparent after only 1 ECS. These results suggest the
of the recovery experience.

Treatment and site	animals	task	trials

1.250 POTTS, 1971

ECS transpinnate	rats	step-through	1
100mA; 300msec		FS	
Ss held in goal		PA	
compartment			
between FS + ECS			

Ss held in
holding compartment
between FS + ECS

It is possible that rats held in goal compartment become less fear-
this explanation is only valid for intervals of 240 sec or longer,
than 120 sec showed impaired retention.

1.251 YAGINUMA AND IWAHARA, 1971

ECS	rats	step-through	1
transpinnate		FS	
28mA; 50Hz; 600msec		PA and CER	

Defecation was used as a measure of the CER. This was increased by
did not occur with defecation. If defecation is a legitimate
has to be concluded the PAR and the CER which were simultaneously

---

1.252 BUCKHOLTZ AND BOWMAN, 1972

ECS	mice	step-through	1
transcorneal		FS PA	

intensity	duration,msec
5mA	100
	400,1600
	100
	400,1600
	100,400,1600

measure of retention	time of treatment	test	retention
STL (30 sec)	1-30 min	24 hr	RA
	1-30 sec		RA
	1 min-30 min		no RA
			(temporally graded)

ful of it because of association, with absence of shock, but
since rats given FS-only but held in goal compartment for more

---

measure of retention	time of treatment	test	retention
STL (300 sec)	20 sec	24 hr	complete RA
no. fecal	40 sec		RA
boli	80 sec		RA
	4 min		RA
	15 min		no RA
	60 min		no RA

FS but the gradient in RA shown with different FS-ECS intervals
measure of conditioned emotionality in this situation, then it
produced by the FS, were differentially affected by ECS.

---

measure of retention	time of treatment	test	retention
STL (600 sec)		24 hr	
	10 sec		no RA
			RA
	100 sec		no RA
			less RA
	1000 sec		no RA

Treatment and site	animals	task	trials

1.252   (Continued)

	mice	step-through	1

intensity   duration, msec
20mA   100,400,1600
            100,400,1600
            100,400,1600

80mA   100,400,1600
            100,400,1600
            100,400,1600

There was no gradient of incubation in this study, the FS-noECS
Conversely, there was a gradient of RA, from maximum at 10 sec to
simply the arrest of an incubation gradient. Increases in both
not from intermediate to high values, produced RA. Increases in

---

1.253   SHINKMAN AND KAUFMAN,   1972

Hippocampal	rats	CS paired	days 1-4
ES, daily		with FS	4 sessions
		CER	daily

threshold to
produce orienting
response
60Hz; 50–180μA
for 30 sec

higher stim-	same rats	CER	days 14-18
200μA for	extinguished	new CS-	4 sessions
10sec		FS pairing	daily

---

measure of retention	time of treatment	test	retention
STL (600 sec)		24 hr	
	10 sec		complete RA
	100 sec		less RA
	1000 sec		no RA
	10 sec		complete RA
	100 sec		less RA
	1000 sec		no RA

groups all showed perfect retention at 10,100 and 1000 sec.
no RA at 1000 sec. Thus the RA gradient in this study was not
ECS intensity and duration from low to intermediate values, but
ECS duration were most effective only at the low ECS intensity.

---

suppression of licking on CS presentation no. licks day 5, no CS day 6, CS	after each session—	days 5,6	
	immediate		slight RA
	10 sec		slight RA
	immediate	day 19	complete RA
	10 sec		partial RA
	20 sec		partial RA
	30 sec		partial RA
	40 sec		partial RA
	120 sec		no RA

Treatment and site	animals	task	trials

2.1 WEISSMAN, 1965

| ECS plus diphenylhydantoin subcutaneous | rats | skinner box FS | 1 |

phenacemide

phenobarbital

These anticonvulsant drugs fail to protect against RA induced by component of ECS.

2.2 ESSMAN, 1966

| ECS plus trycyanoaminopropene (TCAP) i.p. | mice | step-through FS   PA | 1 |

Tricyanoaminopropene presumably accelerates RNA synthesis. The reduction and specifically as a reduction in the magnitude of RNA animals. The data suggest that an acceleration of RNA synthesis

2.3 ESSMAN, 1967(a)

| ECS plus: 5HTP   3.12 mg/kg | mice | step-through PA | 1 |

5HT   100 mg/kg
serotonin antagonists:
DMBC   45 mg/kg
Reserpine   2.5 mg/kg

Saline

5-hydroxytryptophan (5HTP) is a precursor of the transmitter 5-aminoethyl-N-benzyl-methoxy-cinnamide (HCL) is a selective

time of treatment		test	retention
ECS	Other		
5 min	40 min before ECS	24 hr	more RA
5 min	150 min before ECS		RA
5 min	90 min before ECS		RA

ECS, even though they protect against tonic-extension seizure

---

immediate	every day for 3 days before training	24 hr	no RA

effect of ECS on RNA concentration was generally seen as a
concentration differences above base levels in non-convulsed
with TCAP serves to facilitate memory trace formation.

0-60 min	1 hr before	24 hr training	no RA
0-60 min			RA
0-60 min			no RA
0 min			RA
30-60 min			no RA
0 min			RA
30-60 min			no RA

hydroxytryptophamine (5HT) or serotonin. DBMC (Dimethoxy-
serotonin inhibitor.

Treatment and site   animals   task   trials

2.3 (Continued)

With serotonin antagonists or precursors, memory was less severely
after training when ECS was given. The serotonin treated animals
when it was given as long as 1 hour after training, more than a
a depletion of RNA following ECS occurred. In general, ECS
RNA. This suggested that brain serotonin, as well as RNA inter-
which, with such events as ECS, serve as a possible basis in

2.4 ESSMAN, 1967(b)

ECS   mice   conditioned
                                              avoidance
                                              response

5HTP 3.12 mg/kg i.p.

ECS 10mA - transcorneal
    20mA

Inhibition of tryptophan hydroxylation by
P-Chlorophenylalanine
DBMC

no ECS
5HTP 25-100 mg/kg

2.5 ESSMAN, 1968(a)

ECS plus   mice   step-through   1
DBMC 4.5 mg/kg i.p.   FS PA

ECS

time of treatment		test	retention
ECS	Other		

disrupted and disruption was less obvious as a function of time
showed highly impaired retention from post-training ECS, even
doubling of the whole brain concentration of 5HT after ECS; and
produced an elevation in brain serotonin and a lowering of brain
dependency, may serve as a basis for the biochemical alteration
accounting for the amnesic effect produced.

within 30 min		24 hr	100% RA
60 min	60 min before conditioning		80% RA

10 minutes after ECS, brain serotonin levels were 42% above
controls.

			12% RA
			34% RA

28% elevation of brain 5HT

			30% RA
			25% RA

20% elevation of brain 5HT following ECS

			100% RA with 100 mg/kg

32% elevation of brain 5HT. The data, in general, suggest a
functional role for brain serotonin metabolism in memory
consolidation.

within	1 hr	24 hrs	reduced RA
5 sec	before		no RA
30-60 sec	conditioning		complete RA
5 sec			no RA
30-60 min			

Treatment and site   animals   task   trials

2.5   (Continued)

Brain RNA and serotonin concentrations were negatively correlated
animals showed a longer brain serotonin turnover time. With ECS
over rate was increased. The results support the hypothesis that
shock and the rate of memory consolidation are significantly
at 10 or 60 minutes following ECS.

2.6 ESSMAN, 1968(b)

ECS plus   mice   step-through   1
amitriptyline   FS   PA
-antidepressant

nialamide
-MAO inhibitor

pipradol
- stimulant of
5HT synthesis

saline

The drugs alone with no ECS did not affect responses. ECS increases
of the amnesic effect of ECS is apparently accomplished by providing
blocked and there is no elevation of serotonin levels.

2.7 ESSMAN, STEINBERG AND GOLOD, 1968

ECS   mice   step-through
                                                  FS
                                                  PA
ECS plus
nicotine
1.00 mg/kg i.p.

ECS plus
nicotine

The hypothesis was that a change in brain serotonin resulting from
the brain serotonin alteration produced by ECS. In saline treated
nicotine treated animals - serotonin levels were decreased by 6% in
were decreased by 8%.

time of treatment		test	retention
ECS	Other		

in DBMC(a specific serotonin antagonist) treated mice and these
brain serotonin concentration was slightly elevated and turn-
the central changes in serotonin and RNA resulting from electro-
affected by DBMC. No differences were observable in MAO activity

10 sec	1 hr before ECS	24 hr	38% RA
10 sec			31% RA
10 sec			52% RA
10 sec			80% RA

brain serotonin levels and this may account for RA. Antagonism
for conditions wherein this ECS-induced serotonin change is

10 sec		24 hr	RA
	15 and 30 min before training		less RA
	45 and 60 min before training		even less RA
10 sec	every 24 hr for 3 days	24 hr	less RA than saline(=60 min above)

nicotine treatment could impose rate-limiting conditions upon
animals - ECS elevated brain serotonin levels by 12%, in
1 hour and in ECS and nicotine treated animals serotonin levels

Treatment and site   animals   task   trials

2.7 (Continued)

While the relationship between ECS induced elevation in whole brain
observation that attenuation of the amnesic effects of ECS and
nicotine treatment does lend support to the argument that those
attending cerebral electroshock also minimize its amnesic affect.

2.8 ESSMAN AND GOLOD, 1968

ECS transcorneal   mice   step-through   1
10mA   FS
20mA

Tricyanoaminopropene (TCAP)
20mg/kp i.p.
plus ECS 10mA
        20mA

TCAP 40 mg/kg i.p. plus
ECS 10mA
    20mA

RA was markedly attenuated in TCAP treated animals. Analysis of
mice, suggesting the possibility that TCAP-induced acceleration of
effects of electroshock which account for retrograde amnesia.

2.9 BIVENS AND RAY, 1967.

ECS 10   rats   step-down   10
1/day   FS   1/day
strychnine SO4

low dose 0.16 mg/kg

high dose 0.33 mg/kg

Strychnine seems to facilitate learning by accelerating the
ECS.

2.10 KOPP, BOHDANECKY AND JARVIK, 1967

ECS plus   mice   step-through   1
scopolamine
ECS

Scopolamine increased the latency of step-through performance at
dose depressed the temporal gradient of RA to ECS. It was concluded
is increased or that the rate of memory consolidation is susceptible

---

time of treatment		test	retention
ECS	Other		

serotonin level and ECS-induced RA is not necessarily causal, the
reversal of serotonin accompanying ECS, as brought about by
conditions that prevent at least one of the neurochemical changes

ECS	Other	test	retention
immediate		24 hr	RA more RA
immediate	every 24 hr for 3 days	24 hr	no RA no RA
immediate	every 24 hr for 3 days	24 hr	no RA slight RA

brain tissue revealed a slight elevation in RNA for TCAP-treated
brain RNA synthesis may be one factor which reduces the central

---

ECS	Other	test	retention
15 sec	15 min before learning trial	24 hr	facilitation
30 sec			RA
30 sec			no RA

consolidation process and it reduces the disruptive effect on

ECS	Other	test	retention
10-160 sec	20 min before ECS	24 hr	RA
10-80sec	-		RA
160sec			no RA

0.5 and 1.0 mg/kg; whereas 0.1mg/kg had no effect. The latter
that either the disrupting effect of ECS on memory consolidation
to drug action.

Treatment and site	animals	task	trials

2.11 ADAMS, HOBLIT AND SUTKER, 1969

ECS 4	rats		

ECS 3		step-through FS	20

eserine (anticholinesterase)

scopolamine (anticholinergic)

ECS increases brain AChE activity levels as well as causing a
ACh but in a different manner than ECS, results in an increase
Scopolamine, which decreases ACh levels, partially eliminates the

2.12 DAVIS, THOMAS AND ADAMS, 1971

ECS	rats	step-through FS	1
ECS plus PS 0.3 mg/kg SCOP 1.0 mg/kg			
ECS plus PS SCOP			
no ECS PS SCOP			
no ECS PS SCOP			

The results suggested that physostigmine (PS) prior to the learning
protected memory from the normally disruptive effects of ECS. In
physostigmine alone before the retention trial had a disruptive

---

2.13 MUSACHIO, JUNLOU, KETY AND GLOWINSKY, 1969

ECS 2/day for 1 week	rats		

---

time of treatment		test	retention
ECS	Other		

ECS caused increases in AChE levels which return to pre-ECS levels within 96 hours.

time of treatment		test	retention
within 30 min		4 hr	RA
within 30 min of training	30 min before retention		more RA
			no RA

release of bound ACh. Eserine, which results in an increase in that is similar to ECS, at least on a short term basis. effects of ECS.

time of treatment		test	retention
immediate		4 hr	RA
immediate	30 min before learning trial		no RA RA
immediate	30 min before retention trial		RA no RA
	30 min before learning trial		no RA RA
	30 min before retention trial		RA no RA

trial or scopolamine (SCOP) prior to the retention trial addition, scopolamine alone before the learning trial or effect on retention.

There was an increased turnover of norepinephrine coupled with an increased concentration of tyrosine hydroxylase, the enzyme that appears to be rate limiting in norepinephrine synthesis. Results showed an increase in activity in brain stem (24%) and cortex (20%).

Treatment and site	animals	task	trials

2.14 STEIN AND BRINK, 1969

ECS	rats	step-down	1
Mg pemoline		FS	
		PA	

High dose of Mg pemoline, not followed by ECS disrupted performance
ECS-produced neural suppression by maintaining ongoing nervous

ECS alone
$Mg(OH)_2$ + ECS

The action of Mg pemoline suggests an interaction between Mg and

pemoline + ECS

The mechanism by which Mg pemoline facilitates learning is not yet
acts as a mild stimulant.

2.15 BUCKHOLTZ AND BOWMAN, 1970

ECS transcorneal	mice	step-through	1
12 or 20mA; 200msec		FS (varied-	
plus TCAP		1.2mA; 800msec;	
20 mg/kg i.p.		3mA; 2sec;	
		0.6mA; 500msec)	

In this study TCAP had no effect at any point along the RA gradient
not alter the whole brain content of RNA nor the uptake of H^3-
conditions TCAP does not affect retrograde amnesia produced by ECS,
memory consolidation.

---

time of treatment		test	retention
ECS	Other		
immediate	30 min before ECS	24 hr	no RA

but not retention, the results suggest that pemoline retards
activity at a level sufficient for storage to occur.

		24 hr	RA
		24 hr	RA
		10 days	RA

pemoline as by themselves they do not protect against RA.

		24 hr	RA
		10 days	RA

clear, it has been suggested that it increases RNA synthesis and

---

9-11 sec	once daily	24 hr	RA
15 sec	for 3 days 60-90 min before training on day 3		equal to saline controls and nearly complete
15,30 60 sec	as above	24 hr	linear gradient of RA not affected by TCAP
0.25 min 1-16 min		24 hr	RA partial RA
0.25-16 min	as above	24 hr	no difference between ECS and ECS + TCAP

when ECS was given at 9-960 sec after training. TCAP also did
cytidine into RNA. It was concluded that under a variety of
thus suggesting that it has no general effect on the rate of

Treatment and site	animals	task	trials

2.16 OTT AND MATTHIES, 1971

ECS	rats	optical discrimination	

ECS plus orotic acid
100 mg/kg i.p. (single dose)

ECS plus 4 injections of
orotic acid 100 mg/kg i.p.

There was also a prolongation of extinction after orotic acid. An
of orotic acid leads to an improved consolidation of memory,
metabolism.

2.17 RIEGE, 1971

transcorneal ECS	rats	step-down FS	1

p-Chlorophenylalanine
200 mg/kg i.p. (2 injections)

Two injections of the serotonin-depleting drug p-Chlorophenylalanine
but not those of norepinephrine. The same drug treatment protected
ECS.

2.18 LEWIS AND BREGMAN, 1972

transpinnate ECS	rats	step-down PA	1 (3 pre-training)

ECS plus
prostigmine 0.04 mg/kg i.p.
physostigmine 0.5 mg/kg
scopolamine 1.0 mg/kg

The ECS induced RA was not affected by any drug at any interval.
or scopolamine described effects when animals were tested 30 min to
on current behaviour or memory recall, not on memory formation.
given 24 hours after learning which is not in accord with Weiner &

---

time of treatment		test	retention
ECS	Other		
2 hr or less		24 hr	RA
2 hr or less	10 min before training	24 hr	RA
2 hr or less	over 4 days before training	24 hr	no RA

explanation of these findings may be that repeated administration
possibly via some changes in the central nucleotide and/or RNA

---

within 30 sec		1 hr, 1 or 4 days	RA
within 30	2 days and 3 hr before training	1 hr, 1 or 4 days	no RA

decreased the regional brain concentrations of serotonin by 60%
the performance of an avoidance task from the amnesic effect of

---

immediate	-	24 hr after drug injection	RA
	1hr,1 or 7 days		RA
	1hr,1 or 7 days		RA
	1hr, 1 or 7 days		RA

Previous reports of modification of ECS amnesia by physostigmine
4 hours after drug injection. They therefore reflect drug actions
The only drug to have amnesic action by itself was physostigmine
Deutsch, 1968 (3.9).

Treatment and site	animals	task	trials

2.19 MILLER AND SPRINGER, 1972

ECS	rats	step-through	1

ECS plus strychnine sulphate
i.p. 2.0 mg/kg

In this situation strychnine did not attenuate amnesia, this

---

time of treatment		test	retention
ECS	Other		
immediate		24 hr	RA
15 sec			less RA
15 sec	1 min after ECS	24 hr	less RA

observation is supported by the flat dose-response curve.

Treatment and site	animals	task	trials

3.1 PAZZAGLI AND PEPEU, 1964

Treatment and site	animals	task	trials
Scopolamine hydrobromide i.p. 0.5mg/kg	rats	maze- 3 double choices	3
		overtrained	9
i.p. 10mg/kg		overtrained	9
			3

The intensity of the amnesic effect was proportional to the decrease
scopolamine on performance is maximal at 90 minutes. After 3 hours
closely parallels the effect on behaviour with a maximum at 90
and amphetamine antagonized the effects of scopolamine on the
of brain ACh while amphetamine blocks only the amnesic effect.

3.2 MEYERS, 1965

Treatment and site	animals	task	trials
Scopolamine (subcutaneous) methscopolamine	rats	platform descents	
scopolamine			no. over 10 days
methscopolamine			

The effect of scopolamine was not due to dissociation of learning
can produce response disinhibition. Since methscopolamine was
the central nervous system.

3.3 DEUTSCH, HAMBURG AND DAHL, 1966

Treatment and site	animals	task	trials
DFP (diisopropyl-fluorophosphate) hippocampal injection 40mg	rats	discrimination Y-maze escape	no. to 10/10
NOTE injections made under nembutal anaesthesia			

Controls showed that this result was not due to normal forgetting.
differentially susceptible to disruption.

time of treatment		test	retention
Before	After		
	x	50 min	RA
	x	50 min	no RA
	x	50-120 min	RA
	x	120-240 min	RA

of brain ACh. There was a decrease in ACh.   The effect of
the rats perform almost normally. The effect on brain ACh
minutes; 3 hours after injection the content is normal. Eserine
behaviour but they differ since eserine also blocks the decrease

---

25 min		30 min	impaired acquisition no effect on acquisition
	9 days	10 days	RA
			no RA

nor to tolerance. These results seem to suggest that scopolamine
without effect, it was concluded that the site of action is in

---

	30 min	24 hr	RA
		2 days	partial RA
		5 days	no RA
	0 min	24 hr	RA
	3 days	24 hr	no RA
	5 days	24 hr	some RA
	14 days	24 hr	RA

The memory process may have two biochemical phases which are

Treatment and site	animals	task	trials

3.4 DEUTSCH, 1966

DFP hippocampal injection	rats	discrimination Y-maze overlearned	45
		less well learned	25

Larger quantities of ACh are produced with over-learned habits,

puromycin

The same dip in retention at 3 days as seen with DFP; this suggested

3.5 DEUTSCH AND LEIBOWITZ, 1966

DFP hippocampal injection	rats	Y-maze discrimination escape	to 10/10 (45-50)

control (peanut oil)

30
45-50
45-50

Controls were injected with peanut oil. At 28 days, an otherwise
Whereas at 14 days, DFP caused amnesia for an otherwise well
reversal of the change in synaptic conductance which occurs on

3.6 DEUTSCH AND LUTEKY, 1967

DFP hippocampal injection	rats	Y-maze discrimination (more difficult)	30 70 110

The greater the number of original trials the greater the degree of
with this drug. There was more facilitation by DFP in animals which
more within each group.

time of treatment		test	retention
Before	After		
	14 days	24 hr	more RA
			less RA

therefore an anti-cholinesterase will have a greater effect.

	5 days	24 hr	RA
	3 days		no or very little RA
	30 min		RA

that puromycin is affecting the ACh-CHE balance.

	14 days	24 hr	RA
	28 days	24 hr	no RA
	14 days	24 hr	remembered
	28 days	24 hr	forgotten
	14 days	24 hr	no RA
	14 days	24 hr	RA
	14 days	5 days	slight RA

forgotten habit becomes well remembered with an injection of DFP.
remembered habit. It was suggested that forgetting lies in a
learning.

	5 days	24 hr	enhanced recall
			no RA
			slight RA

forgetting with DFP and the smaller the enhancement of recall
had learned less, and more impairment in those who had learned

Treatment and site   animals   task   trials

3.7 DEUTSCH AND ROCKLIN, 1967

scopolamine   rats   Y-maze   45-50
hippocampal   discrimination
injection   escape

An anti-cholinergic drug would block synapses where the ACh
by learning, seem to vary, even without further learning, simply

3.8 HAMBURG, 1967

physostigmine   rats   Y-maze   no.
i.p. injection   discrimination

3.9 WIENER AND DEUTSCH, 1968

DFP   Y-maze   30-36
hippocampal   discrimination
injection   appetitive

peanut oil

scopolamine

The authors concluded that the physiological basis of forgetting is

3.10 DEUTSCH, 1969

physostigmine   Y-maze, trials
                                         during retest- spaced:
                                                        massed:

(ROCKLIN AND DEUTSCH - UNPUBLISHED)   Y-maze
                                         reversal:
                                         massed trials
                                         spaced trials

time of treatment		test	retention
Before	After		

	30 min	24 hr	RA

	1 day		more RA
	3 days		RA
	7 days		no RA
	14 days		no RA

concentration is low. Changes in conductance, once initiated
as a function of time.

	30 min	30 min	slight RA
	1-3 days	30 min	no RA
	5-7 days	30 min	RA max
	14 days	30 min	RA max

	30 min	21 hr	no RA
	1 day		no RA
	3 days		no RA
	7 days		RA
	14 days		no RA
	21 days		no RA
	1-7 days		no forgetting
	18-21 days		less retention
	30 min		no RA
	1-3 days		RA
	7-14 days		no RA
	18 days		partial RA

a decrease in synaptic conductance.

- no RA
- RA

acquisition
- easier
- harder

Treatment and site   animals   task   trials

3.10 (Continued)

Reversal was easier when there is no memory of the original habit.

(LEIBOWITZ DOCTORAL THESIS)   task   constant
DFP   difficulty
                                             varied:
                                             easy task
                                             difficult task

In controls the easier the task was learnt better than the
suggested that the conductance in a set of synapses increased with

3.11 HUPPERT AND DEUTSCH, 1969

                                 rats   Y-maze
                                             escape

                                             undertrained

These results parallel those previously found for the differential
They provide further evidence that memory strength increases with

3.12 DEUTSCH AND WIENER, 1969

physostigmine   rats   appetitive
i.p. injection   maze habit
                                             extinction (E.)
                                             after learning
                                             E. 3 days
                                             E. 6 days

                                             reversal
                                             training
                                             E. 3 days
                                             E. 6 days

If extinction is a separate habit it should be possible to leave it
original habit is unavailable. A rat in this condition should
habit on retest than pre-injected control rats, or rats extinguished
both memory of original learning and of extinction should be blocked.
opposes the performance of the initially rewarded habit. The
ing stimuli.

time of treatment   test   retention
Before   After

RA
strong facilitation

difficult task at the end of the same number of trials. It was
degree of training.

30 min-
5 days   poor retention

7-10 days   better retention

14-17 days   decrement in
                        retention

susceptibility of cholinergic drugs on habits of different age.
time up to a point, and then gradually decreases.

7 days

RA
less RA

no RA
RA

intact, so that it should be remembered on retest while the
therefore find it much more difficult to relearn the original
soon after learning. In rats extinguished soon after learning,
Therefore during extinction a separate habit is learned which
opposing habit is probably an aversion to the initially reward-

Treatment and site	animals	task	trials

3.13 WIENER, 1970

ECS multiple treatments	rats	Y-maze discrimination	no.

Facilitation of relearning was found with both single or multiple
multiple ECS treatments, not single ECS.
physostigmine
0.5mg/kg i.p.
plus single ECS

scopolamine
1.0 mg/kg i.p.
plus single ECS

The effects of ECS were potentiated by physostigmine 5 minutes after
31 days after learning. It was suggested that ECS interferes with
eliminated by scopolamine and potentiated by physostigmine.

3.14 WIENER & MESSER, 1972

hemicholinium 0.4 mg/rat hippocampal injection	rats	step-through passive avoidance	not clear unless rat remained in lighted compartment 120 sec

The drug has no effect at 6 hours after training,or at 3 or 7 days,
action is compatible with probable time course of inhibition of ACh

---

3.15 BOHDANECKY AND JARVIK, 1967

d-amphetamine intraperitoneal	mice	step-through passive avoidance	1
physostigmine intraperitoneal			

| time of treatment | | test | retention |
Before	After		
	5 min	24 hr	RA
	30 min		RA
	1 day		no RA
	3 days		no RA
	5 days		no RA
	7 days		RA
	14 days		RA
	31 days		facilitation of relearning

ECS treatments, whereas the other data was found only with

| time of treatment | | test | retention |
Before	After		
30 min before testing	5 min	24 hr	more RA
30 min before testing	14 days	24 hr	no RA
	31 days		no RA

learning. Scopolamine eliminated effects of a single ECS 14 and performance by elevating ACh levels as the ECS effects were

| time of treatment | | test | retention |
Before	After		
	immediate	6 hr	no RA
		18 hr	RA
		24 hr	RA
		30 hr	RA
		48 hr	RA
		3 days	no RA
		7 days	no RA

apparent amnesia at intervening times. The time course of synthesis. There were no biochemical controls.

| time of treatment | | test | retention |
Before	After		
20 min		24 hr	no facilitation seen, impaired performance
8 min		24 hr	impaired performance

Treatment and site   animals   task   trials

3.15   (Continued)

Animals taught under saline and tested under amphetamine showed
sensitive to cholinergic than to adrenergic disturbance. No
and tested under drugged states.

3.16   DILTS AND BERRY,   1967

(injections   mice   step-down   1
subcutaneous)   passive
                                         avoidance

scopolamine hydrobromide 0.03 - 10.0 mg/kg

scopolamine methyl bromide 0.1-10.0 mg/kg

atropine sulphate 0.3-30.0 mg/kg

atropine methyl bromide 0.3-30.0 mg/kg

physostigmine salicylate 0.003-0.3 mg/kg

neostigmine methyl sulphate 0.1-0.3 mg/kg

mecamylamine hydrochloride 0.1-10.0 mg/kg

hexamethonium bromide 0.3-30.0 mg/kg

Negative results were obtained with corresponding quarternary drug
cross the blood-brain barrier. This indicates that the peripheral
the test results.

scopolamine
atropine
physostigmine
mecamylamine

It was thought unlikely that dissociation played an important role
found no evidence of a state-dependent passive avoidance learning

---

time of treatment		test	retention
Before	After		

impairment just during testing. Passive avoidance test is more
'dissociation' of learning was seen when animals were taught

---

30 min		24 hr	RA
30 min			no RA
30 min			RA
30 min			no RA
20 min			RA
20 min			no RA
60 min			RA
20 min			no RA

derivatives which are just as potent peripherally but do not
effects of the drugs examined do not contribute materially to

	immediate	24 hr	no RA
	immediate		no RA
	immediate		no RA
	immediate		no RA

in these experiments but Meyers (3.2) and Stark (3.17) have
using doses comparable to those used here.

Treatment and site	animals	task	trials

3.17 STARK, 1967

scopolamine i.p.   mice   step-down
<u>trained</u>   <u>tested</u>   passive
scop   saline   avoidance   1/day
                                                         for 2 days

saline   scop

scop   scop

saline   saline

Analysis of data did not reveal evidence of state dependent learn-
the drug on day 1 were impaired in the acquisition of the response.

3.18 EVANS AND PATTON, 1968

scopolamine
i.p. injection 1 mg/kg   rats   fear   1
                                           conditioning
                                           tone + FS
<u>train</u>   <u>test</u>   paired
saline saline
saline scop
scop   saline
scop   scop

Fear conditioning under scopolamine reduces lick response rates
under scopolamine is state dependent and that retention tests take
absence of a drug.

3.19 SLATER, 1968

triethylcholine   rats   multiple T   no.
-intraventricular   maze - FS
                                           for incorrect
hemicholinium-3   choice

N-(4 diethyl
amino-2-butynyl)-
succinimide

These drugs reduce brain ACh content by 64%. Scopolamine produces
correlation between score in the maze and the reduction of brain
amnesic effects of atropine and scopolamine are due to reduced

time of treatment		test	retention
Before	After		

30 min training and/or testing		24 hr	impaired acquisition no RA no RA
			impaired acquisition no RA
			no RA

ing, rather it provided evidence that all mice which received

30 min		2 days	
			good retention good retention RA no RA

under scopolamine but not otherwise. Suggest that learning account of altered stimulus conditions when testing in the

---

	immediate	5 min	no RA
		30 min	no RA
	immediate	30 min	no RA
	immediate	30 min	no RA

amnesia under the conditions of this experiment. There was no ACh-levels. This tends to rule out the possibility that the levels of brain ACh.

Treatment and site   animals   task   trials

3.20 BERGER AND STEIN, 1969

drug or saline (i.p.)   rats   drinking tube   1
                                           FS and CS
Train   Test   paired
scop   saline   fear conditioning
scop   scop
saline   saline
saline   scop

This result was attributed to dissociation of learning and a drug
scopolamine-saline sub-group.

scop.   saline
methyl
nitrate

CPZ   saline

The negative results with methyl scopolamine suggests that
by blockade of central cholinergic synapses. The negative results
important role than cholinergic ones in fear conditioning.

3.21 SUITS AND ISAACSON, 1969

scopolamine   rats   step-through   2
intraperitoneal   passive
                                           avoidance

These results cannot be readily attributed to dissociation effects

---

time of treatment		test	retention
Before	After		
30 min training and/or testing		3 days	
			RA
			no RA
			no RA
			no RA

induced impairment of learning which act in concert only in the

			no RA
			no RA

scopolamine impairs the acquisition of conditioned suppression
with chlorpromazine suggest that adrenergic synapses play a less

---

Before	After	test	retention
30 min		30 min	no RA
	x	30 min	no RA
30 min		48 hr	RA
	x	48 hr	less RA
30 min		48 hr under scop	no RA
	x	48 hr under scop	no RA

alone.

Treatment and site	animals	task	trials

3.22 WARBURTON, 1969

Treatment and site	animals	task	trials
neostigmine 0.0125-0.05 mg/kg i.p.	rats	spontaneous activity skinner box alternation schedule	480 trials /day
atropine 20-60 ug intraventricular			
physostigmine 0.1-0.5 mg/kg i.p.			
physostigmine 2.1-7 ug intraventricular			

Atropine had a slight effect on maintenance of response, the other
and more so by atropine; extinction similarly affected. Both
physostigmine which increases available acetylcholine by inhibition
investigated here. Opposite pharmacological actions may both
peripheral cholinergic systems had no measurable effect.
included and showed inhibition of AChE activity.

3.23 RUSSELL, WARBURTON, VASQUEZ, OVERSTREET AND DALGLISH, 1971

Treatment and site	animals	task	trials
DFP injection in peanut oil 1.0 mg/kg followed by 0.5 mg/kg every 3rd day	albino rats	spatial (water maze)	10
		skinner box appetitive	1 hr test session
		PA of FS	10
		discriminated avoidance	2 hr acquisition

time of treatment	test	retention
Before After		
Before daily training sessions (time not specified)	daily	no RA
		RA acquisition delayed ·
		no RA acquisition delayed
		no RA acquisition delayed

drugs had no effect. Acquisition was delayed by physostigmine
atropine which blocks muscarinic cholinergic receptor sites and
of anti-cholinesterase have similar actions on the behaviour
result in synaptic blockade. Atropine or neostigmine acting on
Biochemical controls for central effects of physostigmine were

DFP injection every 3rd day	24 hr	no effects
	240 hr	at any time
	528 hr	of injection
	24 hr	RA total correct + total trials lower
	240 hr	RA intertrial responses increased
	528 hr	no RA
	24 hr	no effects,no errors
	240 hr	
	528 hr	
	24 hr	deficit
	240 hr	increase in response latency
	528 hr	normal

Treatment and site   animals   task   trials

3.23 (Continued)

The effect of this treatment is to lower brain AChE levels to about
some measures of appetitive and discriminated avoidance learning were
effect is on performance in general as it occurs regardless of
to peripheral action of DFP. Recovery occurs even though brain

---

3.24 SQUIRE, 1970

physostigmine   mice   T-maze   no. to 3/4
i.p. 0.4 mg/kg   spatial
15 min before   discrimination
retention   FS intensity
                                        0.4mA

The controls had forgotten at 14 days.

3.25 SQUIRE, GLICK AND GOLDFARB, 1971

saline i.p.   mice   T-maze   no.(3-12)
                                        spatial
                                        discrimination
                                        FS intensity
                                        0.5mA

physostigmine
0.4 mg/kg
15 min before
retest

A dose dependent effect found with 0.1, 0.2 and 0.4 mg/kg

methscopolamine
0.6 mg/kg
and physostigmine
0.4 mg/kg
15 min before
retest

Methscopolamine antagonized both the impairment by physostigmine
after training.

physostigmine
0.4 mg/kg plus
methscopolamine 0.05-0.6 mg/kg or
scopolamine 0.05-0.6 mg/kg

time of treatment		test	retention
Before	After		

¼ of normal, but also affects peripheral AChE. Deficits in
seen at 24 hours but there is recovery later on. Suggest major
nature of learning or reinforcement and therefore may be due
AChE levels remain depressed.

---

30 min	45 min	no RA
1 day	1 day	no RA
3 days	3 days	no RA
7 days	7 days	RA
14 days	14 days	no RA

1 day	1 day	normal
7 days	7 days	normal
14 days	14 days	forgotten
1 day	1 day	RA
7 days	7 days	no RA
14 days	14 days	no RA

physostigmine 1 day after training.

1 day	1 day	no RA
7 days	7 days	no RA

1 day after training and facilitation by physostigmine 7 days

1 day	1 day	no RA
1 day	1 day	no RA

Treatment and site   animals   task   trials

3.25   (Continued)

Dose dependent effects for both drugs were observed. At the
of physostigmine.

methscopolamine 0.6 mg/kg

scopolamine 0.6 mg/kg

neostigmine 0.33 mg/kg

With physostigmine 1 day after training relearning was impaired and
observed depend on specific conditions of training (footshock) and
likely to be entirely peripheral since neostigmine did not show these
either since methscopolamine, a peripherally acting muscarinic block-
scopolamine were equipotent, it is not likely that the methscopolamine
centrally than methscopolamine. Therefore, methscopolamine antagonized
peripheral action. So physostigmine acts both centrally and peripherally.

3.26 GLICK AND ZIMMERBERG, 1971

Scopolamine   mice   step-through   1
1-20 mg/kg i.p.   passive
                                              avoidance

phencyclidine
1-20 mg/kg i.p.

ketamine
1-40 mg/kg i.p.

scopolamine
10 mg/kg i.p.

Even with scopolamine the median latency to step-through on retest is
scopolamine alone without FS not given (Human premedication dose of

3.27 GLICK AND ZIMMERBERG, 1972

Scopolamine 10 mg/kg   mice   step-through   1
                                              passive
methyl scopolamine 10 mg/kg   avoidance

physostigmine 1 mg/kg
plus scopolamine
(route of administration not specified each
time but probably i.p.)

time of treatment		test	retention
Before	After		

highest dose both drugs fully antagonized the disruptive effect

1 day	1 day		no RA
7 days	7 days		no RA
1 day	1 day		no RA
7 days	7 days		RA
1 day	1 day		no RA

7 and 14 days after relearning was facilitated. Thus the effects
are not fixed (cf. 3.24). The effects of physostigmine are not
effects with an equimolar dose. They are not entirely central
ing agent antagonized them. Because methscopolamine and
effects were due to central action. Scopolamine is more effective
the behavioural effects of physostigmine by opposing its

12 min		24 hr	RA
	immediate		RA
12 min		24 hr	RA
	immediate		no RA
12 min		24 hr	RA
	immediate		no RA
	immediate	24 hr	RA
	1 hr		RA
	6 hr		no RA

still 300 sec and training latencies were not given. Effect of
hyoscine (scopolamine) is 0.5 mg for 70 kg man.)

15 min		24 hr	RA
	immediate		RA
	immediate		no RA

Physostigmine whether
given before or after
training reduced amnesic
effect of scopolamine

Treatment and site   animals   task ·   trials

3.27 (Continued)

Scopolamine has similar amnesic effect when administered prior to
or 7 days after learning.

3.28 SCHNEIDER, KAPP AND SHERMAN, 1970

Treatment and site	animals	task	trials
saline i.p.	rats	step-down passive avoidance	1
atropine sulphate		step-down	1

This anticholinergic drug with peripheral and central actions

Physostigmine		step-down	1

This anticholinesterase drug decreased test latencies at 15 and 120
acquisition.

atropine methylate

This anticholinergic drug with peripheral action only increased

neostigmine

This anticholinesterase drug had no effect on step-down latencies.
due to the synaptic blocking action of high levels of stress-
to give longer step-down latencies. Because (a) atropine, decreas-
(b) physostigmine, increasing ACh levels, reduced step-down
on performance. Physostigmine is not acting peripherally, but

---

time of treatment   test   retention
Before   After

learning, at various levels of FS and when memory tested 1,2

		SDL-
10-20 min	5 sec	3.1 sec
	15 sec	9.6 sec
	120 sec	12.7 sec
10-20 min	5 sec	12.1 sec *
	15 sec	9.8 sec
	120 sec	8.1 sec

increased step-down latencies at 5 seconds.

10-20 min	5 sec	3.2 sec
	15 sec	4.7 sec *
	120 sec	4.3 sec *
	24 hr	12.8 sec

seconds. No effect at 24 hours, therefore it is not affecting

5 sec	8.2 sec *
15 sec	7.6 sec
120 sec	13.2 sec

test latencies at 5 seconds.

5 sec	4.5
15 sec	7.9
120 sec	9.4

With saline, the short step-down latencies are throught to be
induced ACh that subsequently decrease, releasing the blockage
ing ACh levels, increased step-down latencies at 5 seconds;
latencies at 15 and 120 seconds. The atropine effect could be
could effect performance-related processes producing disinhibition.

Treatment and site   animals   task   trials

3.29 GOLDBERG, SLEDGE, HEFNER AND ROBICHAUD, 1971

scopolamine   mice and   spout
6.25-40 mg/kg i.p.   rats   activity

Mecamylamine   active   15
6.25-40 mg/kg i.p.   avoidance
                                          FS
                                          passive   1
                                          dark
                                          avoidance
                                          FS

4(1-naphthyl vinyl)   conditioned   1
pyridine (NVP) i.p.   fear FS
up to 200 mg/kg   suppression
                                          of eating

Mecamylamine and NVP depress spontaneous activity. Scopolamine had
avoidance to all drugs but it is argued that the effect is more
activity. Since only scopolamine affects conditioned fear they argue
involved in avoidance but only muscarinicreceptors in fear. The data
ities but it is not clear what aspects of the drugs action are

---

3.30 KRAL, 1971

Scopolamine   rats   taste   1
1 mg/kg i.p.   aversion
                                          LiCl 0.4M
                                          given 30
                                          min after
                                          sweet water

Scopolamine injection 5 minutes asfter a learning experience acts

---

| time of treatment | | test | retention |
Before	After		
			active avoidance impaired by all drugs with NVP the least effective
30 min or 1 to 2 hr before learning		acquisition impairment	
			passive avoidance impaired with a dose 7 times greater than active avoidance
			conditioned fear impaired by scopolamine

little effect. Active avoidance was more susceptible than passive
pronounced than would be expected from effects on spontaneous
that both muscarinic and nicotinic cholinergic receptors are
do show that the 3 kinds of learning show different susceptib-
responsible.

---

5 min after drinking 25 min before aversant		72 hr	scopolamine as effective an aversant as LiCl

as a UCS to inhibit recent behaviour.

Treatment and site	animals	task	trials

3.31 STAHL, ZELLER & BOSHES, 1971

| L-DOPA 10^{-5}-10^{-4}M in tank water | goldfish | shuttle box active avoidance | 30 min |

Pargyline 10^{-6}-10^{-5}M
in tank water

Biochemical estimation showed pargyline blocked the activity of
epinephrine and serotonin levels increased. L-DOPA increases
explained by effects on brain amines.

___

3.32 RANDT, QUARTERMAIN, GOLDSTEIN AND ANAGNOSTE, 1971

| DDC (diethyldithiocarbamate) 250 mg/kg subcutaneous | mice | step-through passive avoidance | 1 |

Biochemical controls show brain norepinephrine levels lowered and
DDC. DDC has been shown to improve retention 1 min after learning,
performance when injected 30 min prior to retest 24 hr after
expected by a reduction in spontaneous activity which is reduced by

___

3.33 DISMUKES AND RAKE, 1972

| Reserpine 2.5 mg/kg 1.5 mg/kg | mice | shuttle box active avoidance | 30 |

Reserpine (1.5 mg/kg) plus
DOPA (NE precursor)
5HTP (5HT precursor)
Amphetamine (releases NE and
            blocks re-uptake)

time of treatment Before After	test	retention
before and perhaps during learning time not specified	24 hr	acquisition enhanced no RA
	24 hr	RA
	48 hr	RA

monoamine oxidase after 24 hours exposure. Norepinephrine, norepinephrine levels. The behavioural results are not easily

---

30 min	1 min	better retention
	5 min	no RA
	1 hr	RA
	6 hr	RA
	24 hr	RA
immediate		RA
2 hr		no RA
30 min before retest		RA

synthesis stopped between 30 min and 4½ hours after injection of impair retention from 1 hr to 24 hr after learning and impair learning. This last effect is the opposite of that to be about 30%.

---

1 min	8 days	RA
24 hr		no RA
1 min		
1 min		no RA
1 min		RA
1 min		RA

Treatment and site   animals   task   trials

3.33   (Continued)

DOPA   mice   shuttle box   30
5HTP   active
Amphetamine   avoidance
p-Chlorophenylalanine (depresses
                    5HT levels)

Diethydithiocarbamic acid (DEDTC) (lowers NE without
                                affecting dopamine) (1400mg/kg)

Dichloroiso-proterenol(DCT) (blocker of β NE receptors) 75 mg/kg

Since reinforcement was apparently used in testing and the scoring
distinguish retention from relearning. The authors conclude that
the formation of long-term memory.

3.34   MADDEN AND GREENOUGH,   1972

Eserine 0.5 mg/kg   rats   Y-maze   up to 80
chlorpromazine 1.5 mg/kg   active
amphetamine 2.0 mg/kg   avoidance
intraperitoneal

Only one dose level used. No description of effect of drugs on
injection. The effects on maze performance were all small and
chlorpromazine at various times after learning (compare with

---

time of treatment		test	retention
Before	After		
	1 min	8 days	no RA
	1 min		no RA
	1 min		no RA
3 days			no RA
	1 min	8 days	RA
	24 hr		no RA
	1 min		RA
	24 hr		no RA

system does not reveal the original data it is not possible to
normal levels of one of the catecholamines are necessary for

	1,3,7 and 28 days	30 min after injection	retention very slightly improved (i.e. 8/10 correct vs 7/10 correct) after all drugs except amphetamine 28 days after learning

general activity at the time of testing which was 30 min after
there was no change in effectiveness of eserine or
4.47)

Treatment and site	animals	task	trials

4.1 RANSMEIER AND GERARD, 1954

ether or	hamsters	maze	no.
nembutal			
repeated treatments			

Neither nembutal nor ether anaesthesia, achieved by 1-2 min after

---

4.2 LEUKEL, 1957

thiopental	rats	14 unit	no.
intraperitoneal		water maze	

4.3 LEUKEL AND QUINTON, 1964

CO_2 exposure	rats	step-through	31
full anaesthesia		passive	1/day
60 sec		avoidance	

The CO_2 treatment impaired acquisition of the avoidance response acting as a negative reinforcer for the habit.

partial anaesthesia			
(10 sec)			31
full anaesthesia		extinction	31
		trials followed	
		by treatment	
partial			
anaesthesia			

Extinction trials,where negative reinforcement and interruption of indicated that the CO_2 treatment acted as a negative reinforcer.

time of treatment		test	retention
Before	After		
	1-2 min		no RA

learning interfered with memory.

| | 1 min | 30 days | acquisition was slowed, no RA |
| | 30 min after each daily trial | | no effect on acquisition, no RA |

| | 10 sec | 14-31 days | impaired acquisition |
| | 5,30,60 min after 1st 15 trials | | no impairment in acquisition |

either by interrupting the consolidation of the habit or by

	10 sec	14-31 days	inferior acquisition
	10 sec	14-31 days	extinction not impaired
			extinction not impaired

consolidation should lead to different consequences in behaviour,

Treatment and site	animals	task	trials

4.4 QUINTON, 1966

CO_2 inhalation 30%	rats	skinner box	1
50%		footshock	

duration-
2,7,15 min; 30% CO_2

2,7,15 min; 50% CO_2

4.5 PEARLMAN, SHARPLESS AND JARVIK, 1959

ether	rats	skinner box	1
inhalation		footshock	

pentobarbital
intravenous
pentylenetetrazol (PTZ)
intravenous

The results with ether and pentobarbital support the consolidation
qualitatively different.

4.6 ESSMAN AND JARVIK, 1960

ether	mice	step-down	1
inhalation		passive	
		avoidance	

Anaesthesia following electric shock (FS) diminishes, but does not

4.7 PEARLMAN, SHARPLESS AND JARVIK, 1961

ether exposure	rats	skinner box	1
(10 min)		footshock	
pentobarbital			1
intravenous			
PTZ (pentylenetetrazol)			1
intravenous			

time of treatment		test	retention
Before	After		
	10-30 sec		RA
			greater RA
			increasing RA - with increasing duration of anaesthesia
			same RA

---

	immediate	24 hr	RA
	5 min		RA
	10 min		no RA
	immediate- 5 min		less RA than ether
	10 min		no RA
	immediate- 8 hr		RA
	4 days		slight RA

hypothesis but the effects of pentylenetetrazol seem to be

	immediate	24 hr	partial RA

eliminate the inhibiting effect of the shock.

	0-5 min	24 hr	slight RA
	10 min		no RA
	0-10 min	24 hr	RA
	20 min		no RA
	0-8 hr	24 hr	complete RA
	4 days	5 days	partial RA

Treatment and site	animals	task	trials

4.7 (Continued)

The hypothesis was that the consolidation process is dependent on
markedly reduces this activity the authors proposed that this is
pentylenetetrazol seem to be qualitatively different to the effects

4.8 ABT, ESSMAN AND JARVIK, 1961

ether exposure	mice	step-down passive avoidance	1

4.9 ESSMAN AND JARVIK, 1961

diethyl ether exposure 36 sec	mice	step-down passive avoidance	1

Etherization one hour post-conditioning had no apparent effect on
of control subjects with no FS.

4.10 PEARLMAN, 1966

ether exposure 1 min	rats	step-down passive avoidance	1

4.11 BOHDANECKY, KOPP AND JARVIK, 1968

Flurothyl inhalation	mice	step-through (300 sec cut off)	1
ECS			1

Compared with ECS- flurothyl showed an effect longer after training
for the degree of amnesia.

4.12 ESSMAN, 1968

PTZ (pentylenetetrazol) intraperitoneal	mice	step-through passive avoidance	1

RA was associated with a reduction in RNA concentration of 4.5%

lidocaine and PTZ	mice		1

Lidocaine blocked the overt convulsion and there was no RNA

time of treatment		test	retention
Before	After		

electrical activity in the CNS. Since general anaesthesia
the means of disrupting consolidation. The effects of
of ether and pentobarbital.

0-20 min	24 hr	RA
24 hr	48 hr	no RA

5 sec	24 hr	RA
1 hr		no RA

the retention, and ether anaesthesia did not alter the response

1-10 min	21 hr	RA
15 min		no RA

0-1 hr	24 hr	marked RA
6 hr		slight RA
12 hr		no RA
0-1 hr	24 hr	RA
6-12 hr		no RA

than did ECS. The two curves run parallel and are similar except

0 min	24 hr	RA

0 min	24 hr	RA

reduction (only 0.4%).

Treatment and site	animals	task	trials

4.13   GLICK, NAKAMURA AND JARVIK,   1970

sham operation (skin incision plus wound clip) under ether	mice		
(sham-ether)		1	step-through passive
sham-no ether ether			avoidance
sham-ether sham- no ether ether			

Ether anaesthesia was obtained by placing mice in a beaker con-
this study indicate that stress, as induced by a sham operation
the memory of a recently learned event. Ether apparently
combination of the sham operation and ether will disrupt memory at

---

4.14   BUREŜ AND BUREŜOVÁ,   1963

ether anaesthesia exposure for 5 min	rats	step-through passive avoidance	1

4.15   OVERTON,   1964

pentobarbital intraperitoneal	rats	T-maze drug	no.
		no drug	
		drug	
		no drug	

State-dependent learning occurred. In both cases, performance of
condition present during training. The amount of transfer of
inversely proportional to the size of the drug dose used to establish

---

time of treatment		test	retention
Before	After		

	1 hr	24 hr	most RA
	1 hr		RA
	1 hr		no RA
	6 hr	24 hr	RA
	6 hr		no RA
	6 hr		no RA

taining volatile ethyl ether at 23°C for 45 sec. The results of
without anaesthia, is a potent enough stimulus to interfere with
potentiates the effect of this interference such that the
a time when the sham operation alone will not.

---

	1 min	24 hr	no RA

---

		24 hr	
15-45 min		no drug	RA
		drug	RA
		drug	no RA
		no drug	no RA

the response was dependent upon the reinstatement of the drug
training between non-drug and drug states was shown to be
the drug state.

| Treatment and site | animals | task | trials |

4.16 DOTY AND DOTY, 1964

Chlorpromazine (CPZ) intraperitoneal after each daily trial	30 day old rats	active avoidance	30
	120-365 day old rats		
	600 day old rats		

It was postulated that the interval required for memory to adults .

4.17 CHERKIN AND LEE-TENG, 1965

| halothane exposure to 3% for 5 min | chickens | inhibition of pecking | 1 |

4.18 CHERKIN, 1969

Flurothyl 0.43% v/v for 1-16 min	chickens	inhibition of pecking	1
0.85% v/v for 4,8 + 16 min			
1.7% v/v for 4,8 + 16 min			
3.0% v/v			

The longest intervals at which significant differences were observed was increased by increasing either the concentration of the flurothyl retard rather than block memory consolidation, so that post-treatment later and leads to variable consolidation gradients.

time of treatment		test	retention
Before	After		
	10 sec–1 hr	every 24 hr	RA
	2 hr		no RA
	10 sec		RA
	30 min 2 hr		no RA
	10 sec–2 hr		RA

consolidate is longer among immature and aged rats than in young

---

	1 min	4 or 18 hr	RA
	1.5 hr		no RA
		24 hr	
	4,64 min		no RA
	4 min		complete RA
	64 min		RA
	256 min		less RA
	1440 min		no RA
	4,64 min		complete RA
	256,1440 min		RA
	2880 min		no RA
	256 min		RA

depended on the flurothyl treatment parameters. The RA observed
or the duration of the exposure. Incomplete amnesic treatments
consolidation inflates the retention scores measured 24 hours

Treatment and site	animals	task	trials

4.19   CHERKIN,   1970

1.7% v/v flurothyl for 8 min	chickens	inhibition of pecking	1

Flurothyl had a nonspecific effect in the first 2 hours following pecking target i.e. no training.

flurothyl	chickens	inhibition of pecking	1

Retrograde amnesia induced with flurothyl persisted for at least 9 and did not diminish with increased treatment-training interval or consolidation hypothesis but not with a retrieval hypothesis.

4.20   CHERKIN,   1972

strong flurothyl treatment 1.7% v/v flurothyl vapour for 8 min	chickens	inhibition of pecking of lamp	1(MeA) on T_1 retention test: - visual R - visual and oral R (MeA/400)

Neither a visual reminder (R) (distilled water on lamp) nor an oral training with 100% MeA in chicks made amnesic by strong flurothyl

moderate flurothyl treatment 0.85% flurothyl vapour for 8 min			1(MeA) 2 hr after T_1: - no R-(dry lamp) - R-MeA/400 on lamp
moderate flurothyl			1 (MeA) 24 hr after T_1: R-MeA/400 on lamp

time of treatment		test	retention
Before	After		

	4 min	1 day	RA
		2 days	RA
		9 days	RA
	4 min	1 hr	no RA
		2 hr	some RA
		4,24 + 48 hr	complete RA

treatment in control chicks not given methylanthranilate on the

48 hr		4 or 24 hr	no RA
24 hr		4 or 24 hr	no RA
4 hr		4 or 24 hr	no RA
2 hr		4 or 24 hr	no RA

days. Anterograde amnesia did not parallel retrograde amnesia training-testing interval. The results are compatible with the

	4 min	(T_1) 24 hr	RA- 94%
		48 hr	RA
		48 hr	RA

reminder (diluted MeA on lamp) restored the memory of strong treatment.

	136 min	(T_1) 24 hr	RA- 63%
		48 hr	RA
		48 hr	weak reminder effect
	256 min	(T_1) 24 hr	RA- 61%
		48 hr	weak reminder effect

Treatment and site	animals	task	trials

4.20 (Continued)

moderate flurothyl treatment	chickens		1(MeA) 2 hr after T_1: -R-MeA/400 on bead - no R-dry bead

The weak, variable reminder effect was interpreted as reflecting
from partial consolidation of the original training and the second
this interpretation, restoration of learned performance by a
exceed the threshold for retrieval. The reminder effect supports
weak engram that confounds interpretation of RA experiments.

4.21 TABER AND BANUAZIZI, 1965

CO_2 inhalation	mice	step-through passive avoidance	1

Repeated exposures to CO_2 immediately after punished trials spaced
shown by controls.

4.22 TABER AND BANUZIZI, 1966

CO_2 exposure 10 sec	mice	step-through (180 sec cut off)	1

The "amnesic" effect was not the result of a debilitating effect

---

4.23 HERZ, PEEKE AND WYERS, 1966

ether inhalation 40 sec at $31^{\circ}C$ 70 sec at $31^{\circ}C$ 120 sec at $22^{\circ}C$	mice	step-through passive avoidance	1

ECS

time of treatment		test	retention
Before	After		

		(T$_1$) 24 hr	RA- 68%
	96 min		

		48 hr	RA
			more RA (N.S.)

the cumulation of two sub-threshold engrams, the first resulting
resulting from information input on the reminder treatment. By
reminder occurs when the two cumulated sub-threshold engrams
the argument that RA treatments are often incomplete and leave a

	up to		
	30 min	24 hr	RA

at 90 minute intervals prevented the sharp increase in latencies

	0-5 min	24 hr	RA complete
	15-30 min		less RA
	60-120 min		no RA

produced either by shock, anaesthesia or a combination of the two.

---

	immediate	22 hr	
			partial RA
			complete RA
			no RA
	10 sec	22 hr	complete RA

Treatment and site	animals	task	trials

4.24 HERZ, 1969

| diethyl ether exposure at 30–35°C | mice | chamber with cul-de-sac shock | 1 |
| | | appetitive learning | 1 |

4.25 BOVET, McGAUGH AND OLIVERIO, 1966

strychnine i.p.
    0.15–0.3mg/kg
    0.60 mg/kg
    0.30 mg/kg
picrotoxin
    0.30–0.60 mg/kg
    1.20 mg/kg
	mice	shuttle box active avoidance	100

PTZ 5.00–10.00mg/kg			
N$_2$O 50% anaesthesia			50 50 100

The authors concluded"it seems from these results that the influences
the day following the administration. If this was the case greater
It appears increasingly likely that the drugs directly influence

4.26 McGAUGH AND ALPERN, 1966

| ether exposure | mice | step-down passive avoidance | 1 |

4.27 ALPERN AND KIMBLE, 1967

| indoklon (flurothyl) -exposure (convulsant ether) | mice | step-through passive avoidance | 1 |

potentiated ether
exposure at 100°F

ether at room temp.75°F
The results indicate that the severity of treatment may extend the

---

| time of treatment | | test | retention |
Before	After		
	20 sec-15 min	22 hr	no RA
	20 sec	22 hr	slight RA
	15 min		no RA

---

	5 min	over 5 days	acquisition:
			-enhanced
			- no effect
	60 min		- no effect
	5 min		- facilitation
			- no effect
	5 min		- no effect
	5 min	24 hr	RA
	15 min		no RA
	5 min		no RA

of these drugs on memory are not due to performance effects on
effects would be expected in the delayed administration groups.
memory consolidation processes".

	0-25 sec	24 hr	no RA
	0-4 hr	24 hr	RA
	0-24 hr	24 hr	RA
	0-1 hr	24 hr	no RA

duration of the amnesic effect

Treatment and site	animals	task	trials

4.28 PAOLINO, QUARTERMAIN AND MILLER, 1966

CO_2 exposure 25 sec	rats	step-through passive avoidance	1

exposure 15 sec
exposure 10 sec

	mice		

ECS and CO_2 may produce RA via different mechanisms.

The ECS gradient does not extend as far as the CO_2 gradient.

4.29 BLACK, SUBOSKI AND FREEDMAN, 1967

ether exposure at room temp for 60 sec 100 sec	rats	2 choice T-maze FS	1

4.30 SUBOSKI, LITNER AND BLACK, 1968

ether exposure at 100°F	rats	2 choice T-maze	1

A decreasing gradient was found with both free and forced choice
concluded that "Ether anaesthesia as a highly aversive stimulus
disrupts the memory consolidation".

4.31 WEISSMAN, 1967

pentylenetetrazol (PTZ)i.p. injection 27-35mg/kg subconvulsive dose	rats	skinner box	1

45-74 mg/kg convulsive dose

time of treatment		test	retention
Before	After		

	2 sec-4min	24 hr	RA
	5-30 min		no RA
	2sec-1 min		RA
	3 min		no RA
	3 min		RA
	5 min		no RA

---

	5 min	24 hr	no RA
	5 min		no RA
			increased latencies
	100 sec	24 hr	no RA
	3160 sec	24 hr	decreased latencies
			"RA"

testing. Ether apparently improved discrimination. The authors
accounts for the results better than the hypothesis that ether

---

	5 min	1-3 days	no RA
			RA
			(-less RA than with ECS)

Treatment and site	animals	task	trials

4.31 (Continued)

strychnine SO_4 1.2-3.0 mg/kg	rats	skinner box	1

picrotoxin 3.0mg/kg
       5.0-8.4mg/kg

caffeine 30-100mg/kg
     150-225 mg/kg

amphetamine 3mg/kg
      20-50 mg/kg

aminophylline 30mg/kg
nicotine 1.8mg/kg

ethyl ether
inhalation 4.4cc/1
hexobarbital-i.p. 125mg/kg
pentobarbital 40mg/kg
secobarbital 50mg/kg
chlorpromazine 30mg/kg

4.32 KINCAID, 1967

metrazol (PTZ)	rats	step-down	1
intraperitoneal injection		passive	
		avoidance	

Permanent RA was produced by metrazol.

4.33 AHMAD AND ACHARI, 1968

PCA9 (1-(β-phenylethyl) triazolo			
(4,5-c) pyridine HCl	rats	2 compartment	1
i.p. 25mg/kg		box	

chlorpromazine
i.p. 1mg/kg

reserpine
i.p. 0.5mg/kg

NOTE: All the drugs suppressed retrieval of the passive avoidance

| time of treatment | | test | retention |
Before	After		
	`5 min	1-3 days	acquisition possibly enhanced no RA no RA RA
	5 min	1-3 days	no RA RA
			no RA RA
			no RA no RA
	5 min	1-3 days	no RA
			no RA no RA no RA no RA

---

	5 min	24 hr 21 days retest	RA RA

---

15 min		learning trial	learning impaired
1 hr			learning impaired
3 hr			learning impaired

response.

Treatment and site	animals	task	trials

4.33   (Continued)

PCA9 chlorpromazine reserpine	rats	2 compartment box	1
PCA9 chlorpromazine reserpine			
PCA9 chlorpromazine reserpine			

4.34   FRANCHINA AND MOORE,   1968

strychnine i.p. 0.2-0.0125 mg/kg	rats	hurdle-cross	2
0.2,0.1,0.05 mg/kg		passive avoidance	
0.025 mg/kg			
0.0125 mg/kg			

There were no reliable differences among doses, except for the
hurdle. Strychnine had no effect on hurdle crossing with no shock.
by the strychnine.   Strychnine dosage determined both the initial

---

4.35   FRECKLETON AND WAHLSTEN,   1968

CO_2 exposure	american cockroach	step-through FS passive avoidance	4 1/day

---

time of treatment Before	After	test	retention
15 min		retention	retrieval impaired
1 hr		24 hr after	retrieval impaired
3 hr		learning	retrieval impaired
	immediate	learning	consolidation impaired
immediate		consolidation	consolidation impaired
30 min			consolidation impaired
	24 hr	48 hr	no effect on
	24 hr	after	permanent
	24 hr	learning	memory trace

	15 min	24 hr	better retention than controls
	15 min	1/day for 7 days	inhibition of acquisition over all test trials
	15 min	for 7 days	inhibition of acquisition delayed after trial 1
	15 min	for 7 days	no inhibition of acquisition

lowest dose, they showed reliabily longer delays in crossing the
Presumably memory traces of the shock experience were enhanced
appearance and the apparent maintenance of response inhibition.

	15 sec	5th day	RA

Treatment and site   animals   task   trials

4.36 GARG AND HOLLAND, 1968

pentobarbital   rats   Hebb-   1/day
intraperitoneal   Williams
                                       maze

It was suggested that this depressant drug disrupted learning by

---

4.37 IWASAKI, KATAYAMA AND IWAHARA, 1968

chlorpromazine   rats   step-through for 3 min
intraperitoneal   -escapable
                                         shock

                                       -confinement
                                         shock

A slight but non-significant drug-learning dissociation appeared in
clear cut differences were found in open field activity, either
chlorpromazine treatments.

4.38 IWAHARA, IWASAKI AND HASEGAWA, 1968

chlorpromazine   rats   step-through 5 min
2mg/kg intraperitoneal   passive   inescapable
homofenazine   shock at
2mg/kg intraperitoneal   one or two
                                                     min

CPZ and HFZ inhibited passive avoidance i.e. more time was spent
when stronger FS used. On a second and third retest at 24 hour
showed same behaviour as on first retest. The authors claim that the
deficit, locomotor inhibition, drug-learning dissociation and loss

time of treatment		test	retention
Before	After		
	2 min daily	1/day for 10 days	acquisition slower and more errors made than controls

decreasing the rate of the consolidation process.

| 30 min | | 2 days | no RA |

| 30 min | | 2 days | RA |

the 'confinement' shocked rats. 17 minutes after training no
between the two types of treatment or between saline and

| 30 min before retest | | 24 hr | RA |
| 30 min before retest | | | RA |

in previously punishing compartment. Both drugs had less effect
intervals after the first but without drug injection the rats
results could not be explained by such factors as sensory
of attention due to the drug injection.

Treatment and site	animals	task	trials

4.39 PALFAI AND CORNELL, 1968

metrazol (PTZ) injection -convulsive dose -sub-convulsive dose nembutal	rats	classically conditioned FS	1
		general activity	
chlorpromazine metrazol (PTZ) (convulsive dose)			
		skinner box footshock	

No amnesia was seen for subconvulsive doses of metrazol, indicating a single metrazol convulsion does not independently affect

4.40 PALFAI AND CHILLAG, 1971

| metrazol (PTZ) 50mg/kg intraperitoneal | rats | step-through passive avoidance FS intensity 13mA 45mA FS | 1 |

Amnesia following metrazol convulsions is dependent upon the Sharpless and Jarvik, (1961, 4.7).

4.41 WIMER, 1968

| ether (room temp) reserpine 0.96mg/kg i.p. | mice C57BL/6J strain | step-up active avoidance | |

ether plus reserpine

Reserpine treatment increases escape latency and this effect is

time of treatment		test	retention
Before	After		
	within 10 sec	24 hr	
			RA
			no RA
			no RA
			no RA
24 hr	24 hr	no RA	
within 10 sec	24 hr	RA	
	1 week	more RA	
within 10 sec		RA	

that a seizure may be necessary to produce amnesia. Unlike ECS,
behaviour that is indicative of fear.

	immediate (10 sec)	24 hr	RA
	20 min		RA
	60-240 min		no RA
	immediate		RA
	20-240 min		no RA

interval between learning and injection, in contrast to Pearlman,

---

	immediate	1 day after training	no RA
for 2 days			RA (increased escape latencies)
2 days	immediate		less RA

partially counteracted by post-trial etherization.

Treatment and site   animals   task   trials

4.41 (Continued)

Post-trial etherization has been shown to have a facilitative
upon mice of strain C57BL/6J. Pretreatment of mice of strain
norepinephrine, dopamine, and γ-aminobutyric acid) resulted in
unaffected strain. This result suggests that ether facilitation in
release of brain norepinephrine, dopamine, or γ-aminobutyric acid.

4.42 BALDWIN AND SOLTYSIK, 1969

methohexitone	goats	delayed	no.
intracarotid		response	
		task	

4.43 GROSSMAN, 1969

PTZ (pentylenetetrazol)	rats	T-maze	1/day
hippocampal		discrimination	
injection			
5-10 μg		reversal	1/day

There was no reliable drug effect on general activity.

4.44 JOHNSON, 1969

chlorpromazine	mice	step-through	1
intraperitoneal		passive	
		avoidance	

time of treatment		test	retention
Before	After		

effect upon retention in mice of strain DBA/2J, but no effect
C57BL/6J with reserpine (a drug which reduces brain levels of
appearance of the ether facilitation effect in this hitherto
strain DBA/2J may be due to stimulation by ether of increased

---

during 10min delay period		10 min	no RA

---

5 min		every 24 hr	acquisition: facilitated
	1 min		more facilitation
5 min		every 24 hr	more facilitation
	1 min		facilitation

	0.5 min	24 hr	RA
	2 min		no RA
	10 min		no RA

Treatment and site	animals	task	trials

4.45   JOHNSON,   1970(a)

| chlorpromazine
i.p. 0.5mg/kg | mice | step-through
passive
avoidance | 1 |
| 2.0mg/kg | | | 1 |

Drug action has a duration of less than 4 hours. At 6 and 3 minutes
action on processes occurring after learning, i.e. memory, because
minute. There is no performance index depression but significant

4.46   JOHNSON,   1970(b)

| chlorpromazine
intraperitoneal
0.5, 2.0 and
3.5 mg/kg | mice | step-through | 1 |

This apparent amnesia was dose but not time dependent.

| before learning | | | 1 |
| before testing | | | |

There was no state dependent dissociation of learning. Test
expression followed by more rapid extinction.

4.47   JOHNSON,   1971

| chlorpromazine
2mg/kg intraperitoneal | mice | step-through
passive
avoidance
black or white
compartments
extinction | 1 |

time of treatment		test	retention
Before	After		
	0.5 min	24 hr	RA
	2 min		no RA
	10 min		no RA
6 hr		24 hr	no effect on acquisition, no RA
2 hr, 8 min			acquisition blocked, no retention
6 min			acquisition reduced, partial RA
3 min			acquisition reduced partial RA
	1 min		partial RA
	1.5 min		no RA
	20 min		no RA

before learning, the partial effect on retention may be due to
the effects are identical to post shock injections of 0.5 and 1
and submaximal depression of extinction and learning indices.

time relative to testing

10 min		24 hr	RA
90 min			RA
3 hr			RA
10 min		24 hr	no RA
10 min		48 hr retest	no RA

performance under chlorpromazine is compounded of reduced initial

10 min before testing		24 hr	RA

faster

Treatment and site   animals   task   trials

4.47 (Continued)

Retention was affected by chlorpromazine and extinction was faster
preceeded extinction tests. This paper is interesting for its
closely related can affect some aspects of conditioned avoidance

---

4.48 NACHMAN AND MEINECKE, 1969

Treatment and site	animals	task	trials
CO_2 exposure	rats	drinking	1
		task with	
		shock	3

Repeated treatments proved ineffective as with ECS. This could be

---

4.49 ELIAS AND SIMMERMAN, 1971

Treatment and site	animals	task	trials
ether	mice	water maze	30
(temperature	two strains		1/day
not specified)	DBA/2J		
	& C57BL/6J		

More errors were made by mice treated after learning than controls.
faster swimming times than controls. This paper is very hard to
as Fig 2, only the captions are different.)

4.50 GRUBER, 1971

Treatment and site	animals	task	trials
ether	mice	step-through	1
various depths of		passive	
anaesthesia were		avoidance	
controlled by time of		tested in same	
administration or		or in different	
temperature of		apparatus	
vapourization			

Mice received passive avoidance training followed by etherization
different levels of anesthesia were reached. Twenty-four hours

time of treatment		test	retention
Before	After		

after chlorpromazine but not if the relevant T-maze learning had
demonstration that previous learning experiences even if not
behaviour.

---

	4 sec	24 hr	RA
	4 sec	48 and 72 hr	no RA

due to the accumulation of partial consolidation with each trial.

8-10 min each day		daily	
	"immediate"		RA

Pretrial etherization had no effect on errors, but mice showed
understand either from the text or the figures (Fig 1 is the same

---

	60 sec		RA
	4 hr		no RA

at different temperatures, shock-ether intervals, and until
later the mice received generalization testing.

| Treatment and site | animals | task | trials |

4.50 (Continued)

Etherization 4 hours after learning results in longer crossing different apparatus. Similar effects are produced by increasing

Depending upon the technique of administration, ether produced induced changes in the generalization slopes were similar to those

---

4.51 MAYSE AND DeVIETTI, 1971

Treatment and site	animals	task	trials
pentobarbital 12 or 25 mg/kg intraperitoneal	rats	water T-maze FS	to criterion of 4 correct successively
			reversal of T-maze choice

This experiment was done in conjunction with ECS (1.245) to produce a state-dependent learning relative to pentobarbital. produced state-dependency in the no drug-drug order but not in the

---

4.52 PENROD AND BOICE, 1971

Treatment and site	animals	task	trials
halothane anaesthesia	rats	step-through passive avoidance	1

| time of treatment | | test | retention |
| Before | After | | |

latencies in same apparatus but no change in performance in shock. Ether 60 sec after learning produced retrograde amnesia.

retrograde amnesia or a facilitative effect on learning. Ether-resulting from changes in the reinforcement level.

Before	After	test	retention
15-20 min before training		3 days	no RA
	15-20 min before re-training		RA
15-20 min before training	15-20 min before retraining		no RA
15-20 min before training			no RA
	15-20 min before retraining		RA
15-20 min before training	15-20 min before retraining		no RA

compare the efficacy of ECS and ECS preceded by footshock to Pentobarbital injected just prior to either training or retraining drug-no drug order.

Before	After	test	retention
	20 sec	1 day	RA
	30 min		less RA
	20 sec	4,7 days	no RA
	30 min	4 days	most RA
		7 days	RA
2 days			

Treatment and site   animals   task   trials

4.52   (Continued)

The 24 hour retention replicated the usual gradient of retrograde
scores did not exhibit the similarity to Day 1 scores predicted by
retention were marked but did not appear to be due to drug

4.53   SCHMALTZ,   1971

Penicillin plugs   white rats   active   up to 400
in hippocampus   avoidance
                                          shuttle box

Acquisition of avoidance was slowed but not prevented by penicillin
hippocampus.

5.54   AHLERS AND BEST,   1972

pentylenetetrazol   rats   discriminated   2
40mg/kg intraperitoneal   taste-aversion   CS-US
                                          US-apomorphine   interval
                                          CS-saccharin   15 min

Due to the nature of the discriminated-avoidance paradigm used, the
the RA treatment or general disinhibition. The data indicate that
which is due to the disruption of the CS trace (because RA was

---

4.55   ANGEL, BOUNDS AND PERRY,   1972

halothane   mice   step-through   1
anaesthesia   FS
1.5% for 5 min

halothane 5%
for 5 min

Although the differences in retention were apparent, (with a greater
significant. A similar experimental design was utilized to test the
in rats. A parallelism between the degree of disruption of brain
different concentrations of halothane was shown.

---

time of treatment   test   retention
Before   After

amnesia (but there were no significant differences) 4 and 7 day
the consolidation theory. The effects of pre-anaesthesia on
dissociation.

---

up to
one month

in hippocampus. It was not slowed by bilateral destruction of

---

before US   24 hr   more RA

             2 hr after
             US   RA

RA could not be explained in terms of the punishing effects of
an amnesic treatment causes a memory deficit, at least part of
greater when induced before the US).

---

             immediate   24 hr   slight RA
             (30-60 sec)

             immediate   slightly more RA
             (25 sec)

deficit for the greater halothane concentration), these were not
effect of different concentrations of halothane on blood-brain barrier
barrier function and the trend towards amnesia production by

Treatment and site	animals	task	trials

5.1 JONES, 1943

immersion in water; body temperature maintained 20- 25°C for 24 hr	rats	14 unit maze	no. until criterion 2 correct

---

5.2 RANSMEIER AND GERARD, 1954

body temperature reduced to 5°C maintained for as long as 12 hr	hamsters	maze learning	no.

Body temperatures of $5°C$ did not disturb memory, although they cortex. Such temperatures were attained 40 min after the training

5.3 GERARD, 1955

cooling ECS cooling during ECS interval	hamsters	maze learning	no.

Cooling and the resultant cessation of electrical activity in the consolidation period as determined to susceptibility to ECS.

5.4 CERF AND OTIS, 1957

heat narcosis 36.5°- 37 C	goldfish	shuttle box	10

Disruption of electrical activity occurs with heat narcosis. It recently acquired association is reminiscent of the retroactive interference factors are liable to affect various processes in the activity could underly, at least partially, their similar action on

---

time of treatment		test	retention
Before	After		
	immediate	24 hr to 1 month	no RA

| | attained 40 min after training | | no RA |

eliminated electrical activity in the hypothalamus, thalamus and
experience and were maintained for as long as 12 hours.

		every 24 hr	no RA
	15 min		RA
	1 hr		RA

brain did not destroy memory but cooling did prolong the

	0-15 min	24 hr	RA
	60 min		partial RA
	4 hr		no RA

was concluded that this deleterious effect of narcosis on a
inhibition on learning caused in mammals by ECS. Both
brain; but their common disruptive effect of electrical
memory.

Treatment and site	animals	task	trials

5.5 ESSMAN AND SUDAK, 1962

Immersion in water	mice	water	3
20°C; given		maze	
2,4-D (2,4-dichlorophenoxyacetic acid)		escape	
		learning	3

It was suggested that moderate sustained hypothermia interferes (2,4-dichlorophenoxyacetic acid) was given intraperitoneally.

5.6 ESSMAN AND SUDAK, 1963

decrease of body	mice	step-down	1
temperature by		escape	
2.8°C		response	

2,4-D i.p. gave
a reduction of
9.3°C

5.7 SUDAK AND ESSMAN, 1964

body temperature	rats	stepping	1
25.2°C		response	
2,4-D-28.6°C			

5.8 MROSOVSKY, 1963

| Deep body | rats | shuttle box | 6 |
| temp. reduced to 2°C | | | |

The treatment did not significantly affect retention or unlearning

---

5.9 DAVIS, BRIGHT AND AGRANOFF, 1965

| ECS (17-19°C) | goldfish | shuttle box | 20 |

cooling to 9°C
cooling to 9°C and ECS

Cooling subjects following trial 20, prolonged the interval during

---

time of treatment		test	retention
Before	After		

hypothermia maintained through acquisition		30 min after treatment	no learning
hypothermia on trials and raised during intervals (15 min)			learning occurred

with consolidation of experience. The thermolytic agent 2,4-D

30 min		30 min after treatment	impaired acquisition
			unimpaired retention

	within 1 min	24 hr	RA
	1-3 hr		no RA
	11 min		no RA

	15 min	13 days	no RA

of this task.

	1-90 min	3 days	RA
	120-360 min		no RA
	120 min	3 days	no RA
	120 min	3 days	RA

which ECS could cause a retention deficit.

Treatment and site	animals	task	trials

5.10   BEITEL AND PORTER,   1968

immersion $2^{o}C$	mice	step-down	1
duration 1/6 min		FS	
5 min		PA	
15 min			
30 min			

$20^{o}C$ for 30 min		T-maze	5/day
$29^{o}C$ for 30 min		simple	for 12 days
$20^{o}C$ for 15 min		discrimination	
20° for 30 min			
$20^{o}C$ for 30 min			

Immersion for 15 min had a transitory effect on acquisition, but cooled for 30 min.

These animals were more deeply chilled or for longer than Riccio Bietel & Porter used more than 1 trial. Partial recovery occurred

---

5.11   RICCIO, GAEBELEIN AND COHEN,   1968

Strychnine SO_4	rats	step-through	1
i.p. 0.33mg/kg		FS	
hypothermia- immersion in $2-3^{o}C$			1
water for 10-12 min colonic temp- $21.5^{o}C$			
strychnine and hypothermia			1

The single hypothermic treatment was not punishing. None of the decrement obtained in rats receiving hypothermia does not appear this situation. Hypothermia, serving as a retrograde amnesic agent

time of treatment		test	retention
Before	After		
	0.5,5,20 min	24 hr	no RA
	0.5,5,20 min		no RA
	20 min		no RA
	0.5, 5 min		RA
	20 min		no RA
	0.5, 5 min		RA
3 days		3 days	acquisition
3 days		after treatment	impaired
3 days			transitory impairment
60 days			partial impairment of acquisition
	30 min		RA
30 min			no RA

acquisition and long-term retention were impaired in groups

and Stikes, (1969,5.13) who found no proactive effect of cooling.
when cooling - training period was extended from 3 to 60 days.

---

15 min		24 hr	no effect on acquisition, no RA
	20 sec	24 hr	RA
15 min (strychnine)	20 sec	24 hr	more RA

shocked groups differed on CER duration, so the performance
to be based on disruption of conditioned motor suppression in
acts primarily on discriminated avoidance behaviour.

   Treatment and site   animals   task   trials

5.12 RICCIO, HODGES AND RANDALL,   1968

immersion   rats   step-through   1
for 10-11 min   FS
colonic temp.
68.5°F

Immersion and retention control showed complete retention.

immersion
duration varied
colonic temp: inescapable   1
60°F   shock
65°F
70°F
80°F
85°F

Inescapable shock was used to show that the effect is not due to
modification of CNS activity plays a major role in producing

5.13 RICCIO AND STIKES,   1969

Immersion in ice water   step-through   1
for 20 min   rats   inescapable
colonic temp   shock
19.8°C

(there is no prograde effect of hypothermia)
This RA was not complete. Controls cooled only, with no shock

5.14 JENSEN AND RICCIO,   1970

Immersion in   rats   step-through   1
2-4°C water   FS
(colonic temp. less   PA
than 20°C)
prior treatment:
HYPO.
EXT.
FAM.

Animals received one of three types of experience over two days
FAM. pre-exposure to training stimuli, familiarization with
EXT. negatively reinforced stimulus experience followed by
HYPO. second training trial-amnesic treatment following an initial

time of treatment		test	retention
Before	After		
	20 sec	24 hr	RA
	5 sec		RA
	15 min		no RA
	60 min		no RA
	30 sec	24 hr	RA
	30 sec		RA
	30 sec		RA
	30 sec		no RA
	30 sec		no RA

fear conditioning in the safe chamber. The conclusion was that
memory impairment.

	20 sec	1 day	RA
	20 sec	5 days	RA
	20 sec	10 days	RA
24 hr		24 hr after treatment	no RA
	20 sec	2 days	RA
	20 sec	2-4 days	no RA

training showed no deficit in retention.

	immediate	24 hr	RA
			less RA
			no RA
			no RA

prior to hypothermic treatment:
apparatus prior to training
extinction (training, extinction, retraining)
RA (training, hypothermia, retraining)

Treatment and site   animals   task   trials

5.14 (Continued)

Each type of prior experience significantly diminished the amount
there is less new information to acquire after each type of prior
It was concluded that these findings are consistent with the idea
the severity of RA.

5.15 JACOB AND SORENSON, 1969

immersion in   mice   step-through   1
cold water   FS
1°C for 10 sec

immersion in
hot water
48°C

Immersion in cold water led to a decrease of 1.0°C in deep colonic
deep colonic temperature. These results, plus the appropriate
stimuli applied to the peripheral nervous system in the absence
of the brain and large changes in body temperature – not hypothermia

---

5.16 KANE AND JARVIK, 1970

heat induced   mice   step-through   1
convulsions   FS PA

heating
without
convulsions

Retention was impaired only in those animals that had heat-induced
normal when they did not produce convulsions, failed to produce
stimulation provided by hyperthermia is not sufficient in itself

---

time of treatment   test   retention
Before   After

of RA produced by hypothermia. It was suggested that because
experience, the amount of consolidation necessary is reduced.
that psychological variables play an important role in modifying

---

0-2 sec   24 hr   RA

10-30 sec   24 hr   graded RA

0 sec   24 hr   RA

temp. Immersion in hot water led to a mean increase of 0.8^{o}C in
controls indicate that memory disruption can be obtained with
of both gross changes in the normal electrical or chemical state
per se.

---

immediate   24 hr   RA

no RA

convulsions. Even elevations of temperature more than 5°C above
amnesia. These results indicate that even the strong
to produce amnesia.

Treatment and site	animals	task	trials

5.17 GROSSER AND PERCY, 1971

Treatment and site	animals	task	trials
Immersion in cold water $1^{\circ}C\pm0.5^{\circ}C$ for 10 sec hot water $48^{\circ}C\pm1.0^{\circ}C$ for 10 sec manner of E releasing Ss onto apparatus, cold water as above	mice	step-through FS	1 1 1

The manner in which the Ss were positioned on the step-through
both learning and retention trials, but not enough to influence the
this experiment failed to support the contentions of Jacobs and
of immersion in hot or cold water.

5.18 MISANIN AND HOOVER, 1971

Treatment and site	animals	task	trials
Hypothermia by immersion duration constant,depth- 0-0.5,$5^{\circ}C$ $10^{\circ}C$ $15^{\circ}C$	rats	step-down with FS	1

There was a graded impairment of memory for animals cooled in 5-15°C
recovery from hypothermia play a significant role in hypothermia

Depth constant,duration-
rapid recovery
slow recovery

Rate of recovery was a prime determinant of hypothermia produced
rather than to disruption of memory consolidation.

5.19 MISANIN, NAGY, KEISER AND BOWEN, 1971

Treatment and site	animals	task	trials
Immersion $1-4^{\circ}C$	rats (9 days old)	escape task FS	25

(colonic temp. $16-22^{\circ}C$)

time of treatment		test	retention
Before	After		

	immediate	24 hr	no RA
	immediate	24 hr	no RA
			no RA

apparatus did influence the measured step-through latencies on retention with a 300 sec cut-off latency. It is concluded that Sorenson (1969, 5.15) with regard to the memory disrupting role

---

	immediate	24 hr	
			RA
			less RA
			no RA

water. These results suggest that depth of and/or rate of produced amnesia.

	immediate	24 hr	RA
			no RA

forgetting. These results were attributed to retrieval failure

	immediate	1 hr	no RA
	23 hr	1 hr	no RA
	immediate	24 hr	RA
1 hr			same as control
			no immersion gp.
	0,5 min	24 hr	complete RA
	15 min		partial RA
	6 hr 45 min,23 hr		no RA

Treatment and site   animals   task   trials

5.19 (Continued)

Rats first show signs of retention of an escape response over 24
memory because it was selectively impaired by hypothermia.

5.20   SMITH AND MISANIN,   1972

ECS   rats   step-down   1
transpinnate   FS

hypothermia-immersion in
0.5^{o}-3.0^{o}C water for 10 min

ECS plus hypothermia

These results were interpreted in terms of hypothermia-induced
memory-retrieval-failure interpretation of ECS-produced amnesia.

---

time of treatment		test	retention
Before	After		

hours at 9 days of age. This memory was called long-term

---

	immediate	24 hr	slight RA
	immediate		less RA
	immediate		no RA

attenuation of sensory input following ECS and lend support to a

---

Treatment and site	animals	task	trials

6.1 HAYES, 1953

ECS; anoxia - compression of chest	rats	T-maze	10

Anoxia appears to produce much the same effects as ECS

6.2 RANSMEIER AND GERARD, 1954

Hypoxia	hamsters	maze learning	no.

Convulsion (ECS) and hypoxia were both disturbing when administered
degree of disturbance decreased along characteristic curves with

---

6.3 THOMPSON AND PRYER, 1965

Anoxia - decompression chamber 10 min at simulated altitude of 20,000 ft	rats	discriminated avoidance T-maze	no.

6.4 THOMPSON, 1957

Anoxia -decompression chamber 10 min at simulated altitude of 20,000 ft 30,000 ft	rats	discriminated avoidance	no.

ECS and anoxia
30,000 ft

Anoxia plus ECS failed to cause a greater deficit in memory than

time of treatment		test	retention
Before	After		

| | 1 hr
after each
trial | every
24 hr | RA |

| | "some
minutes" | | RA |
| | 12 hr | | RA |

some minutes to 12 hours after the training experience. The
increasing intervals between training and treatment.

| | 30 sec-
2 min | 48 hr | temporally
graded RA |
| | 15 min-
4 hr | 48 hr | no RA |

| | 60 sec | 24 hr | RA |
| | 60 sec | 24 hr | more RA
-comparable to ECS |

| | 60 sec | 24 hr | RA |

caused by a single ECS.

Treatment and site   animals   task   trials

6.5 PENNINGTON, 1958

Anoxia   rats   vertical-   30
- exposure for 1 hr   horizontal
at 27,000 ft   discrimination

ECS
ECS and anoxia

It was suggested that the anoxia causes some brain damage, but
animals receiving anoxia alone.

6.6 BALDWIN AND SOLTYSIK, 1966

Cerebral   goats   classical   1/day
ischaemia by   conditioning
cutting off blood
supply

There was temporary abolition of both cortical and subcortical
following the application of the ischaemic procedure. Cerebral
"consolidation" of the learning had occurred in less than 65

6.7 BALDWIN AND SOLTZSIK, 1969

Cerebral   goats   delayed   no.
ischaemia by   response
cutting off blood   task
supply

A period of unconsciousness and temporary flattening of EEG
of the goats. Assuming that isoelectric EEG implies absence of unit
memory involved in delayed response tasks does not require pro-
intraneuronal chemical change.

6.8 TABER AND BANUAZIZI, 1966

Nitrogen gas inhalation   mice   step-through   1

It was concluded that anoxia is not a major factor in producing

---

time of treatment		test	retention
Before	After		
3 weeks		2 days	no effect on acquisition or retention
	30 sec		RA
3 weeks	30 sec		more RA

this was not apparent in learning or relearning scores of

| | 20 sec | 1.5 min | no RA |

EEG activity – which was isolectric 25-45 seconds
ischaemia was in itself not aversive. It was concluded that
seconds after each learning trial.

| during 10 min delay period | | 10 min (treatment did not exceed 10 min delay) | no RA |

occurred during the delay period,did not impair the performance
neuronal activity it was concluded that the type of recent
longed reverberatory neuronal activity but depends on some

| | 0-60 min | 24 hr | no RA |

amnesia.

Treatment and site	animals	task	trials

6.9 VACHER, KING AND MILLER, 1968

Hypoxia - exposure to 9% oxygen	rats	step-through	1
nitrogen gas			
ECS			
hypoxia - exposure to 6.1% oxygen for 10 min		2 choice discrimination	to 9/10

Hypoxia itself produced no difference in performance. Failure to
necessary severity of intracellular hypoxia rapidly enough. They
between results of 6.3 and 6.4 and these.

6.10 CHERKIN, 1971

Hypoxia - exposure to oxygen: nitrogen mixtures of 6.6%, 7.9% or 10% oxygen for 30 hr	chickens	inhibition of pecking	1
Hyperoxia - exposure to 99.9% oxygen			

Hypoxia has been suggested as a mechanism for the RA action of ECS,
produce RA in this situation where ECS and flurothyl have been

---

6.11 ERKERT AND VIERCK, 1971

Hyperbaric oxygen twice a day for 10 days; with convulsions	rats	Lashley III maze	to 9/10 15/day
Hyperbaric oxygen as above	rats	T-maze position training	to 10/11

time of treatment		test	retention
Before	After		
	immediate	24 hr	no RA
	immediate	24 hr	no RA
	immediate	24 hr	RA
	immediate	48 hr	no RA

produce RA may have been due to inability to produce the
suggested a strain difference to account for discrepancy

---

	immediate	48 hr	no RA
	immediate	48 hr	no RA

chemoconvulsants, anaesthetics and cerebral trauma but did not
shown to do so.

---

24 hr		11 days	deficit in retention
24 hr		11 days	no RA,controls had no training and treatment

Treatment and site   animals   task   trials

6.11 (Continued)

The results suggest that the Lashley III maze deficit was
deficiency.

6.12 GIURGEA, LEFEVRE, LESCRENIER AND DAVID-REMACLE, 1971

Treatment and site	animals	task	trials
Atmosphere of 96.5% nitrogen gas 10 min	rats	skinner-box white light CS	daily for 30 min (40 stimulations per session)

No particularly aversive learning effect was seen after delayed
blocked learning during the period examined, the authors attributed
consolidation of daily learned acquisition.

Hypoxia (as above)
plus piracetam
10mg/kg
100+500mg/kg

Piracetam was used as a possible protective agent against the
normal EEG-tracing after hypoxic-hypoxia. The higher doses of
amnesic effects.

6.13 SARA AND LEFEVRE, 1972

sudden hypoxia-nitrogen gas 96.5% for 10 min	rats	step-through FS PA	1
piracetam (100mg/kg)			1
piracetam plus hypoxia			1

Hypoxia produced RA for the one trial passive avoidance response
this hypoxia-induced amnesia.

Progressive hypoxia induced gradually for 25 min	rats		1

These results do not support the hypothesis of Vacher, King and
was due to the establishment of the hypoxic conditions being

---

time of treatment		test	retention
Before	After		

produced by alterations in activation and not by a memory

	30-60 sec	daily for 3 days	RA
	7 hr		no RA

hypoxia. The influence of "immediate" hypoxia which practically
to a hypoxia-induced retrograde amnesia which interferes with the

	30 min daily	30-60 sec	RA no RA

hypoxia-induced amnesia since it facilitates recuperation of a
piracetam were effective in preventing the hypoxia-induced

	immediate	24 hr	RA
30 min		24 hr	normal retention
30 min	immediate	24 hr	no RA

24 hours after learning. Piracetam protected the animals from

	immediate	24 hr	RA

Miller (1968, 6.9) that the failure of hypoxia to produce RA
too slow.

Treatment and site	animals	task	trials

7.1 PEARLMAN AND JARVIK, 1961

| KCl 25%; bilateral spreading depression (SD) | rats | step-down FS | 1 |

7.2 PEARLMAN, 1966

| KCl 25%; bilateral SD | rats | step-down FS | 1 |

Ether anaesthesia and KCl appear to have similar effects on

7.3 BUREŠ AND BUREŠOVÁ, 1963

KCl; cortical SD	rats	Y-maze discrimination	1
		reversal	1
		step-through FS	1

7.4 KUPFERMAN, 1965

| KCl 25%; -bilateral SD | rats | discrimination task | no. |

The training and injection took a total of 20 minutes.

7.5 BLACK, SUBOSKI AND FREEDMAN, 1967

| KCl, SD | rats | 2 choice T-maze FS | 1 |

---

time of treatment		test	retention
Before	After		
	10 min	24 hr	RA
	1-10 min	21 hr	RA
	15 min	21 hr	no RA

consolidation in this situation.

---

	1 min	24 hr	RA less than ECS
	2-6 hr	24 hr	no RA
	1 min	24 hr	RA slightly less effective than ECS

| | 0 min | 24 hr | no RA |

| | 5 min | 24 hr | slight RA (decreased latencies) |

Treatment and site	animals	task	trials

7.6 AVIS AND CARLTON, 1968

KCl 25% bilateral hippocampal injection	rats	conditioned suppression of drinking CS-FS pairing	1

Tone was paired with FS and presented during drinking and results learning, neither performance nor the ability to relearn was

---

7.7 DAVIS AND KLINGER, 1969

KCl -intracranial 600 μg	goldfish	shuttle box	20

KCl injection produced immediate seizures. Convulsive swimming The KCl-produced amnesia develops in 6-12 hours.

ITE-KCl			20

The rate of development of the amnesia produced by the ITE-KCl 24 hours after injection (day 3). The fish showed a retention 48 hours after injection, indicating that the amnesia developed more slowly than when it was given immediately post trial.

7.8 HUGHES, 1969

KCl-25% posterior hippocampal injection	rats	conditioned suppression of drinking CS-FS pairing	4 CS-FS pairings

Hippocampal EEG indicated that KCl produced marked attenuation of

---

| time of treatment | | test | retention |
Before	After		
	24 hr	4 days	RA and EEG depression
	24 hr	4 days	no RA and no EEG depression

compared with EEG activity. All animals were capable of re-
permanently impaired by the injection.

---

	1 min-18 hr	3 days	RA
	24 hr	3 days	no RA
	1 min	6 hr	no RA
		12-18 hr	RA

movements diminished in intensity over a period of 1-2 hours.

	24 hr	48 hr	less RA
		72 hr	RA

treatment (see 8.35) on day 2, was estimated by retraining fish
defect significantly smaller than the defect for fish retrained
over a period of 24-48 hours. KC1 thus produced amnesia 2-3 times

---

	1,3,7 or 21 days	4 days after injection	RA
	1 day	4 or 7 days after injection	RA
		21 days	no RA - but not complete recovery

EEG.

    Treatment and site   animals   task   trials

7.9 REED AND TROWILL, 1969

KCl
- unilateral SD   rats   active   40
without shifting   avoidance
depressed   step-through
hemispheres
10,15 or 20%
KCl concentrations:
Training Test
15%   15%
15%   10%
15%   20%
20%   10%
10%   20%

Any change in SD conditions from one session to another is a
decrement.

_____

7.10 KAPP AND SCHNEIDER, 1971

Hippocampal-
crystals of KCl   rats   CER   4
                                        drinking
                                        response
                                        FS and tone

cortical-
crystals of KCl

Criterion for treatment was disruption of ongoing electrical
so differences do not reflect thirst or impairment of motor
both storage and retrieval effects produced, at least in part, by

_____

7.11 PAOLINO AND LEVY, 1971

Cortical spreading   rats   step-through   1
depression (CSD) for   FS
4 hr with 25% KCl   PA

2nd treatment with
reinstatement of CSD
after 16 min without CSD

| time of treatment | | test | retention |
Before	After		
15 min		24 hr under CSD	

no RA
RA⎫
RA⎭ same amount
RA⎫-acquisition was
RA⎭ proportional to concentration

stimulus change which can also account for a performance

---

	10 sec	4 days	RA
		21 days	RA
	24 hr	4 days	RA
		21 days	no RA
	10 sec	4 days	no RA
	24 hr	4 days	no RA

activity for at least 30 min. Controls treated with NaCl,
ability. Results suggest that the interference is related to
disruption of neural activity in the hippocampus.

---

	immediate	24 hr	no RA
	16 min		RA
	256 min		no RA
	immediate and 16 min after removal of first CSD	24 hr	RA

Treatment and site   animals   task   trials

7.11 (Continued)

The U-shaped function of amnesia for the disruptive effects of
an initial subcortical memory trace localization, which is
eventual permanent storage involving cortical participation.
confinement rather than in permanent fixation of the trace at

ECS- subcutaneously at base
of each ear; 100mA; 500msec

CSD immediate and ECS

CSD immediate for 4 hr
and ECS

The reasoning for this experiment was - (i) if immediate CSD does
form, and (ii) ECS produces memory impairment by disruption of
possible to extend the short temporal gradient of retrograde
by CSD.

* This lack of RA was explained by partial premature release of
interaction.

_____

time of treatment   test   retention
Before   After

CSD induced by potassium chloride was interpreted as indicating
followed within a few minutes by a release of the trace for
Immediate induction of CSD appears to result in a temporary
subcortical levels.

4 sec	24 hr	RA
16 min		no RA
256 min		no RA
4 sec	24 hr	RA
16 min		RA
256 min		no RA*
16 min after	24 hr	no RA
removal of CSD		

confine the memory trace at the subcortical level in a labile
this labile trace at the subcortical level, then it should be
amnesia produced with ECS by using the memory trace confinement

the subcortically confined trace with subsequent cortical

Treatment and site	animals	task	trials

8.1 DINGMAN AND SPORN, 1961

Treatment and site	animals	task	trials
8-azaguanine intra-cisternal	rats	well-learned maze	no.
		new maze	

8-azaguanine inhibits RNA synthesis, producing a non-functional
No attempt was made to measure retention in the classical type of

---

8.2 FLEXNER, FLEXNER, STELLAR, de la HABA AND ROBERTS, 1962

Treatment and site	animals	task	trials
Puromycin subcutaneous 0.42 mg/gm	mice	hurdle box	no.to 9/10
83% inhibition		Y-maze	no.to 9/10 no.to 3/4
		Y-maze reversal	

This dose of puromycin injected subcutaneously produced 83%
cerebral administration sufficient to produce 97% inhibition of
learning or retention.

8.3 FLEXNER, FLEXNER AND STELLAR, 1963

Treatment and site	animals	task	trials
Puromycin 80% inhibition·bilateral injections each of 0.09 mg into T; T+V+F F; V; V+F	mice	Y-maze FS	to 9/10

Temporal injections of puromycin will disrupt memory when the
multiple injections are necessary, involving most of the remaining

time of treatment		test	retention
Before	After		
	30 min	45 min	no RA
x		15 min	acquisition retarded

RNA. (STM could still be present if the drug had any effect). experiment, i.e. 24 hours after learning.

1-7 hr		24 hr	no RA
	24 hr	2-8 hr	no RA
	24 hr	2-8 hr	no RA
2-8 hr		24 hr	no RA
	0 min	4 days	no RA
	24 hr	4 days	no RA
	24 hr	5 weeks	no RA

inhibition of protein for 6 hours. With subcutaneous plus protein synthesis there was disorientation incompatible with

	1 day	3 days	RA
	1 day	3 days	no RA

injections are made 1 day later. Whereas at longer intervals cortices: Temporal (T), Ventricular (V) and Frontal (F).

Treatment and site   animals   task   trials

8.3 (Continued)

T+V+F
T;V;F
V+T; V+F; T+F

T
T

T   Y-maze
                                             reversal 3
                                             weeks after
                                             original
                                             learning

The enlarged locus of longer term memory becomes effective in 4-
given reversal training 3 weeks later, reverted to the original
that the effect of puromycin in destroying a recent habit is not
conclusions were drawn that the hippocampal zone is the site of
with longer term memory storage. Puromycin hydrolyzed at the

8.4 FLEXNER, FLEXNER, ROBERTS AND de la HABA, 1964

Chloramphenicol   mice   Y-maze   to 9/10
bitemporal injections   FS
60,260,520 μg

The chloramphenicol injections produced 50% inhibition of protein
cerebral chloramphenicol to affect memory can be related to their
protein synthesis. Loss of recent memory by puromycin can be

8.5 FLEXNER, FLEXNER AND STELLAR, 1965

Puromycin   mice   Y-maze   to 9/10
T+V+F-   FS
inhibition   dose μg
93%   180
93%   90
71,72%   48,24

Temporal
97,90%   180,120
80%   60
72, 48%   30,16

As the concentration of puromycin was reduced, it became
trend in its effect on degree and duration of inhibition of

time of treatment		test	retention
Before	After		
	18-43 days	3 days	RA
	11-38 days		no RA
	28-43 days		no RA
	2-3 days	3 days	RA
	5-6 days	3 days	no RA
	1 day	3 days	RA (original retention retained)

6 days depending on the individual animal. Mice trained and then
response when injected with puromycin. This is strong evidence
due to disorganization or incapacitance of the animal. The
recent memory and an extensive part of the neocortex is concerned
glycoside bond is without effect on memory.

	1 day	3-6 days	no RA

synthesis. The failure of subcutaneous puromycin and intra-
inadequate effect on the degree and duration of inhibition of
related to degree and duration of inhibition of protein synthesis.

	11-60 hr	3 days	
			RA
			impaired retention
			no RA
	25 hr	3 days	RA
			impaired retention
			no RA

progressively less effective in destroying memory with a similar
protein synthesis.

Treatment and site   animals   task   trials

8.6 FLEXNER, FLEXNER, de la HABA AND ROBERTS, 1965

Hydrolyzed puromycin   mice   Y-maze
            T   FS
          T+V+F

Aminonucleoside
            T
          T+V+F

L-Phenylalanyl
puromycin
            T
          T+V+F

D-Phenylalanyl
puromycin
            T
          T+V+F

As with recent memory, destruction of longer term memory of simple
of inhibition of cerebral protein synthesis in appropriate areas
puromycin to affect memory is correlated with their inadequate

"It is tentatively concluded that maintenance of memory depends

8.7 FLEXNER AND FLEXNER, 1966

AXM   mice   Y-maze   to 9/10
T,120 or 240μg   FS
T+V+F 90 or 180μg

AXM plus puromycin
T 240 μg each
T+V+F
48 or 90 μg AXM
180 μg puromycin

Intracerebral injections of AXM caused profound inhibition (100%)
of simple maze learning in mice. Intracerebral injections of a
destructive effects of puromycin when injected alone. This is
the formation of peptidyl puromycin. They suggest that memory

8.8 FLEXNER, FLEXNER AND ROBERTS, 1966

AXM 120 μg   mice   1.Y-maze   to 9/10
bitemporal   32.4
                                                        (difficult)

time of treatment		test	retention
Before	After		
	1 day		no RA
	7 days		no RA
	1 day		no RA
	7 days		no RA
	1 day		no RA
	7 days		no RA
	1 day		no RA
	7 days		no RA

maze performance appears to be related to the degree and duration
of the brain. The failure of several substances related to
effect on degree and duration of inhibition of protein synthesis.

upon the continuing synthesis of protein."

1 day	several days		no RA
12-35 days	several days		no RA
1 day	several days		no RA
14 days	several days		no RA

of cerebral protein synthesis but were without effect on memory
mixture of AXM and puromycin protected memory against the
explained in terms of AXM preventing loss of mRNA and preventing
loss with puromycin is due to loss of new mRNA.

2-4 hr		period 1	no RA
		period 2	impaired retention
		period 3	no RA

Treatment and site	animals	task	trials

8.8   (Continued)

	mice	2. Y-maze reversal	1
		3. Y-maze (mice tested more than once)	to 9/10 12.6
		4. Y-maze (single test)	to 9/10
AXM and ECS		5. Reversal training	1

This dose of AXM produced 90% inhibition for 10 hours. The
intermediate period in which memory was apparently lost and a final
that protein synthesis is not necessary for learning. (Note that
protein synthesis in this period but not enough for expression).
hr in (2) and 14 hours in (3) and (4). Reverberatory action
intermediate period protein synthesis seems to be necessary for

It was concluded that mRNA required for the ultimate establishment
conserved throughout in the presence of AXM.

8.9   FLEXNER, FLEXNER AND ROBERTS,   1967

| Puromycin T+V+F | mice | Y-maze | to 9/10 |

Both recent and longer term memory are maintained for 10-20 hrs

| | | overtraining on Y-maze | to 9/10 plus 60 |

Mice trained to criterion and then given 60 additional runs are

8.10   FLEXNER AND FLEXNER,   1967

Puromycin 180 µg	mice		
T		Y-maze	to 9/10
T+V+F			

time of treatment		test	retention
Before	After		
2-3 hr		1-3 hr	no RA
		5-14 hr	RA
		29-96 hr	no RA
	5 min	14 hr	no RA
		17-36 hr	impaired retention
		40-96 hr	no RA
	5 min	5-14 hr	no RA
		17-48 hr	impaired retention
		58-96 hr	no RA
2-3 hr	(ECS) 1 hr	4 days	no RA

results show an initial period in which memory was retained, an
period during which expression of the memory returned. It appears
training takes 15 min and injection 5 min; so there could be some
The initial stage is independent of protein synthesis lasting 5
(prolonged by the drug) is ruled out by using ECS (5). In the
expression. For the final period protein synthesis is restored.

of a long-term memory is formed during the first period and

| | 24 hr | 10-20 hr | no RA |
| | 24 hr | 3 months | RA |

after injection of puromycin and then disappear permanently.

| | 24 hr | | no RA |

not affected by puromycin.

		after treatment :	
	1 day	6-13 hr	RA
		33-78 hr	RA
	13 days	13-15 hr	RA
	7-14 days	33-50 hr	RA

Treatment and site	animals	task	trials

8.10   (Continued)

| Puromycin, T 24 hr after training. Saline injected T after puromycin | mice | Y-maze | to 9/10 |

Puromycin
T+V+F 13-15 days
after training

Puromycin T 24 hours
after training
2nd injection of
puromycin

Puromycin
T+V+F 13-15 days
after training
2nd injection of
puromycin

When all of the above groups were retested 1-2 weeks after testing groups had memory of this relearning at a high level.

The conclusion was drawn that puromycin blocks expression of maintains the basic memory trace. Therefore the abnormal peptides the characteristics of neuronal synapses.

8.11   FLEXNER AND FLEXNER,   1968(a)

H^3-puromycin was injected bilaterally into temporal areas. It was 58 days after the injection.

8.12   FLEXNER AND FLEXNER,   1968(b)

| Puromycin bitemporally | | Y-maze then reversal | to 9/10 |

Saline injected
5 days after
puromycin

| Puromycin bitemporally | mice | Y-maze | to 9/10 |

time of treatment		test	retention
Before	After		

	saline injection after puromycin		
	4-10 hr		no RA
	12-20 hr		impaired retention
	30 hr		no RA
	2-12 days		impaired retention
	30-40 days		impaired retention
	60 days		no RA
	3-18 days		no RA
	puromycin after puromycin		
	1-9 days		RA
	30-60 days		impaired retention
	puromycin after puromycin		
	2-12 days		RA

there was no RA. A retention test of relearning showed all

memory in mice without substantially altering the process which
formed in the presence of puromycin alter in a reversible way

shown that peptidyl-puromycin lasts in the brain for at least

5 hr		10 days	RA
5 hr		10 days	less RA
	4-8 min	10 days	RA impaired retention

Treatment and site   animals   task   trials

8.12   (Continued)

Saline injected   mice   Y-maze   to 9/10
5 days after
puromycin

Treatment with puromycin either before or immediately after train-
basic memory trace.

8.13   GAMBETTI, GONATAS AND FLEXNER,   1968(a)

Electron microscopic studies of mouse entorrhinal cortex injected
(a)   Abnormalities were not observed in presynaptic terminals and
      swollen mitochondria.
(b)   Dispersion of polyribosomes into single units or condensation
      ness was noted in a few neurones 7-27 hours after puromycin
(c)   Cytoplasmic aggregates of granular or amorphous material were
(d)   Mitochondria in many neuronal perikarya and dendrites were
      Mitochondria in axons, presynaptic terminals and glial cells

8.14   GAMBETTI, GONATAS AND FLEXNER,   1968(b)

Electron microscopic studies of mouse brain injected with
      Puromycin produces swelling of neuronal mitochondria. AXM
      and AXM together produce minimal swelling and a decrease of
      alone. Therefore the swelling of neuronal mitochondira in
      protein synthesis per se, but is related to a specific action
      complexes are responsible for the mitochondrial swelling.

8.15   FLEXNER AND FLEXNER,   1969(a)

Puromycin   mice   Y-maze   to 9/10
bitemporal

Saline
bifrontal
2 days after
puromycin

Saline injected into the frontal cortex 3 days after training did
area. However, saline 6 and 11 days after training did release
puromycin. Therefore, the memory trace appears widely in the
hippocampus.

time of treatment   test   retention
Before   After

          4-8 min   10 days   less RA than
                                          above

ing interfered with the process responsible for establishing the

---

bitemporally with puromycin revealed the following:
synaptic clefts; many post-synaptic dendrites or somas contained

of ribosomes into irregular aggregates with loss of distinctive-
treatment.
frequently noted within otherwise normal perikarya.
swollen, which disappeared 36 hours after the injection.
were unaltered.

antibiotics revealed that-
fails to produce swelling of neuronal mitochondria. Puromycin
peptidyl-puromycin complexes to 30% of that seen with puromycin
the presence of puromycin is not due to inhibition of cerebral
of puromycin on ribosomal protein synthesis. Peptidyl-puromycin

          1 day   6 days   RA

          saline given   after training
          3 days   8 or 11 days   RA
          6 days   11 days   no RA
          11 days   16 days   no RA

not release the puromycin blockage of memory in the hippocampal
memory in mice whose recent memory had been suppressed by
cortex despite the suppression of recent memory in the

Treatment and site   animals   task   trials

8.16 FLEXNER AND FLEXNER,   1969(b)

Puromycin neutralized   mice   Y-maze   15
with various cations
bitemporal 180-300 μg

NaOH
KOH
Ca(OH)2
MgO
Li_2O_3
T+V+F, 180 μg
KOH

Animals treated with Na^+ lose their excitability and give reliable
longer. It is possible that K^+,Li^+, Ca^{++},Mg^{++}, protect memory by
exclusion of sufficient peptidyl-puromycin to make it ineffective

8.17 FLEXNER AND FLEXNER,   1970(a)

Puromycin   mice   Y-maze   to 9/10
bitemporal 180-300 μg   (15)
substances injected (T)
4 days after puromycin
KCI
LiCl
$CaCl_2$
$MgCl_2$
Ultrafiltrate of
mouse blood serum (UF)
H_2O
sham injection

Puromycin T+V+F 180 μg
substances injected (T+V+F)
8 days after puromycin
KCl
LiCl
$CaCl_2$
$MgCl_2$
UF
H_2O

Memory was recovered after intracerebral injections of the
blood serum (UF) and of water, whereas sham injections were

time of treatment		test	retention
Before	After		

		days after training	
	1 day	6	RA
		11	no RA
		11	no RA
		8	no RA
		11	no RA
	9 days		no RA

maze performance 5 days after treatment. The other cations take
binding to anionic sites of neuronal membranes with the resultant
in blocking memory.

	24 hr	9 days	RA
			no RA
			partial RA
			no RA
			partial RA
			no RA
			no RA
			RA
	14-19 days		
		+ 16 days	
			no RA
			no RA
			no RA
			no RA
			no RA
			no RA

chlorides of several cations, of an ultrafiltrate of mouse
ineffective.

Treatment and site   animals   task   trials

8.18   FLEXNER AND FLEXNER,   1970(b)

Adrenalectomy and
puromycin   mice   Y-maze   to 9/10

T
T+V+F

T; T+V+F
T; T+V+F

T

Adrenalectomy alone had no effect on retention and puromycin after
after training had no effect on puromycin-induced suppression of
effect on puromycin-induced RA in trained mice, and adrenalectomy

The author's conclude that adrenalectomy before training modifies
makes puromycin ineffective in blocking expression of the memory.
epinephrine turnover increasing after adrenalectomy.

8.19   ROBERTS, FLEXNER AND FLEXNER,   1970

Puromycin T;180-240 μg+   mice   Y-maze   to 9/10
Reserpine 2.5 mg/kg i.p.
L-dopa 175 mg/kg i.p.
Imipramine 100 mg/kg i.p.
Tranylcypromine 25 or 12.5 mg/kg
subcutaneous
D-amphetamine 25 or 12.5 mg/kg i.p.
Saline i.p.

The reason for selection of these drugs was the similarity of the
to norepinephrine (NE) and various mescalin-like drugs. It is
to adsorption of peptidyl-puromycin to adrenergic sites and that
were chosen in an attempt to restore memory blocked by puromycin.

Reserpine releases NE from storage vesicles.
L-dopa or its metabolic products, dopamine or NE might displace
Imipramine blocks synaptic uptake by competing with NE.

time of treatment		test	retention
Before	After		

1-2 weeks

Adrenalectomy before training	Puromycin after training		retention
5 days	–		no RA
1-13 days	1 day		no RA
5-13 days	1 day		no RA
–	1 day		complete RA
1 day after	2 or 9 days		complete RA

Puromycin after training	Adrenalectomy after training		retention
1 day	2 or 7 days		RA
–	1 or 6 days		no RA

adrenalectomy was ineffective in suppressing memory. Adrenalectomy
memory. Adrenalectomy either before or after puromycin had no
alone after training had no effect on retention.

factors responsible for the expression of memory. This alteration
This could possibly be due to ACTH increases in the plasma or nor-

1 day			
8 days	18 days		partial RA
8 days	18 days		partial RA
8 days	18 days		no RA
8 days	18 days		no RA
8 days	18 days		no RA
8 days	18 days		RA

chemical structure of the O-methyl tyrosine moiety of puromycin
suggested that the blockage of memory caused by puromycin is due
these sites may be involved in the memory trace. The above drugs

puromycin bound to adrenergic receptor sites.

Treatment and site	animals	task	trials

8.19 (Continued)

Tranylcypromine is a MAO inhibitor which raises NE levels. It
re-uptake of NE.
D-Amphetamine causes marked changes in CNS possibly by mimicking
All these drugs had no effect on memory in the absence of puromycin.

8.20 FLEXNER, GAMBETTI, FLEXNER AND ROBERTS, 1971

H^3-puromycin	mice	Y-maze	to 9/10
120 μg/injection			

Peptidyl-puromycin persists for long periods in subcellular
When memory is restored by intracerebral injection of water or
puromycin concentration in the synaptosomal fraction but not in the

8.21 SEROTA, 1971

AXM 40 μg			
bitemporal	rats	Y-maze	to 6/7
		brightness	(16 to 18)
		discrimination	
		FS	

There was no evidence of AXM interference with memory consolidation,
suggested that this deficit may be due to a deficiency of

8.22 FLEXNER AND FLEXNER, 1971

ACTH (cortrophin	mice	Y-maze	to 9/10
gel) CG		FS	(10-14)
subcutaneous			
T or T+V+F			

time of treatment   test   retention
Before   After

may discharge NE and act like imipramine in interfering with

NE, inhibiting MAO, releasing NE or inhibiting re-uptake of NE.

24 hr		21 days	RA
	24 hr		
	saline 16 days	21 days	no RA

fractions of synaptosomes (nerve endings) and also in mitochondria.
tranylcypromine, there is a significant reduction in peptidyl-
mitochondrial fraction.

5 hr	24 hr	RA
5 hr	7 days	no RA

but rather a transient deficit in the retrieval phase. It was
neurotransmitters.

CG(ACTH) before training	Puromycin after training	1-2 weeks	
1 hr	-		no RA
-	(T)1 day		RA
30 min-			
3 days	(T) 1 day		only slight RA
5 days	(T) 1 day		RA
3 hr	(T+V+F) 1 day		slight RA

CG(ACTH) after training	Puromycin after training		
0-16 hr	(T) 1 day		no RA
18-20 hr	(T) 1 day		impaired retention
24 hr	(T) 1 day		RA
24 hr	Saline		no RA

| Treatment and site | animals | task | trials |

8.22   (Continued)

Treatment and site	animals	task	trials
Subcutaneous T or T+V+F	mice	Y-maze	to 9/10 (10-14)

Treatment with cortrophin gel or gelatin had no effect on
memory if CG was injected 0.5 hours to 3 days before training.
16 hours after training; 1 or more days after treatment with

8.23   SEROTA, ROBERTS AND FLEXNER,   1972

Treatment and site	animals	task	trials
AXM 40 µg bitemporal	rats	Y-maze FS	to 6/7 (16)

Metaraminol (MA) 0.3 mg i.p.

AXM + MA

AXM + MA

AXM + d-amphetamine (AMP)
2.5 mg i.p.

Metaraminol, a false transmitter which displaces norepinephrine
before testing, prevents AXM induced amnesia. D-amphetamine,
results indicate that an increase in the availability of
during consolidation, or at the time of testing protect against
reducing the available amount of norepinephrine.

(* The authors show a figure of 20% savings as good retention,

8.24   LANDE, FLEXNER AND FLEXNER,   1972

Treatment and site	animals	task
ACTH (highly purified corticotropin) subcutaneous in saline or gelatine Desglycinamide vasopressin (DGVP) 1 mg in gelatine	mice	T-maze

time of treatment		test	retention
Before	After		

Puromycin 1 day after training	CG 1-6 days after puromycin		RA

retention. Puromycin was largely ineffective in suppressing
Puromycin also failed to block memory if CG was injected up to
puromycin injection of CG failed to protect memory from puromycin.

Before	After	test	retention
5 hr		24 hr	RA
		6 days	no RA *
30 min		24 hr	no RA
AXM 5 hr		24 hr	RA
AXM 5 hr + MA 30 min		24 hr	good retention
AXM 5 hr		24 hr	RA
AXM 5 hr	MA 0-2 hr	24 hr	good retention
AXM 5 hr	MA 2.5-21.5 hr	24 hr	RA
AXM 5 hr	MA 22-23.5 hr	24 hr	no RA
	MA 2-2.5 hr	24 hr	partial RA
	MA 21.5-22 hr	24 hr	partial RA
AXM 5 hr	AMP 0-2 hr	24 hr	no RA

and inhibits its uptake given either before or after training or
injected soon after training also prevents the amnesia. The
norepihephrine at the time of training or for the first 2 hours
the amnesia. They suggest that AXM produces its effect by

which is presumably a misprint.)

ACTH before training	Puromycin after training		
20 hr	1 day		RA
1 and 20 hr	1 day		RA
5 hr	1 day		less RA
DGVP before training	Puromycin after training		
1,5& 20 hr	1 day		no RA

Treatment and site	animals	task	trials

8.24   (Continued)

	mice	T-maze	

Protection of memory from puromycin-induced amnesia was not found
"Purified Cortrophin Gel" 8.22) but DGVP was found to be effective.
corticotropin and vasopressin contamination of the commercial
previously reported (8.22).   The authors suggest that vasopressin
that the "expression" of memory becomes insensitive to puromycin.

8.25   CHAMBERLAIN, ROTHSCHILD AND GERARD,   1963

8-azaguanine	rats	conditioned	25
50 mg/kg i.p.		avoidance	
		Hebb-Williams	
		maze	

8-azaguanine prolongs the critical fixation time for the
from 45 to 70 minutes.   Animals receiving 150 or 200 mg/kg showed
receiving 50 mg/kg did not. The drug had no effect on acquisition.

8.26   AGRANOFF AND KLINGER,   1964

Puromycin	goldfish	shuttle box	20
90 µg intracranial			
Puromycin aminonucleoside			
Puromycin			to 80% correct
ECS			20

Puromycin did not affect performance or retention in naive or
80% of leucine incorporation into protein 3 hours after injection.

time of treatment   test   retention
Before   After

DGVP after Puromycin
training   after training
0 and 12 hr 2 days   no RA
24 hr   2 days   RA
-            1 day   RA

after administration of highly purified corticotropin (cf
Pressor-peptides appear to be more protective than
preparation was probably responsible for the protective effects
and its congeners modify memory consolidation in such a way

_____

4 hr   1+2 days   no RA

4 hr   1-11 days   no RA

persistence of an assymmetry after section of the spinal cord
reduced activity when placed in an activity wheel. Animals

_____

            immediate   3 days   RA
3 days   3 days   no RA

            immediate   3 days   no RA

            immediate   3 days   no RA

            immediate   3 days   RA

overtrained fish. Puromycin produced a maximum inhibition of

Treatment and site	animals	task	trials

8.27 DAVIS, BRIGHT AND AGRANOFF, 1965

| ECS | goldfish | shuttle box | 20 |

Puromycin
90 μg intracranial

The effect of puromycin resembles that of ECS extremely closely in
shock had no significant effect.

8.28 AGRANOFF, DAVIS AND BRINK, 1965

Puromycin	goldfish	shuttle box	20
intracranial			
10-50 μg			
90 or 130 μg			
170 or 210 μg			
170 μg			20
90 μg			20
90 μg			20
170 μg			
90 μg			20
170 μg			

Memory on day 1 (during training) is not disrupted by puromycin but
administering puromycin at different times during the hour follow-
puromycin and the drug acts specifically on the fixation process in
moiety) does not impair memory.

8.29 DAVIS AND AGRANOFF, 1966

Puromycin	goldfish	shuttle box	20
intracranial			
170 μg			

Time between training
and treatment in:
home tank
shuttle box

time of treatment		test	retention
Before	After		
	1-90 min	3 days	RA
	120-360 min	3 days	no RA
	1-30 min	3 days	RA
	60-360 min	3 days	no RA

the parameters of RA it produces in the goldfish. Subconvulsive

	1-5 min	3 days	no RA
	1-5 min		partial RA
	1-5 min		complete RA
	1 min	3 days	RA
	30 min		RA
	60 min		no RA
	90 min		no RA
	1-30 min	3 days	less RA
	60,90,360 min		no RA
1 min		3 days	partial RA
1 min			complete RA
	20 min	3 days	no RA
	20 min		partial RA

memory on day 4 can be completely or partially blocked by
ing trial 20 on day 1. Short term memory is unaffected by
which long term memory is formed. Methyl tyrosine (a puromycin

	1 min	1-6 hr	no RA
	1 min	1 day	partial RA
	1 min	2-3 days	complete RA
	60 min	3 days	no RA
	60 min	3 days	RA

Treatment and site   animals   task   trials

8.29 (Continued)

The RA develops over 6-24 hours after training and puromycin.
the period where puromycin can interfere with memory formation.
initiate the fixation process.

8.30 BRINK, DAVIS AND AGRANOFF, 1966

Intraperitoneally injected H^3-leucine is incorporated into
When puromycin or AXM is injected intracranially, there is a
which lasts for days. The inhibitory effect of Actinomycin D on
after injection.

8.31 AGRANOFF, DAVIS AND BRINK, 1966

Acetoxycycloheximide   goldfish   shuttle box   20
0.1 μg intracranial

8.32 AGRANOFF, DAVIS, CASOLA AND LIM, 1967

Actinomycin D   goldfish   shuttle box   20
2 μg intracranial

AXM
0.2 μg intracranial

Actinomycin D inhibits DNA mediated RNA synthesis to 65% inhibition.
is not blocked for several hours.

8.33 CASOLA, LIM, DAVIS AND AGRANOFF, 1968

Cytosine   goldfish   shuttle box   20
arabinoside
100 μg intracranial

AXM
0.2 μg intracranial

Cytosine arabinosine produces 95% inhibition of DNA synthesis, thus
was no deficit in learning when AXM was given before training, but

time of treatment		test	retention
Before	After		

Keeping the goldfish in the shuttle box after training prolongs
The removal from the training environment serves as a trigger to

goldfish-brain protein; the maximum being reached in 4 hours.
rapid onset of inhibition of incorporation of labelled leucine
protein synthesis occurs more slowly and becomes maximal a day

1 min		3 days	RA
6 hr		3 days	no RA
1 min		3 days	RA
1 hr			partial RA
3 hr			no RA
1 min		3 days	RA
1 hr			RA
3 hr			no RA

Actinomycin D blocked memory at a time when protein synthesis

4 hr		3 days	no RA
	1 min		no RA
	24 hr		no RA
4 hr		3 days	RA
	1 min		more RA
	24 hr		no RA

the formation of memory does not depend on DNA synthesis. There
there was RA 3 days later.

Treatment and site	animals	task	trials

8.34 DAVIS, 1968

(1) Puromycin   goldfish   shuttle box   30
    intracranial
    pre-injection time (intertrial environment I.T.E.)
    in home tank
    170 μg

    210 μg

(2) I.T.E. in dark
    shuttle box
    no injection

    puromycin 170 μg

(3) I.T.E. in lighted
    shuttle box
    no injection

    puromycin 170 μg

(4) I.T.E. in home
    tank with water
    from shuttle box
    no injection
    puromycin 170 μg

Memory fixation was suppressed when fish were kept in the inter-
shuttle box greatly impaired retention of the avoidance habit.
not when the overhead light was turned on (normally turned on to

It was postulated that arousal or excitement evoked during train-
arousal after training. Substances released into water by the
Visual stimuli are the primary agents in postponing fixation.

8.35 DAVIS AND KLINGER, 1969

Intracranial injections   goldfish   shuttle box   30
I.T.E.*
I.T.E.
I.T.E.-KC1
I.T.E.-puromycin
I.T.E.- ECS
I.T.E.- AXM

(* see page 422)

time of treatment Before	After	test	retention
	1-90 min	3 days	RA *
	3-6 hr		no RA
	1 min	3 days	complete RA
	6 hr		no RA
	(1-90 min)	3 days	normal retention
	(3.5-48 hr)		poor retention
	1 min-48 hr	3 days	RA*
			(equal to RA* at 1 min)
	(90 min)	3 days	normal retention
	90 min	3 days	RA*
	(90 min)	3 days	normal retention
	90 min	3 days	RA*

trial conditions up to 3.5 hours, longer intervals in the
Fixation occurred when S was removed from the shuttle box and
remove fish).

ing inhibits fixation and stimuli in the shuttle box maintain
fish do not play a role in suppressing memory fixation (4)

		test	retention
		3 days	normal retention
		7 days	normal retention
	24 hr	3 days	RA
		3 days	no RA
		7 days	moderate RA
		3 days	no RA
		7 days	moderate RA
		3 days	no RA
		7 days	no RA

Treatment and site	animals	task	trials

8.35 (Continued)

| Intracranial injections | goldfish | shuttle box | 30 |

Puromycin 130 μg
AXM 0.2 μg
KC1 600 μg

* I.T.E. fish were returned to the inter-trial environment in the
of drug 24 hours after training.

Amnesia can be obtained 24 hours after training if the fish are
injection.

8.36 AGRANOFF, 1970

| AXM 0.2 μg | goldfish | shuttle box | 20 |
| intracranial | | | |

AXM, 3 treatments

KC1 600 μg
intracranial

KC1 and AXM

Memory formation in goldfish is susceptible to KC1 for longer than
also much faster for KC1 than antibiotics. It was hypothesized that
term memory as well as for the formation of long-term memory. This
following antibiotics. It was suggested that short-term memory
supported with repeated injections of AXM. AXM also appears to
temporally. The results support the concept that STM is converted
and puromycin plus AXM in mice whose memory is susceptible to
synthesis obtained with large doses of AXM may have prevented STM
an amnesic effect.

8.37 LIM, BRINK AND AGRANOFF, 1970

| Intracranial | goldfish | shuttle box | 20 |
| AXM 0.2 μg | | | |

Puromycin 180 μg
AXM and puromycin
Puromycin
AXM and puromycin

AXM did not protect against the effect of puromycin. Controls were
of the drugs, and sickness alone could not have accounted for the

time of treatment		test	retention
Before	After		
	24 hr	7 days	no RA
	24 hr	7 days	no RA
	24 hr	3 days	no RA

shuttle box for 5 minutes (with no shock) before the injection

replaced in the I.T.E. for a brief period just prior to

	immediate	4-6 hr	no RA
		1 day	no RA
		2 days	RA
		3 days	complete RA
	0,24,48 hr	3 days	partial RA
	immediate	4-6 hr	RA
		1 day	complete RA
		3 days	complete RA
	immediate	1 day	RA
		3 days	complete RA

to antibiotics. The short-term memory decay following KCl is
protein synthesis might be required for the decay of short-
could account for the prolonged decay of short-term memory
remains until normal protein synthesis is restored. This was
retard the KCl-mediated short-term memory decay, but only
to LTM. This may explain the reported lack of effect of AXM
puromycin alone. The severe, prolonged block of protein
from decaying; retraining in this circumstance would not reveal

	1 min	7 days	RA
	1 min	7 days	RA
	1 min	7 days	more RA
	24 hr	7 days	no RA
	24 hr	7 days	slight RA

carried out for possible sickness resulting from the injection
behavioural deficit.

Treatment and site	animals	task	trials

8.38 GOLUB, CHEAL AND DAVIS, 1972

Puromycin, 170 μg intracranial	goldfish	operant conditioning appetitive	well-established response pattern

(see ECS table 1 for results with ECS (1.112)).
Intracranial administration of puromycin immediately following a
established operant response.

8.39 SCHOEL AND AGRANOFF, 1972

Puromycin intracranial 195 μg 62% inhibition	goldfish	conditioned heart rate deceleration	20
			10

Puromycin did not block retention of conditioned cardiac

8.40 BARONDES AND JARVIK, 1964

Actinomycin D intracerebral 20 μg	mice	shock for crossing 2 plates	1± 1.6

The injection of Actinomycin D produced decreased activity and

8.41 COHEN AND BARONDES, 1966

Actinomycin D 60 μg intracerebral T+V+F	mice	Y-maze	to 9/10
		2 choice T-maze	to 9/10

The effect of Actinomycin D on memory at intervals greater than
No specific role for RNA synthesis in brain function was

time of treatment		test	retention
Before	After		
	immediate	7,8,9 days	no effect
	19.5 hr	7,8,9 days	no effect

training session did not disrupt the performance of a well-

	immediate	2 days	no RA
	4 hrs	2 days	no RA
30 min		3 days	no RA
	24 hr	3 days	no RA
	immediate	3 days	no RA
	24 hr	3 days	no RA

deceleration in this experiment.

---

4 hr		1-3 hr	no RA

subsequent illness, followed by death 48 hours later.

4.5 hr		1 hr	no RA
		4 hr	no RA
		2 hr	no RA

4 hours after learning was unobtainable because of illness.
demonstrated.

Treatment and site	animals	task	trials

8.42 BARONDES AND COHEN, 1966

| Puromycin | mice | Y-maze | to 9/10 |
| bitemporal 180 μg | | | (18) |

Frontal 180 μg
Temporal 180 μg

At a time when animals have forgotten what they learned 3 hours
is retained.

8.43 COHEN, ERVIN AND BARONDES, 1966

Hippocampal electrical activity was recorded 5 hours after 200 μg
strikingly abnormal - very low amplitude and no rhythmic activity.
200 μg of cydoheximide were indistinguishable from mice injected

8.44 COHEN AND BARONDES, 1967(a)

Within the first few hours after intracerebral injection of
showed frequent seizure activity which was not apparent from
less frequent seizure activity.

The susceptibility to pentylenetetrazol seizures was observed in
puromycin were more prone to developing seizures 5 min, 1,5 and 24
plus CXM or hydrolyzed puromycin.

| Diphenylhydantoin | mice | T-maze | to 3/4 |
| (DPH) and puromycin | | | |

puromycin
DPH and AXM

DPH protects memory from the effect of puromycin, but does not
may be due to occult seizures.

8.45 BARONDES AND COHEN, 1967(a)

Puromycin:	mice	T-maze	to 9/10
T+V+F, 450 μg			
bitemporal 120 μg			

CXM:
T+V+F, 450 μg
T   200 μg
T+V+F, 450 μg
T+V+F, 450 μg

| time of treatment | | test | retention |
Before	After		
5 hr		15-45 min	no RA
		90 min	slight RA
		3 hr	RA
5 hr		3 hr	no RA
8 hr		15 min	no RA

before, their capacity for learning and "short-term" memory

of puromycin was injected bitemporally. Records obtained were
Records obtained from mice injected in the same manner with
with saline alone.

puromycin electrical recordings from the hippocampal region
observation of behaviour. With cycloheximide there was far

the presence of various drugs. Mice injected with 200 µg of
hours after injection than with saline, 20 µg AXM; puromycin

5 hr		3 hr	partial RA
5 hr		6 hr	more RA
5 hr		6 hr	RA

prevent AXM induced amnesia. The puromycin effect on memory

5 hr		3 hr	RA
5 hr		70 hr	complete RA
5 hr		3 hr	no RA
5 hr		70 hr	no RA
5 hr		13 hr	no RA
	1 hr	9 hr	no RA

Treatment and site	animals	task	trials

8.45   (Continued)

AXM   360 μg   mice   T-maze   to 9/10
T+V+F
ECS

Puromycin T.200 μg
Puromycin plus CXM   T,
50,100,150 or 200 μg

Cycloheximide inhibited cerebral protein synthesis more
after injection, but did not produce RA.   Therefore, puromycin
with synthesis of a protein required for memory storage.   The
the amnesic effects of puromycin.

8.46   BARONDES AND COHEN,   1967(b)

AXM bitemporal
20 μg   mice   T-maze   to 3/4 (6)

120 μg
20 μg

120 μg   to 9/10 (16)
                                                               to 3/4 (6)

2 injections of 20 μg

Actinomycin D   to 3/4 (6)
20 μg
ECS

There was no inhibition of protein synthesis at time of training
produced by AXM would be present.   There was no effect on retention.
synthesis if necessary had occurred before the drug diffused
prior to training is necessary to demonstrate its amnesic effect.
Increasing the dose of AXM does not abolish the amnesic effect

The impairment of performance observed in mice trained while under
but rather to some effect of the drug on memory storage processes.
the ECS study it appears that long term processes apparently are
STM persists for between 3 and 6 hours.

time of treatment		test	retention
Before	After		
5 hr		3 hr	no RA
	15 min	3 hr	no RA
5 hr		3 hr	RA
5 hr		3 hr	less RA decreasing with increasing dose of CXM

extensively than puromycin in the interval between 5 and 8 hours
effects 3 hours after training may not be due to interference
addition of cycloheximide to the puromycin solution diminished

18 hr		1 day	no RA
5 hr			RA
	1 min		no RA
	1 min	4 days	no RA
	4 days	5 days	no RA
5 hr		3 hr	no RA
5 hr		6hr-6 weeks	RA
5 hr		4 and 7 days	no RA
5 hr		1-7 days	RA
5 hr		3 days	no RA
5 hr	4 days	4 days & 5 hr after 2nd injection	RA
5 hr			no RA
	15 min		no RA

when AXM was given 18 hours before, but any abnormalities
With injection of AXM immediately after training, protein
significantly to interfere. The administration of the drug
Overtraining can overcome the amnesic effect of the drug.
with brief training.

the influence of AXM is not due to "state-dependent learning"
Nor is it due to systemic illness produced by the drug. From
established within 15 minutes of training, yet retrieval of

Treatment and site	animals	task	trials

8.47   COHEN AND BARONDES,   1967(b)

AXM   mice   T-maze   to 9/10
bitemporal 120 μg
(95% inhibition)   to 3/4

AXM
subcutaneous
20 μg   to 3/4
(79% inhibition)
bitemporal 20 μg   to 3/4

        120 μg

Prolonged repetition of the correct solution to a task may obscure
highly potent, may not completely obliterate a critical process in

8.48   BARONDES AND COHEN,   1968(a)

AXM 240 μg   mice   T-maze   to 5/6 (13)
subcutaneous

There was 90% inhibition of cerebral protein synthesis 10-15 min
protein synthesis during training or within a short period of time
the subsequent illness which the drug produces is not.

8.49   COHEN AND BARONDES,   1968(a)

AXM 20 μg   mice   T-maze   to 5/6(14.6)
bitemporal   light/dark
                                            discrimination

                                                          to 9/10
                                                          (22.6)

| time of treatment | | test | retention |
Before	After		
5 hr		3 hr	no RA
		1+7 days	no RA
5 hr		3 hr	RA
		1+7 days	no RA
5 hr		1 day	no RA
18 hr		1 day	no RA
	1 min	1 day	slight RA
	1 min	4 days	no RA

the amnesic effect of a pharmacological agent which, although
an extremely redundant nervous system.

| time of treatment | | test | retention |
Before	After		
30 min		3 hr	no RA
30 min		6 hr	RA
	1 min	6.5 hr	RA
	30 min	7 hr	no RA
5 hr		7 days	RA
30 min		7 days	RA
5 min		7 days	RA
0 min		7 days	less RA
	0 min	7 days	less RA
	5 min	7 days	less RA
	30 min	7 days	no RA
	24 hr	7 days	no RA

after subcutaneous injection of AXM. Inhibition of cerebral
thereafter, is correlated with the amnesic effect of AXM, whereas

| time of treatment | | test | retention |
Before	After		
5 hr		3 hr	no RA
5 hr		6 hr	RA
5 hr		24 hr	RA
5 hr		7 days	RA
5 hr		1 day	RA
5 hr		7 days	RA

Treatment and site	animals	task	trials

8.49   (Continued)

AXM 20 μg bitemporal	mice	T-maze light/dark discrimination	to 15/16 (36.3) to 5/6

95% inhibition of protein synthesis was maintained for at least
to simpler task where no RA occurred, the light-dark discrimination
extensive training is given; but very prolonged training can

8.50   COHEN AND BARONDES,   1968(b)

CXM subcutaneous 500 μg	mice	appetitive T-maze	to 3/4(9)

Between 30 min+1 hr after injection there was 90% inhibition of
sustained inhibition of cerebral protein synthesis than AXM. This
interference with cerebral protein synthesis which could impair

8.51   BARONDES AND COHEN,   1968(b)

CXM 0.12 mg/kg	mice	T-maze	to 5/6
CXM			non-contingent FS (NCFS) after training
CXM and d-amphetamine (A) or corticosteroids (C) 1 mg/kg			

time of treatment		test	retention
Before	After		
5 hr		1 day	no RA
30 min		7 days	slight RA
	1 min	7 days	no RA

8 hours and established 3 hours after injection of AXM. Compared
task is more susceptible to the amnesic effect of AXM even when
antagonize its amnesic effect.

30 min		3 hr	no RA
30 min		6 hr	RA
30 min		7 days	RA
	1 min	7 days	less RA
	30 min	7 days	no RA
	24 hr	7 days	no RA

cerebral protein synthesis. Cycloheximide produces less
allows less time for the possible development of a non-specific
behaviour.

30 min		3 hr	no RA
30 min		6 hr	RA
30 min		7 days	RA

CXM	NCFS		
30 min	3 hr	7 days	no RA
30 min	6 hr	7 days	RA

CXM	A or C		
30 min	3 hr	6 hr	partial RA
30 min	3 hr	7 days	partial RA
30 min	6 hr	9 hr	RA
30 min	6 hr	7 days	RA
30 min	7 days	7 days + 3 hr	RA

A or C			
30 min		7 days	RA

Treatment and site	animals	task	trials

8.51 (Continued)

Treatment and site	animals	task	trials
AXM 8 mg/kg and amphetamine (A)	mice	T-maze	to 5/6
CXM 0.12 mg/kg and amphetamine (A)			
CXM, amphetamine (A) and pentobarbital (P) 40 mg/kg			
CXM and amphetamine (A)		T-maze appetitive	

CXM administered subcutaneously produced 95% inhibition of
Long-term memory was not formed despite marked recovery of the
term memory remained. A single FS without any additional
lead to the establishment of LTM. This is probably associated
is given at a time when cerebral protein synthesis inhibition is
STM has terminated is ineffective. The re-establishment of
Sedation obliterates the action of amphetamine. The inhibitors
producing sedation. If the establishment of "long-term" memory
administered prior to training, the LTM will not subsequently
STM concurrent with marked recovery of the capacity for cerebral
will lead to the development of LTM. Therefore, cognitive
protein synthesis capacity are insufficient for the production
specifically direct the establishment of LTM also seems

8.52 ROSENBAUM, COHEN AND BARONDES, 1968

Treatment and site	animals	task	trials
Saline bitemporal	mice	T-maze light-dark discrimination	to 9/10
Puromycin 100 μg			
AXM 10 μg			
Saline Puromycin 100 μg			

| time of treatment | | test | retention |
Before	After		
AXM 30 min	AXM + A 2.5 hr	7 days	RA
CXM 30 min	CXM + A 2.5 hr	7 days	RA
CXM 30 min	A + P 3 hr	7 days	RA
CMX 30 min	A	7 days	RA
30 min	3 hr	7 days	partial RA
30 min	6 hr	7 days	RA

protein synthesis within 30 minutes and 19% at 3 to 3.5 hours.
capacity for cerebral protein synthesis at a time when short-
discriminative training, if given while STM persisted, could
with arousal. If amphetamine (to produce a "state of arousal")
slight and STM remains, LTM is formed. Administration after
protein synthesis inhibition antagonized the amphetamine effect.
of protein synthesis do not antagonize the amphetamine effect by
is prevented by inhibitors of cerebral protein synthesis
develop spontaneously despite persistence of the information in
protein synthesis. However, manipulations producing "arousal"
information acquired from training and an intact cerebral
of LTM. An appropriate state of arousal which appears to
necessary.

Before	After	test	retention
	1 day	8 days	normal retention
	1 day + saline 3 days	8 days	normal retention
	1 day	8 days	RA
	1 day + saline 3 days	8 days	partial RA
	7 days	14 days	no RA
5 hr		8 days	RA
5 hr	saline 2 days	8 days	RA
	1 day	8 days	no RA
	1 day	8 days	normal retention
	1 day	8 days	RA
	1 day + saline 3 days	8 days	no RA

Treatment and site   animals   task   trials

8.52   (Continued)

The puromycin effect when injected one day after training is
injection of puromycin 7 days after training is ineffective.
not effective 1 day after training. This work with puromycin and
and shows the AXM effect is not influenced by saline injections.

8.53 GELLER, ROBUSTELLI, BARONDES, COHEN AND JARVIK, 1969

CXM 150 mg/kg
subcutaneous   mice   step-through   1
                                        PA

There was 95% inhibition of protein synthesis in the 30 minutes
longer gradient than observed with CXM in T-maze run for water
RA was not complete. They suggested that under conditions in
synthesis was enough to permit some retention. Here the task was
carry much of the information necessary for its successful

8.54 SQUIRE AND BARONDES, 1970

Actinomycin D   mice   2 choice
temporal   discrimination to 2
1 or 30 μg   escape   successive
1 μg frontal   correct
                                                        (3.4)

They do not believe the loss of memory was due to a lack of RNA
cerebral RNA synthesis by 14% or 18% 3 hr or 27 hr after injection.

8.55 SQUIRE, GELLER AND JARVIK, 1970

CXM 150 mg/kg
subcutaneous   mice   measured   10 min
                                        activity   session

                                        habituation   10 min
                                        of exploratory
                                        activity

                                                        5 min
                                                        1 min
                                                        10 min

| time of treatment | | test | retention |
| Before | After | | |

antagonized by intracerebral injection of saline. Temporal
Saline has no effect on the amnesia produced by AXM. AXM is
saline confirms that done by Flexner et. al. (8.12, 8.15, 8.17)

30 min		7 days	RA
	immediate		RA
	10 min		RA
	30 min		less RA
	2 hr		no RA
	6 hr		no RA

after injection, this falls to 54% 3 hours later. There was a
reinforcement, and with AXM in a discriminated avoidance task.
which animals received prolonged training, the remaining protein
very simple and the 5% protein synthesis may be sufficient to
retention.

3 hr		1 day	RA
	1 day	2 days	RA
	7 days	8 days	no RA
	1 day	2 days	no RA

synthesis. The low dose of Actinomycin D inhibited whole
Actinomycin D did not effect acquisition.

0-30 min			
45min-3 hr			
24 hr			
10 min		2 days	no RA
0 min			no RA
	0 min		no RA
	0 min	2 days	no RA
	0 min		no learning
	0 min	4 days	no RA
		7 days	no RA
		14 days	no RA

Treatment and site   animals   task   trials

8.55   (Continued)

The activity was increased during 0-30 min after CXM injection
later was normal. CXM had no measurable effect on the habituation
forgetting of the habituated response occurred at the same rate
habituation is not vulnerable to cycloheximide.

8.56   SEGAL, SQUIRE AND BARONDES, 1971

CXM 200 μg   mice   T-maze   to 5/6
intracerebral   and
                                         activity
                                         measures

1SO-CXM   to 5/6

CXM when injected subcutaneously or intracerebrally produced an
followed by decreased activity 1 to 4 hours after injection.
effects on activity but it did not produce inhibition of cerebral
antagonize the amnesic effect of CXM (Amphetamine 1 mg/kg 45 min and
activity.   Effects of CXM on activity do not appear to be

8.57   GELLER, ROBUSTELLI AND JARVIK, 1970

CXM 150 mg/kg   mice   step-through   1
subcutaneous   FS
                                        delay of FS
                                        0 sec
                                        30 sec
                                        60 sec
                                        120 sec
                                        240 sec

Delay of punishment was used to obtain conditioned responses of
greater amnesic effect upon the weaker conditioned responses
a proactive effect with the weaker conditioned responses.

8.58   GELLER, ROBUSTELLI AND JARVIK, 1971

CXM subcutaneous   mice   step-through   1
150 mg/kg   FS
Detention in
apparatus for 10 min

CXM
Saline
CXM
Saline

time of treatment		test	retention
Before	After		

and depressed from 1 to 3 hours after. Activity 24 hours
of activity resulting from 10 minutes of exploration. The
with either saline or CXM. The results suggest exploratory

4 hr		3 days	RA

4 hr		3 days	no RA

initial hyperactivity up to 30-40 min after injection, this was
Isocycloheximide injected intracerebrally produced identical
protein synthesis or amnesia. Amphetamine, in doses that can
3 hrs after CXM), does not antagonize the effect of CXM on
responsible for its amnesic action.

	20 sec	1 week	partial RA
	20 sec		partial RA
	20 sec		partial RA
	20 sec		RA
	20 sec		RA

different strengths. CXM given immediately after training had a
obtained with the longer delays of punishment. CXM did not show

	10 min	1 week	RA

	10 min	1 week	more RA
	10 min	1 week	RA
	10 min	1 week	normal retention
	60 min	1 week	no RA
	60 min	1 week	normal retention

Treatment and site	animals	task	trials

8.58   (Continued)

Detention- 10 min	mice	step-through FS	1

Detention- 10 min after treatment

Detention- 10 min before treatment

Detention- 60 min

Detention did not prolong the cycloheximide susceptible phase of provoke a cycloheximide induced amnesia at a time after training summation of the amnesic effects of the two treatments occurred without effect upon the detention experience itself.

8.59   SQUIRE AND BARONDES,   1972

CXM 120 mg/kg subcutaneous 95% inhibition 15-45 min after injection	mice	2 choice object discrimination FS	15 21 27
			15
			21
			15
			21
			15
			21

CXM did not affect acquisition of the discrimination task when training for an additional 21 trials revealed an impairment in the explained by sickness or by known side-effects of CXM on activity. Recovery from CXM induced amnesia seen at 24 hours occurs and

| time of treatment | | test | retention |
Before	After		
SAL –	10 min		RA
CXM –	10 min		most RA
SAL –	60 min		RA
CXM –	60 min		RA
SAL –	60 min		less RA
CXM –	60 min		less RA
SAL –	60 min		most RA
CXM –	60 min		RA

memory formation nor did reexposure to the conditioning apparatus
when, under normal circumstances, none could be demonstrated. A
only at a time when both were effective alone. Cycloheximide was

30 min		24 hr	RA
30 min			RA
30 min			no RA
30 min		10 sec	no RA
		15 min	no RA
		1 hr	partial RA
		3 hr	RA
		24 hr	RA
30 min		10 sec	no RA
		3 hr	partial RA
		6 hr	partial RA
		12 hr	RA
		24 hr	RA
	30 min	4 hr	no RA
		25 hr	no RA
	30 min	25 hr	no RA
30 min		1,2 days	RA
		3,5 days	no RA
30 min		1 day	RA
		2 days	partial RA
		3,7 days	no RA

training was conducted for 15 or 21 trials. However, further
performance of CXM treated mice. This impairment cannot be
Extending training protects mice from the amnesic effects of CXM.
appears to be complete after 3 days.

Treatment and site   animals   task   trials

8.59   (Continued)

The authors suggest that these results are consistent with the
  (i)   a short-term process that is independent of protein synthesis,
 (ii)   a long-term process that is dependent on protein synthesis,
(iii)   a slow-developing memory storage that becomes apparent
        during the days after training.

8.60   GOLDSMITH,   1967

| Actinomycin D | rats | skinner box | 1 |
| intracerebral 25 μg | | +/- footshock | |

Actinomycin D seemed to have produced a change in the punishing
performance but not latency of first bar press. There was no
recovery or non-recovery of bar pressing in experimental group.
the degree of RNA suppression and the extent of the deficit in

---

8.61   KRYLOV,   1967

RNAse	mice	T-maze	no. to
subdural		conditioned	re-establish
intraperitoneal		defence	conditioned
		reflex of	reflex
		running	

DNAse
Actinomycin C

RNAse
DNAse
Actinomycin C

Neither subdural nor intraperitoneal RNAse administration affected
Intraperitoneal administration has a weaker effect possibly due to
brain. Drugs administered before training had less effect the
occurred following the administration of RNAse. The content of
DNAse and Actinomycin C under these conditions. (Actinomycin C
disintegration in the higher levels of the brain effects the
connections and inhibits new conditioning (ii) DNA disintegration
destroy the earlier established conditioned reflexes, but inhibits
disturb the main processes of metabolism. Thus, the function of

---

time of treatment		test	retention
Before	After		

operation of three processes of memory storage:

---

24 hr		24 hr	RA in half of the animals

consequences of footshock but not an amnesia for it. It inhibited
consistent relationship between the degree of RNA suppression and
With the non-suppressed group there was no relationship between
passive avoidance.

---

	x	1/day	suppressed
	x	1/day	suppressed
	x	1/day	normal retention
	x	1/day	normal retention
x			
x			acquisition
x			delayed

the general condition, motor activity or growth of the mice.
some decomposition before it reached the higher level of the
older the animal. Reduction in RNA levels in cerebral cortex
RNA in the brain was only slightly altered under the action of
inhibits RNA synthesis on the DNA matrix). Therefore, (i) RNA
disappearance of the earlier established conditioned
and blockage of the RNA synthesis on the DNA matrix does not
new conditioning. The possibility exists that these agents
formation and storage is disturbed.

Treatment and site	animals	task	trials

8.62 POTTS AND BITTERMAN, 1967

Puromycin 170 μg intracranial (repeated treatments)	goldfish	discriminated avoidance in shuttle box	
			20/day on 6 training days, 1 week apart
			90 trials in one session
			90

The performance of goldfish given puromycin immediately after each
later. There was no difference to start with. These results would
conditioned fear. (Note: repeated injections of puromycin are
consolidation does begin before the animal is removed from the
this with overtraining.) The drug does not depress performance.
interferes with consolidation of conditioned fear.

8.63 SHASHOUA, 1968

Puromycin 120 μg	goldfish	new swimming pattern	no.

The change in RNA base ratios observed with normal learning did
controls and injected fish learned at the same rate indicated

---

8.64 WARBURTON AND RUSSELL, 1968

8-Azaguanine 136 or 272 μg intra-ventricular	rats	skinner box- change in schedules	no.

The transition to the new schedule of training was slowed down in
higher dose suggested that it was due to lack of protein synthesis.

---

time of treatment		test	retention
Before	After		
	1 min	daily	slow improvement
	24 hr		normal retention
	1 min	1 week	no RA
	1 min	3 days	RA

session improved but less than fish given puromycin 24 hours
be obtained if puromycin interfered with the consolidation of
reported to lose their effectiveness). They suggest that
training situation. (Agranoff and Klinger - (8.26) also found
They claim that this is further evidence that puromycin

| 1.5 hr | | 22 hr | RA |

not occur with prior injection of puromycin. The fact that
that the changes were not due to stress or work.

| before | | for next 3 hours | slow |

animals treated with 8-azaguanine. The greater effect with the

---

Treatment and site	animals	task	trials

8.65 MAYOR, 1969

Puromycin intracerebral 180 µg 720 µg	Japanese quail	skinner box discrimination appetitive	to 90% correct
Puromycin aminouncleoside (PANS) 360 µg AXM 36 µg puromycin		reversal of above experiment	
Puromycin 720 µg		trained subjects	

The lack of effect of PANS suggested that the puromycin effect was
Generalized inhibition could not be responsible for the memory
sensory, motor or motivational factors - it seems to act on memory.
electrical activity or by occult seizures. High doses of puromycin
inhibited memory, the basis of its effect appears more likely to be
quantitative inhibition of macromolecular synthesis or by some non-

---

8.66 NAKAJIMA, 1969

Actinomycin D 1 µg hippocampus cortex	rats	T-maze	to 7/8

Spike discharges rather than suppression of macromolecular synthesis

---

8.67 REINIS, 1969

Extract of puromycin-treated brains from untrained mice, i.p.	trained mice		no.

After the injection of the extract of puromycin affected brains, the
decreased almost to the performance of untrained animals. It was
puromycin injection were able to change the activity of nerve cells

| time of treatment | | test | retention |
Before	After		
5 min	3 days	RA	
5 min		RA	
5 min	3 days	no RA	
5 min	3 days	no RA	
5 min		better performance than controls	
1 day	5 hr	no RA	
1 day	3 days	no RA	

not related to chemical structure of protein synthesis.
deficit. Puromycin apparently does not have a toxic effect on
Puromycin does not act on performance by the suppression of
and AXM inhibited RNA and protein synthesis. Since only puromycin
mediated by the action of peptidyl-puromycin rather than by the
specific toxic action.

| 4 days | | 1 day | deficit in acquisition |
| 4 days | | 1 day | no deficit |

appear to be responsible for the deficits.

| x | | 24 hr | "RA" |

performance of the trained mice in the experimental space
suggested that defective polypeptides - pathological products of
- probably a peripheral action.

Treatment and site	animals	task	trials

8.68 REINIS, 1970

| Hydroxylamine 0.5M intracranial | mice | appetitive alimentary conditioning | 150 |

Hydroxylamine acts specifically on activated, derepressed DNA, defective protein is produced.

8.69 REINIS, 1971(a)

| Hydroxylamine 0.5M intracranial | mice | alimentary conditioning | 150 |

| Hydroxylamine 0.5M intracranial | | step-through PA | 1 |

Hydroxylamine injected up to 3 weeks after training on a multiple possible in all groups. Learning of a one-trial task, parallel injection of hydroxylamine.

8.70 REINIS, 1971(b)

| 5-iodouracil intracranial | mice | step-through PA | 1 |

| 2,6-diaminopurine intracranial | | | |

These two antimetabolites do not change motor coordination and hours after acquisition (i.e. at one day) the differences were not

time of treatment		test	retention
Before	After		
2 weeks		1 day and 2 weeks	no RA
1 week			no RA
1 day			no RA
	after 15th session	1 day	RA
	"	1 week	more RA
	"	2 weeks	complete RA

leading to misreading of the code in producing RNA and hence a

4 hr		2 weeks after injection	RA
1 week			RA
2 weeks			most RA
3 weeks			less RA
4,6, & 8 weeks			no RA cf to controls injected- with saline
4 hr-8 weeks		2 days	no RA

trial learning task interferes with retention. Retraining was with the other testing sessions was not affected by previous

48-24 hr		2-7 days	no RA
2 hr		2-7 days	RA
	1 hr	2-7 days	RA
48 hr		2-7 days	no RA
	2-24 hr	2-7 days	no RA
24-2 hr		2-7 days	RA
	1 hr	2-7 days	RA

only slightly decrease exploratory activity. (When tested 24 statistically significant).

Treatment and site	animals	task	trials

8.71   SWANSON, McGAUGH AND COTMAN,   1969

| AXM bilateral | mice | step-through PA | 1 |

The retention tested 2 hours after learning was greatest for the
AXM produced less retention that the other times. The RA increased
trial AXM showed less RA than the pre- or immediately post-trial

---

8.72   HUBER AND LONGO,   1970

| Puromycin intracranial 200 μg | goldfish | shuttle box | 60 |
| | | | 160 |

The time of injection did not alter the amnesic effect of

8.73   QUARTERMAIN AND McEWAN,   1970

CXM 3 mg subcutaneous	mice	step-through FS intensity 1.6mA	1
		0.16mA	
Saline 0.85%		1.6mA 0.16mA	

| time of treatment | | test | retention |
Before	After		
5 hr		2 hr	slight RA
2 hr		2 hr	no RA
	immediate	2 hr	no RA
5-2 hr		6-14 days	RA
	immediate	6-14 days	RA
	15 min-18 hr	2 hr-14 days	less RA

immediately post-trial AXM. 5 hours pre-trial injection with
as testing was delayed from 2 hours to 2 days. Delayed post-
AXM groups tested at the same post-trial interval.

---

	0 hr	3 days	RA
	24 hr	3 days	RA
	48 hr	3 days	RA
	0 hr	3 days	RA

puromycin and with overtraining there was still amnesia.

---

30 min		1 min	no RA
		5 min	no RA
		6 hr	no RA
		24 hr	RA
		48 hr	no RA
30 min		1 min	RA
		5 min	RA
		6 hr	RA
		24 hr	RA
		48 hr	RA
30 min		1 min-48 hr	good retention
30 min		1 min-48 hr	moderate retention

Treatment and site	animals	task	trials
8.73 (Continued)			
CXM 3mg	mice	step-through FS intensity 1.6mA	1
		0.16mA	
CXM 3mg		1.6mA	
		0.16mA	

The aim of this study was to investigate whether habits learned
different rates. With high intensity footshock there was no RA
recovery occurred at 48 hours. Amnesia was found at all testing
memory 6 hours after training with high footshock intensity. With
gradient comparable to that seen with both groups tested at 24

RA present at 24 hours but not at 6 hours for high intensity

^{3}H-leucine studies showed maximum inhibition of protein synthesis

The authors suggest that these results raise the possibility that
necessary for information retrieval rather than exclusively

| time of treatment | | test | retention |
Before	After		
30 min		6 hr	no RA
	immediate		no RA
	1 hr		no RA
	2 hr		no RA
	5.5 hr		no RA
30 min		6 hr	RA
	immediate		RA
	1 hr		RA
	2 hr		RA
	5.5 hr		no RA
30 min		24 hr	most RA
	immediate		most RA
	1 hr		most RA
	2 hr		less RA
	5.5 hr		no RA
30 min		24 hr	most RA
	immediate		most RA
	1 hr		RA
	2 hr		less RA
	5.5 hr		no RA

under different shock levels go into long-term storage at
up to 6 hours but transient RA at 24 hours. Spontaneous
times with the low intensity footshock. There was no loss of
low intensity footshock tested at 6 hours there was a temporal
hours.

footshock.

30 min after CXM, which disappeared over 6 hours.

protein synthesis inhibitors may be interfering with mechanisms
preventing the consolidation of long-term memory.

Treatment and site	animals	task	trials

8.74 QUARTERMAIN, McEWAN AND AZMITIA, 1970

CXM 3 mg subcutaneous	mice	step-through PA (0.16 mAFS)	1

2nd injection of
CXM before T_1
before RS

T_1 and T_2 = retention tests, T_1 - 24 hours after training, T_2 - 24
apparatus) 1 hour after the first retention test T_1 restored the
recovery occurred if T_1 was omitted. Footshock in another
interaction of FS and CXM. No increased latencies with CXM+noFS
memory when the amnesia agent is CXM or ECS (1.25).

8.75 RANDT, BARNETT, McEWAN AND QUARTERMAIN, 1971

CXM 3 mg subcutaneous	mice,strain C57BL/6J	step-through	1
Saline			
CXM 3 mg	mice, strain DBA/2J		
CXM 5 mg			
Saline			

Mice of strain C57BL/6J have poor retention for avoidance tasks
retention 6 hours after learning, which can be blocked by CXM.
there is no retention at 6 hours. Again it is not surprising that
the controls at this time.

time of treatment   test   retention
Before   After

$$C.T_0 \text{------------} T_1 \text{----------} RS \text{-----------} T_2$$
$$\quad\quad 24\ hr \quad\quad 1\ hr \quad\quad 4\ hr$$

30 min	T_1	RA
	T_2	RA
	$T_1;RS;T_2$	no RA
	$RS;T_2$	RA
	$C.T_1;RS;T_2$	RA
	$T_1;C.RS;T_2$	RA

hours after T_1. A reminder shock (RS) given (outside the learn-
memory. T_1 was necessary before the RS to produce amnesia. No
apparatus also gave RA therefore there was no nonspecific
were observed. A reminder shock can restore apparently lost

30 min	1 min	"no RA"
	5 min-1 hr	RA
	6 hr	partial RA
	24-72 hr	RA
30 min	1 min	poor retention
	24 hr	good retention
30 min	1 min	RA
	1 hr	RA
	6-72 hr	no RA
30 min	1 min	"RA"
	5 min	"RA"
30 min	1 min	good retention
	1 hr	no retention
	6-72 hr	no retention

shortly after learning but this develops into good long-term
Strain DBA/2J has good retention up to 1 hour after learning but
at 6 hours and later there is no RA as there was no retention in

Treatment and site   animals   task   trials

8.75   (Continued)

These two strains of mice show other differences-

1.   Time course of inhibition of protein synthesis; with DBA/2J
         required 7 hours.
2.   Strain C57BL/6J had shorter initial latencies. CXM lowered
3.   At 30 min the same dose of CXM produced a greater inhibition

8.76   QUARTERMAIN, McEWAN AND AZMITIA,   1972

Treatment and site	animals	task	trials
CXM 3.0 mg subcutaneous 94% inhibition 30-60 min after injection 0% by 5-7 hr	mice	step-through FS 0.16mA PA	1

The reminder shock (RS) is producing recovery of the CXM-induced
exposure of the amnesic animal to the training apparatus is
not extinguish with repeated trials.

CXM first injection
30 min before T_0

T_1 is necessary for RS to restore memory. Re-exposure to CXM.

time of treatment   test   retention
Before   After

there was a rapid return to control levels in 2-3 hours, C57BL/6J

these but had no effect with DBA/2J.
of protein synthesis in DBA/2J mice.

$(C.T_0$-------T_1--------RS-------T_2-------$T_3)$
　　　24hr　　　1hr　　23hr　　　24hr

30 min T_1 24 hr   RA

                                 T_2 48 hr

                                 T_2;RS;T_2 no RA

                                 T_3;T_4;T_5 no RA

30 min T_1;no RS;T_2 partial RA

                                 T_3;T_4;T_5 no RA

memory loss, in the same manner as ECS-induced memory loss. Re-
sufficient to initiate recovery. Once recovered, the memory does

$(C.T_0$---------- T_1--------RS--------$T_2)$
　　　24 hr　　　　1 hr　　　4 hr

2nd CXM

-                                RS;T_2 RA

-                                T_1;RS;T_2 no RA

30 min before RS T_1;C.RS;T_2 partial RA

30 min before T_1 C.T_1;RS;T_2 RA

30 min before T_1 C.T_1 RA

before RS or T_1 partially prevented the recovery.

Treatment and site	animals	task	trials
8.76 (Continued)			
CXM first injection 30 min before T_0	mice	step-through	1

Reversal of T_1-RS presentation to RS-T_1 also leads to recovery

CXM 3 mg

CXM 5 mg

The higher dose of CXM was not capable of sufficiently suppressing

CXM 30 min before T_0

There is an increase in latency to re-enter between 4 and 8 hours given 30 min before T_1.

It appears that restoration of memory by exposure to T_1 or in of CXM prior to re-exposure to the training apparatus.[1]

time of treatment   test   retention
Before   After

$(C.T_0$ ------------RS--------T_1--------$T_2)$
       24 hr   1 hr   4 hr

2nd CXM

-	$RS;T_1$	RA
-	$RS;T_1;T_2$	no RA
30 min before RS	$C.RS;T_1$	RA
30 min before RS	$C.RS;T_1;T_2$	partial RA
30 min before T_1	$RS;C.T_1$	RA
30 min before T_1	$RS;C.T_1;T_2$	RA

from CXM-induced amnesia.

$(C.T_0$ ---------- T_1---------RS--------$T_2)$
       24 hr   1 hr   4 hr

30 min before T_0	T_1	RA
30 min before T_0	$T_1;RS;T_2$	no RA
30 min before T_0	T_1	RA
30 min before T_0	$T_1;RS;T_2$	no RA (but more than 3 mg)

memory so that T_1 and RS cannot recover it.

$(C.T_0$ -----------T_1---------$T_2)$
       24 hr   4,8or 24hr

30 min before T_0	T_1-T_2 4 hr	RA
30 min before T_0	T_1-T_2 8 hr	partial RA
30 min before T_1	$C.T_1-T_2$ 8 hr	RA
30 min before T_1	$C.T_1-T_2$ 24 hr	partial RA

after exposure to T_1, which is significantly reduced if CXM is

combination with RS is severely attenuated by a second injection

Treatment and site	animals	task	trials

8.77 MARK AND WATTS, 1971

| Cycloheximide 37.5 μg intracranial | chickens | inhibition of pecking PA | 1 |

Chloramphenicol 48.5 μg

It seems that mitochondrial protein synthesis is not involved in

Ouabain 0.365 μg
intracranial

Lithium chloride 245 μg
intracranial

The action of CXM, ouabain and lithium chloride on retention were
after learning. The RA was maintained over 3 days of repeated test-
did it interrupt normal EEG activity in the doses used. It did not

Ouabain-before
training and testing
before training
before testing

Inhibitors of the sodium pump have been found to block the formation
Inhibitors of protein synthesis will prevent long-term memory
appear to be at least two stages in the formation of memory. A
sodium pump inhibitors which leads to permanent storage dependent

8.78 WATTS AND MARK, 1971(a),(b)

| CXM 3.75 μg intracranial | chickens | inhibition of pecking PA | 1 |

37.5-300 μg

37.5 μg

time of treatment		test	retention
Before	After		
30 min		1 day	less RA
15 min			RA
5 min			RA
	10 min		RA
	30 min		no RA
5 min		24 hr	no RA

memory formation.

30 min		1 day	slight RA
15 min			RA
5 min			RA
	10 min		no RA
30 min		1 day	no RA
15 min			no RA
5 min			RA
	10 min		no RA

all dose dependent injected 5 min before and tested 24 hours
ing.   Ouabain had no adverse effects on pecking latencies, nor
cause state dependent learning.

5 min		24 hr	RA
5 min			RA
5 min			no RA

of long-term memory only if present at the time of learning.
formation even if they are administered after learning. There
short-term phase dependent on membrane mechanisms susceptible to
on protein synthesis.

5 min		10-90 min	no RA
		24 hr	no RA
5 min		10 min	no RA
		30 min	slight RA
		60 min	more RA
		90 min	RA
5 min		24 hr	RA almost complete

Treatment and site   animals   task   trials

8.78   (Continued)

At doses of CXM 37.5 μg or greater no increase in RA could be
beyond 37.5 μg CXM was dose-independent and the retention could

Puromycin
90 or 180 μg

Puromycin 90 μg

180 μg

Puromycin injected 3 hours before learning produced a pattern of
before learning it was dose dependent at both concentrations.

Ouabain 0.037 μg

0.37 μg

0.548 μg

Increasing the concentration of the cardiac glycoside-ouabain, a
memory over 90 min.

Copper chloride   0.008 μg Cu^{2+}

0.016 μg Cu^{2+}; 0.333 μg Cu^{2+}

Lithium chloride 32.7 μg

163.5 μg

327 μg

time of treatment		test	retention
Before	After		

achieved, nor any increase in the rate of decay of the STM,i.e. not be reduced completely in 90 min.

3 hr		10-90 min	RA
		24 hr	RA
5 min		10 min	no RA
		60,90 min	increasing RA
		24 hr	RA
5 min		10,60,90 min	more RA
		24 hr	than 90 μg

RA similar to that seen with CXM. However, when injected 5 min

5 min		10-90 min	no RA
		24 hr	RA
5 min		10,30 min	no RA
		60,90 min	RA
		24 hr	RA
5 min		10 min	no RA
		30 min	RA
		60,90 min	complete RA

sodium pump inhibitor produced an increase in the decay of the

5 min		10-90 min	no RA
		24 hr	RA
5 min		10 min	no RA
		30-90 min	RA
		24 hr	complete RA
5 min		10-90 min	no RA
		24 hr	no RA
5 min		6-30 min	RA
		24 hr	RA
5 min		10 min	no RA
		30-90 min	RA
		24 hr	complete RA

Treatment and site   animals   task   trials

8.78   (Continued)

Memory in day-old chickens during the first few hours after learn-
of two classes of drugs. Sodium pump inhibitors in increasing
synthesis inhibitors in increasing doses attain a maximum potency
accelerated by higher doses. Adding a sodium pump inhibitor to the
adding a protein synthesis inhibitor to a sodium pump inhibitor

Therefore within a few minutes of learning a short-term memory
becomes supplemented and eventually replaced by a long-term storage
set by the amount of short-term memory. The short term store could
extrusion from neurons.

8.79   GIBBS, JEFFREY, AUSTIN AND MARK,   1973

In vitro biochemical studies revealed that ouabain does not inhibit
was a correlation between the inhibitions produced by the sodium
ATPase activity (sodium pump) ^{14}C-leucine uptake and the
inhibited leucine-incorporation into protein. In vivo studies
ouabain, much greater than seen in vitro. The results suggest
transport of amino acid between nerve impulse activity and neuronal
and long-term storage of memory.

8.80   CODISH,   1971

Actinomycin D   chickens   imprinting   no.
1.2 µg
hippocampal

The chickens exhibited no behavioural deficits at the time of

---

8.81   DANIELS,   1971(a)

Actinomycin D   rats   appetitive   1
hippocampal   head poke
10 µg
(50% inhibition)

There was no RA with either number of headpokes or general
when compared to controls. RA was possibly obscured by rapid
of same animals. When testing commenced 4 hours after training,
was the same as the controls.

time of treatment		test	retention
Before	After		

ing can be made to decline by the prior intracranial injection
doses cause increasingly rapid loss of memory. Protein
in causing memory decline and the rate may not be further
inhibition of protein synthesis increased memory loss, but
caused no further loss.

of limited time span but independent of protein synthesis
requiring protein synthesis. The amount of long-term store is
be directly dependent on post-activation enhancement of Na^+

ribosomal protein synthesis. In the synaptosomal fraction there
pump blockers used in the previous study (8.77, 8.78),of Na/K
incorporation of ^{14}C-leucine into protein. The antibiotics only
revealed a profound inhibition of leucine incorporation by
that there is a biochemical link involving a sodium pump and the
protein synthesis. This link may also interconvert short-term

---

	30 min	3 days	RA
	24 hr	3 days	no RA

testing.

---

4 hr		4-10 hr	no RA
		8-11 hr	RA

activity as measures of retention 1 to 6 hours after learning
extinction in the control group because of successive testing
there was RA in head poke latencies but the general activity

Treatment and site	animals	task	trials

8.82 DANIELS, 1971(b)

AXM 40 µg hippocampal cannulation	rats	Y-maze brightness discrimination FS	to 4/5 (21)

There was no effect of AXM on recall of short-term or long-term
(a) two memory systems,(b) brain protein synthesis is necessary
and (c) activity in both short and long-term systems is initiated
parallel rather than in series.

8.83 DANIELS, 1972

AXM 40 µg hippocampal cannulation	rats	appetitive head poke	1

The author concluded that-
(1) AXM has similar effects on appetitive and avoidance learning.
(2) AXM administered immediately after acquisition has no effect
         on memory.
(3) 4 hours after acquisition memory is affected by AXM.
(4) Short-term memory is unaffected by AXM and can exist
         independently of long-term memory.
(5) AXM consistently reduces general motor activity.

8.84 QUINTON, 1971

CXM 4 mg subcutaneous 93-95% inhibition at 45 min	mice	step-through FS	1

Controls show the impaired test trial performance observed at 5 hr
secondary non-amnesic effect on CXM on passive avoidance performance.

time of treatment		test	retention
Before	After		
5 hr		3 hr	no RA
		6 hr	RA
		24 hr	RA
		7 days	RA (less)
2 hr		3 hr	no RA
5 hr before retest		6 hr - 7 days	no RA
5 hr before training and			
5 hr before test		7 days	RA
	immediate	6 hr	no RA

memory and no state-dependent effect. The results indicate
for establishment but not for the recall of long-term memory,
during acquisition.   The two memory systems appear to run in

5 hr		1-4 days	RA
		repeated	
	19 hr	24 hr	no RA
	30 sec	1-4 days	no RA
5 hr		(repeated	
		trials)	
		1,2,3, hr	no RA
		4,5,6 hr	RA

---

45 min		1 hr	no RA
		1,5,3 hr	partial RA
		5-72 hr	complete RA
	next day	2.25 or	
		5.75 hr	no RA

in the first study and not at 1.5 hr was not caused by some

Treatment and site   animals   task   trials

8.85 QUINTON, 1972

CXM 3 mg   mice   step-through 1
subcutaneous
ACTH

The author suggests that recall from short-term memory store, but
synthesis, and that this impairment can be overcome by treating
suggest that amnesia develops if initial recall occurs during a
shortly before first recall does not affect the development of
prevent the development of amnesia if the recall is from long-term

---

8.86 OTT, LÖSSNER AND MATTHIES, 1972

Intraventricular injection rats   optical   no.
uridine monophosphate (UMP) 100 μg   discrimination
cytidine   "   (CMP) 100 μg   extinction
adenosine   "   (AMP)
guanosine   (GMP) 100 μg
thymidine   (TMP) 200 μg

None of these nucleotide monophosphates had a significant
reaction. The extinction was affected differently. The
also delayed by UMP or CMP. An injection of UMP, CMP, AMP. or
days of extinction. It was concluded that an increased supply of
of an acquired type of behaviour presumably through RNA-synthesis

| time of treatment | | test | retention |
Before	After		
	CXM 1 hr +	1.5 hr	no RA
	ACTH 75 min	73.5 retest	RA
	ACTH 45 min +	1.5 hr	RA
	CXM 1 hr	73.5 retest	RA
	CXM 1 hr	1.5 hr	RA
		73.5 retest	RA
	CXM 23.5 hr +	24 hr	no RA
	ACTH 23.75 hr	96 hr retest	no RA
	ACTH 23.25 hr +	24 hr	no RA
	CXM 23.5 hr	96 hr retest	no RA
	CXM 23.5 hr	24 hr	no RA
		96 hr retest	RA

not from long-term store, is impaired by inhibition of protein
the animal with ACTH shortly before recall. The data further
period of inhibition of protein synthesis. Treatment with ACTH
amnesia if the recall is from the short-term store, but does
store.

---

delayed extinction
delayed
no effect
no effect
delayed extinction
enhanced extinction

influence on the acquisition of the optical discrimination
extinction of a different conditioned avoidance reaction was
CMP increased the number of positive reactions during the first
pyrimidine-nucleotides is of significance for the consolidation
and its role in the protein synthesis in the nerve cells.

       Treatment and site   animals   task   trials

8.87   OTT AND MATTHIES,   1972

Intraventricular injection of
Orotic acid (OA)   rats   conditioned   no.
Uridine-5-monophosphate (UMP)   avoidance
                                          reaction

6-aza-uridine
(inhibitor of orotidine-5-phosphate
decarboxylase)
6 aza-uridine plus OA

6 aza-uridine plus UMP

These results are compatible with the assumption that orotic acid
transformation into pyrimidine nucleotides which act as precursors

| time of treatment | | test | retention |
Before	After		
30 min		24 hr	relearning
30 min		24 hr	facilitated
30 min		24 hr	no effect
			abolition of OA effect
			no influence on UMP effect

does not directly facilitate retention, but only after a
in brain RNA synthesis.

INTRODUCTION

References

HEBB, D.O.   1949
The Organization of Behaviour.
New York: Wiley

KANDEL, E.R. and SPENCER, W.A.   1968
Cellular neurophysiological approaches in the
study of learning.
Physiol. Rev. 48: 65-134

MÜLLER, G.E. and PILZECKER, A.   1900
Experimentelle Beitrage zur lehre von Gedachtniss.
Z. Psychol. 1: ergbd. 1, 1-288

ROBERTS, R.B. and FLEXNER, L.B.   1969
The biochemical basis of long-term memory.
Quart. Rev. Biophys. 2: 135-173

RUSSELL, W.R. and NATHAN, P.W.   1946
Traumatic amnesia.
Brain 69: 280-300

References

ADAMS, H.E. and LEWIS, D.J.   1962a   1.63
Electroconvulsive shock; retrograde amnesia and
competing responses.
J. comp. physiol. Psychol. 55: 299-301

ADAMS, H.E. and LEWIS, D.J.   1962b   1.64
Retrograde amnesia and competing responses.
J. comp. physiol. Psychol. 55: 302-305

ADAMS, H.E. and PEACOCK, L.J.   1965   1.68
Retrograde amnesia from electroconvulsive shock:
Consolidation disruption or interference?
Psychon. Sci. 3: 37-38

ADAMS, H.E., PEACOCK, L.J. and HAMRICK, D.D.   1967   1.70
ECS and one-trial learning: Retrograde amnesia or
disinhibition?
Physiol. and Behav. 2: 435-437

ALPERN, H.P. and McGAUGH, J.L.   1968   1.35
Retrograde amnesia as a function of duration of
electroshock stimulation.
J. comp. physiol. Psychol. 65: 265-269

ARON, C., GLICK, S.D. and JARVIK, M.E.   1969   1.141
Long-lasting proactive effects of a single ECS.
Physiol. and Behav. 4: 785-789

BANKER, G., HUNT, E. and PAGANO, R.   1969   1.208
Evidence supporting the memory disruption hypothesis
of electroconvulsive shock action.
Physiol. and Behav. 4: 895-899

BARCIK, J.D.   1969   1.207
Hippocampal afterdischarges and memory disruption.
Proc. Am. psychol. Ass. 4: 185-186

BARRETT, R.J., HUGHES, R.A. and RAY, O.S.   1971   1.182
ECS disruption of time-dependent processes in
discriminated avoidance conditioning in rats:
Incubation or consolidation?
J. comp. physiol. Psychol. 74: 319-324

BARRETT, R.J. and RAY, O.S.   1969   1.179
Attenuation of habituation by electroconvulsive shock.
J. comp. physiol. Psychol. 69: 133-135

BENOWITZ, L. and MAGNUS, J.G.   1.172
Memory storage processes following one-trial aversive
conditioning in the chick.
Behavl. Biol. (In Press)

BIVENS, L.W. and RAY, O.S.   1967   1.175
Effects of electroconvulsive shock and strychnine
sulphate on memory consolidation.
Neuropsychopharmacology, (Proc. V. Intern. Congr.
C.I.N.P., Washington, 1966) p. 1030-1034

BLACK, M. and SUBOSKI, M.D.   1971   1.192
Incubation and ECS-produced gradients in one-trial and
multitrial discriminated-avoidance conditioning in rats.
J. comp. physiol. Psychol. 74: 325-330

BOHDANECKY, Z. and JARVIK, M.E.   1966   1.127
Temporal relations of proactive ECS disinhibition.
Fed. Proc. 25: 262

BOVET, D., BOVET-NITTI, F. and OLIVERIO, A.   1969   1.210
Genetic aspects of learning and memory in mice.
Science 163: 139-149

BRADY, J.V.   1951   1.6
The effect of electroconvulsive shock on a conditioned
emotional response: The permanence of the effect.
J. comp. physiol. Psychol. 44: 507-511

BRADY, J.V. and HUNT, H.F.   1951   1.5
A further demonstration of the effects of
electroconvulsive shock on a conditioned emotional
response.
J. comp. physiol. Psychol. 44: 204-209

BRADY, J.V., HUNT, H.F. and GELLER, J.   1954   1.7
The effect of electroconvulsive shock on a conditioned
emotional response as a function of the temporal
distribution of the treatments.
J. comp. physiol. Psychol. 47: 454-457

BRUNNER, R.L., ROSSI, R.R., STUTZ, R.M. and
ROTH, T.G.   1970   1.218
Memory loss following post-trial electrical
stimulation of the hippocampus.
Psychon. Sci. 18: 159-160

BUCKHOLTZ, N.S. and BOWMAN, R.E.   1972   1.252
Incubation and retrograde amnesia studied with
various ECS intensities and durations.
Physiol. and Behav. 8: 113-117

BUREŜ, J. and BUREŜOVÁ, O. 1963   1.58
Cortical spreading depression as a memory disturbing
factor.
J. comp. physiol. Psychol. 56: 268-272

BUREŜOVÁ, O., BUREŜ, J. and GERBRANDT, L.K. 1968   1.60
The effect of an electroconvulsive shock on retention
of a spatial discrimination or its reversal.
Physiol. and Behav. 3: 155-159

CAREW, T.J. 1970   1.219
Do passive-avoidance tasks permit assessment of
retrograde amnesia in rats?
J. comp. physiol. Psychol. 72: 267-271

CAUL, W.F. and BARRETT, R.J. 1972   1.183
Electroconvulsive shock effects on conditioned heart
rate and suppression of drinking.
Physiol. and Behav. 8: 287-290

CHERKIN, A. 1966
Memory consolidation: Probit analysis of retrograde-
amnesia data.
Psychon. Sci. 4: 169-170

CHERKIN, A. 1969
Kinetics of memory consolidation: Role of amnesic
treatment parameters.
Proc. natn. Acad. Sci. U.S.A. 63: 1094-1101

CHEVALIER, J.A. 1965   1.102
Permanence of amnesia after single post-trial
electroconvulsive seizure.
J. comp. physiol. Psychol. 59: 125-127

CHOROVER, S.L. and de LUCA, A.M. 1969   1.607
Transient change in electrocorticographic reaction to
ECS in the rat following footshock.
J. comp. physiol. Psychol. 69: 141-149

CHOROVER, S.L. and SCHILLER, P.H. 1965   1.103
Short-term retrograde amnesia in rats.
J. comp. physiol. Psychol. 59: 73-78

CHOROVER, S.L. and SCHILLER, P.H. 1966   1.104
Re-examination of prolonged RA in one-trial learning.
J. comp. physiol. Psychol. 61: 34-41

COONS, E.E. and MILLER, N.E.   1960   1.20
Conflict versus consolidation of memory traces to explain
"retrograde amnesia" produced by ECS.
J. comp. physiol. Psychol. 53: 524-531

COOPER, R.M. and KOPPENAAL, R.J.   1964   1.90
Suppression and recovery of a one-trial avoidance
response after a single ECS.
Psychon. Sci. 1: 303-304

CORSON, J.A.   1965   1.108
Memory as influenced by a single electroconvulsive
shock.
J. Psychiat. Res. 3: 153-158

COTMAN, C.W., BANKER, G., ZORNETZER, S.F.
and McGAUGH, J.L.   1971   1.57
Electroshock effects on brain protein synthesis:
relation to brain seizures and retrograde amnesia.
Science 173: 454-456

DARBELLAY, D.W. and WINOCUR, G.   1971   1.239
Electroconvulsive shock, stress, and avoidance
conditioning.
Psychon. Sci. 23: 46-47

DAVIS, R.E., BRIGHT, P.J. and AGRANOFF, B.W.   1965   1.109
Effect of ECS and puromycin on memory in fish.
J. comp. physiol. Psychol. 60: 162-166

DAVIS, R.E. and HIRTZEL, M.S.   1970   1.110
Environmental control of ECS-produced retrograde
amnesia in goldfish.
Physiol. and Behav 5: 1089-1092

DAVIS, R.E. and HOLMES, P.A.   1971   1.111
ECS-produced retrograde amnesia of conditioned
inhibition of respiration in cataleptic goldfish.
Physiol. and Behav. 7: 11-14

DAWSON, R.G.   1971
Retrograde amnesia and conditioned emotional response
incubation reexamined.
Psychol. Bull. 75: 278-285

DAWSON, R.G. and McGAUGH, J.L.   1969a   1.39
Electroconvulsive shock effects on a reactivated
memory trace; further examination.
Science 166: 525-527

DAWSON, R.G. and McGAUGH, J.L.   1969b   1.40
Electroconvulsive shock-produced retrograde amnesia:
Analysis of the familiarization effect.
Commun. Behavl. Biol. 4: 91-95

DAWSON, R.G. and McGAUGH, J.L.   1969c
Familiarization and retrograde amnesia: A re-evaluation
re-evaluated.
Commun. Behavl. Biol. 4: 257-259

DAWSON, R.G. and PRYOR, G.T.   1965   1.32
Onset vs recovery in the aversive effects of
electroconvulsive shock.
Psychon. Sci. 3: 273-274

DEADWYLER, S.A. and WYERS, E.J.   1972   1.160
Disruption of habituation by caudate nuclear
stimulation in the rat.
Behavl. Biol. 7: 55-64

DELPRATO, D.J. and THOMPSON, R.W.   1965   1.113
Effect of electroconvulsive shock on passive avoidance
learning with high and low intensity foot-shock.
Psychol. Rep. 17: 209-210

DENTI, A., McGAUGH, J.L., LANDFIELD, P.W.
and SHINKMAN, P.G.   1970   1.42
Effects of posttrial electrical stimulation of the
mesencephalic reticular formation on avoidance
learning in rats.
Physiol. and Behav. 5: 659-662

DeVIETTI, T.L. and KALLIOINEN, E.K.   1972   1.246
ECS-induced retrograde amnesia indicated by a heart-
rate measure of retention.
Psychon. Sci. 27: 35-36

DeVIETTI, T.L. and LARSON, R.C.   1971   1.244
ECS effects: Evidence supporting state-dependent
learning in rats.
J. comp. physiol. Psychol. 74: 407-415

DORFMAN, L.J. and JARVIK, M.E.   1968a   1.132
Comparative amnesic effects of transcorneal and
transpinnate ECS in mice
Physiol. and Behav. 3: 815-818

DORFMAN, L.J. and JARVIK, M.E.   1968b   1.133
A parametric study of electroshock-induced
retrograde amnesia in mice.
Neuropsychologia 6: 373-380

DUNCAN, C.P.   1945   1.1
The effect of electroshock convulsions on the maze
habit in the white rat.
J. exp. Psychol. 35: 267-278

DUNCAN, C.P.   1948   1.2
Habit reversal induced by electroshock in the rat.
J. comp. physiol. Psychol. 41: 11-16

DUNCAN, C.P.   1949   1.3
The retroactive effects of shock on learning.
J. comp. physiol. Psychol. 42: 32-34

ESSMAN, W.B.   1.134
Electroshock-induced retrograde amnesia in seizure-
protected mice.
Psychol. Rep. 22: 929-935

FISHBEIN, W.   1970   1.53
Interference with conversion of memory from short-
term to long-term storage by partial sleep deprivation.
Commun. Behavl. Biol. 5: 171-175

FISHBEIN, W.   1971   1.54
Disruptive effects of rapid eye movement sleep
deprivation on long-term memory.
Physiol. and Behav. 6: 279-282

FISHBEIN, W., McGAUGH, J.L. and SWARZ, J.R.   1971   1.52
Retrograde amnesia: Electroconvulsive shock effects
after termination of rapid eye movement sleep
deprivation.
Science 172: 80-82

GALLUSCIO, E.H.   1971   1.241
Retrograde amnesia induced by electroconvulsive shock
and carbon dioxide anaesthesia in rats: An attempt
to stimulate recovery.
J. comp. physiol. Psychol. 75: 136-140

GALOSY, R.A. and THOMPSON, R.W.   1971   1.115
A further investigation of familiarization effects
on ECS produced retrograde amnesia.
Psychon. Sci. 22: 147-148

GASTAUT, H. and FISCHER-WILLIAMS, M.   1959
The physiopathology of epileptic seizures.
In: Handbook of Physiology, edited by J. Field,
Washington, DC. American Physiological Society, vol.1.

GELLER, A. and JARVIK, M.E.   1968a   1.135
Electroconvulsive shock induced amnesia and recovery.
Psychon. Sci. 10: 15-16

GELLER, A. and JARVIK, M.E.   1968b   1.136
The time relations of ECS induced amnesia.
Psychon. Sci. 12: 169-170

GELLER, A. and JARVIK, M.E.   1970   1.148
Permanence of a long temporal gradient of retrograde
amnesia induced by electroconvulsive shock.
Psychon. Sci. 19: 257-259

GELLER, A., ROBUSTELLI, F. and JARVIK, M.E.   1970   1.147
A parallel study of the amnesic effects of cycloheximide
and ECS under different strengths of conditioning.
Psychopharmacologia 16: 281-289

GELLER, J., SIDMAN, M. and BRADY, J.V.   1955   1.8
The effect of electroconvulsive shock on a
conditioned emotional response
J. comp. physiol. Psychol. 48: 130-131

GERARD, R.W.   1955   1.9
Biological roots of psychiatry.
Science 122: 255-230

GERBRANDT, L.K., BUREŠOVÁ, O. and BUREŠ, J.   1968   1.61
Discrimination and reversal learning followed by a
single electroconvulsive shock.
Physiol. and Behav. 3: 149-153

GERBRANDT, L.K. and THOMPSON, C.W.   1964   1.59
Competing response and amnesic effects of
electroconvulsive shock under extinction and
incentive shifts.
J. comp. physiol. Psychol. 58: 208-211

GLENDENNING, R.L. and MEYER, D.R.   1971   1.233
Motivationally related retroactive interference in
discrimination learning by rats.
J. comp. physiol. Psychol.75: 153-156

GLICKMAN, S.E.   1958   1. 19
Deficits in avoidance learning produced by stimulation
of the ascending reticular formation.
Can. J. Psychol. 12: 97-102

GOLD, P.E., FARRELL, W. and KING, R.A.   1971   1.122
Retrograde amnesia after localized brain shock in
passive-avoidance learning.
Physiol. and Behav. 7: 709-712

GOLD, P.E. and McGAUGH, J.L.   1972
Effect of recent footshock on brain seizures and
behavioral convulsions induced by electrical
stimulation of the brain.
Behavl. Biol. 7: 421-426

GOLDSMITH, L.J.   1967   1.184
Effect of intracerebral Actinomycin D and of
electroconvulsive shock on passive avoidance.
J. comp. physiol. Psychol. 63: 126-132

GOLUB, M.S., CHEAL, M.L. and DAVIS, R.E.   1972   1.112
Effects of electroconvulsive shock and puromycin on
operant responding in goldfish.
Physiol. and Behav. 8: 573-578

GREENOUGH, W.T. and SCHWITZGEBEL, R.L.   1966   1.150
Effect of a single ECS on extinction of a bar press.
Psychol. Rep. 19: 1227-1230

GREENOUGH, W.T., SCHWITZGEBEL, R.L.
and FULCHER, J.K.   1968   1.151
Permanence of ECS-produced amnesia as a function of
test conditions.
J. comp. physiol. Psychol. 66: 554-556

GROSSER, G.S., PERCY, H.E. and PIERCE, L.E.   1971   1.247
Short footshock-electroconvulsive shock intervals and
retrograde amnesia in mice.
Psychon. Sci. 25: 26-28

HARTMAN, A.M. and KLIPPLE, A.G.   1966   1.149
Effect of place of electroconvulsive shock and place
of recovery on conditioned avoidance.
J. comp. physiol. Psychol. 61: 138-140

HERIOT, J.T. and COLEMAN, P.D.   1962   1.62
The effect of electroconvulsive shock on retention of
a modified "one-trial" conditioned avoidance.
J. comp. physiol. Psychol. 55: 1082-1084

HERZ, M.J.   1969   1.155
Interference with one-trial appetitive and aversive
learning by ether and ECS.
J. Neurobiol. 1: 111-122

HERZ, M.J. and PEEKE, H.V.S.   1967   1.153
Permanence of retrograde amnesia produced by
electroconvulsive shock.
Science 156: 1396-1397

HERZ, M.J. and PEEKE, H.V.S.   1968   1.153
ECS-produced retrograde amnesia: Permanence vs recovery
over repeated testing.
Physiol. and Behav. 3: 517-521

HERZ, M.J. and PEEKE, H.V.S.   1971   1.159
Impairment of extinction with caudate nucleus
stimulation.
Brain Res. 33: 519-522

HERZ, M.J., PEEKE, H.V.S. and WYERS, E.J.   1966   1.152
Amnesic effects of ether and electroconvulsive shock
in mice.
Psychon. Sci. 4: 375-376

HINE, B. and PAOLINO, R.M.   1970   1.26
Retrograde amnesia: production of skeletal but not
cardiac response gradient by electroconvulsive shock.
Science 169: 1224-1226

HIRANO, T.   1966   1.161
Effect of hippocampal electrical stimulation on memory
consolidation.
Psychologia 9: 63-75

HOWARD, R.L. and MEYER, D.R.   1971   1.232
Motivational control of retrograde amnesia in rats:
A replication and extension.
J. comp. physiol. Psychol. 74: 37-40

HUDSPETH, W.J., McGAUGH, J.L. and THOMPSON, C.W.   1964   1.30
Aversive and amnesic effects of electroconvulsive shock.
J. comp. physiol. Psychol. 57: 61-64

HUGHES, R.A., BARRETT, R.J. and RAY, O.S.   1970a   1.180
Retrograde amnesia in rats increases as a function of
ECS-test interval and ECS intensity.
Physiol. and Behav. 5: 27-30

HUGHES, R.A., BARRETT, R.J. and RAY, O.S.   1970b   1.181
Training-to-test interval as a determinant of a temporally
graded ECS-produced response decrement in rats.
J. comp. physiol. Psychol. 71: 318-324

HUNT, H.F. and BRADY, J.V.   1951   1.4
Some effects of electroconvulsive shock on a conditioned
emotional response ("Anxiety")
J. comp. physiol. Psychol. 44: 88-89

IRWIN, S., BANUAZIZI, A., KALSNER, S. and
CURTIS, A.   1968   1.100
One trial learning in the mouse. I. Its characteristics
and modification by experimental-seasonal variables.
Psychopharmacologia 12: 286-302

IRWIN, S., KALSNER, S. and CURTIS, A.   1964   1.99
Direct demonstration of consolidation of one-trial
learning.
Fed. Proc. 23: 101

JAMIESON, J.L. and ALBERT, D.J.   1970   1.220
Amnesia from ECS: the effect of pairing ECS and footshock
Psychon. Sci. 18: 14-15

JARVIK, M.E. and KOPP, R.   1967   1.130
Transcorneal electroconvulsive shock and retrograde
amnesia in mice.
J. comp. physiol. Psychol. 64: 431-433

KESNER, R.P.   1971   1.198
ECS as a punishing stimulus: Dependency on retrograde
amnesia, duration of anterograde amnesia, and intensity
of pain.
J. comp. physiol. Psychol. 74: 398-406

KESNER, R.P. and CONNER, H.S.   1972   1.202
Independence of short- and long-term memory: a neural
system analysis.
Science, 176: 432-434

KESNER, R.P. and D'ANDREA, J.A.   1971   1.199
Electroconvulsive shock disrupts both information
storage and retrieval.
Physiol. and Behav. 7: 73-76

KESNER, R.P. and DOTY, R.W.   1968   1.195
Amnesia produced in cats by local seizure activity
initiated from the amygdala
Expl Neurol. 21: 58-68

KESNER, R.P., GIBSON, W.E. and LECLAIR, M.J.   1970   1.196
ECS as a punishing stimulus: Dependency on route of
administration.
Physiol. and Behav. 5: 683-686

KESNER, R.P., McDONOUGH, J.H. and DOTY, R.W.   1970   1.197
Diminished amnesic effect of a second electroconvulsive
seizure.
Expl Neurol. 27: 527-533

KINCAID, J.P.   1967   1.185
Permanence of amnesia after single post-trial treatment
of metrazol or electroconvulsive shock.
Psychon. Sci. 9: 56-60

KINCAID, J.P.   1968   1.186
Different temporal gradients of retrograde amnesia
produced by metrazol or electroconvulsive shock.
Psychon. Sci. 11: 329-330

KING, R.A.   1965   1.116
Consolidation of the neural trace in memory:
Investigation with one-trial avoidance conditioning
and ECS.
J. comp. physiol. Psychol. 59: 283-284

KING, R.A.   1967   1.117
Consolidation of the neural trace in memory: ECS-
produced retrograde amnesia is not an artifact of
conditioning.
Psychon. Sci. 9: 409-410

KING, R.A. and GLASSER, R.L.   1970   1.121
Duration of electroconvulsive shock-induced retrograde
amnesia in rats.
Physiol. and Behav. 5: 335-339

KLEMM, W.R.   1972
Theta rhythm and memory
Science 176: 1449

KOHLENBERG, R. and TRABASSO, T.   1968   1.203
Recovery of a conditioned emotional response after one
or two electroconvulsive shocks.
J. comp. physiol. Psychol. 65: 270-273

KOPP, R.   1966   1.128
The temporal gradient of RA to ECS in mice.
Fed. Proc. 25: 262

KOPP, R., BOHDANECKY, Z. and JARVIK, M.E.   1966   1.129
Long temporal gradients of retrograde amnesia for a
well-discriminated stimulus
Science 153: 1547-1549

KOPP, R., BOHDANECKY, Z. and JARVIK, M.E.   1967   1.131
Proactive effect of a single ECS on step-through
performance on naive and punished mice.
J. comp. physiol. Psychol. 64: 22-25

KOPPENAAL, R.J., JAGODA, E. and CRUCE, J.A.F.   1967   1.94
Recovery from ECS-produced amnesia following a reminder
Psychon. Sci. 9: 293-294

KRAL, P.A.   1970   1.222
Interpolation of electroconvulsive shock during CS-US
interval as an impediment to the conditioning of taste
aversion.
Psychon. Sci. 19: 36-37

KRAL, P.A.   1971a   1.223
Electroconvulsive shock during taste-illness interval:
evidence for induced disassociation.
Physiol. and Behav. 7: 667-670

KRAL, P.A.   1971b   1.224
ECS between tasting and illness: effects of current
parameters on a taste aversion.
Physiol. and Behav. 7: 779-782

LANDFIELD, P.W. and McGAUGH, J.L.   1972   1.55
Effects of electroconvulsive shock and brain stimulation
on EEG cortical theta rhythms in rats.
Behavl. Biol. 7: 271-278

LANDFIELD, P.W., McGAUGH, J.L. and TUSA, R.J.   1972   1.56
Theta rhythm: a temporal correlate of memory storage
processes in the rat.
Science 175: 87-89

LEE-TENG, E.   1966   1.162
Disruption of electroconvulsive shock (ECS) of memory
consolidation in chicks.
Proc. Am. psychol. Ass. 1: 109-110

LEE-TENG, E.   1967   1.164
Retrograde amnesia in relation to current intensity and
seizure pattern in chicks.
Proc. Am. psychol. Ass. 2: 87-88

LEE-TENG, E.   1969   1.166
Retrograde amnesia in relation to subconvulsive and
convulsive current in chicks.
J. comp. physiol. Psychol. 67: 135-139

LEE-TENG, E.   1968   1.165
Presence of short-term memory after immediate post-trial
subconvulsive current in chicks.
Proc. Am. psychol. Ass. 3: 329-330

LEE-TENG, E.   1970   1.169
Retrograde amnesia gradients by subconvulsive and high
convulsive transcranial currents in chicks.
Proc. natn. Acad. Sci. U.S.A. 65: 857-865

LEE-TENG, E. and GIAQUINTO, S.   1969   1.167
Electrocorticograms following threshold transcranial
electroshock for retrograde amnesia in chicks.
Expl Neurol. 23: 485-490

LEE-TENG, E., MAGNUS, J.G., KANNER, M. and
HOCHMAN, H.   1970   1.170
Two separable phases of behaviorally manifest memory for
one-trial learning in chicks.
Int. J. Neuroscience 1: 99-106

LEE-TENG, E. and SHERMAN, S.M.   1966   1.163
Memory consolidation of one-trial learning in chicks.
Proc. natn. Acad. Sci. U.S.A. 56: 926-931

LEONARD, D.J. and ZAVALA A.   1964   1.101
Electroconvulsive shock, retroactive amnesia, and the
single-shock method.
Science 146: 1073-1074

LEUKEL, F.A.   1957   1.17
A comparison of the effects of ECS and anaesthesia on
acquisition of the maze habit.
J. comp. physiol. Psychol. 50: 300-306

LEWIS, D.J.   1969
Sources of experimental amnesia.
Psychol. Rev. 76: 461-472

LEWIS, D.J. and ADAMS, H.E.   1963   1.65
Retrograde amnesia from conditioned competing responses.
Science 141: 516-517

LEWIS, D.J. and MAHER, B.A.   1965
Neural consolidation and electroconvulsive shock.
Psychol. Rev. 72: 225-239

LEWIS, D.J. and MAHER, B.A.   1966
Electroconvulsive shock and inhibition: some problems
considered.
Psychol. Rev. 73: 388-392

LEWIS, D.J., MILLER, R.R. and MISANIN, J.R.   1968   1.72
Control of retrograde amnesia.
J. comp. physiol. Psychol. 66: 48-52

LEWIS, D.J., MILLER, R.R. and MISANIN, J.R.   1969   1.74
Selective amnesia in rats produced by electroconvulsive
shock.
J. comp. physiol. Psychol. 69: 136-140

LEWIS, D.J., MISANIN, J.R. and MILLER, R.R.   1968   1.71
Recovery of memory following amnesia.
Nature, Lond. 220: 704-705

LIDSKY, A. and SLOTNICK, B.M.   1970   1.226
Electrical stimulation of the hippocampus and
electroconvulsive-shock produce similar amnesic effects
in mice.
Neuropsychologia 8: 363-370

LIDSKY, A. and SLOTNICK, B.M.   1971   1.227
Effects of posttrial limbic stimulation on retention of
a one-trial passive-avoidance response.
J. comp. physiol. Psychol. 76: 337-348

LUTTGES, M.W. and McGAUGH, J.L.   1967   1.34
Permanence of retrograde amnesia produced by
electroconvulsive shock.
Science 156: 408-410

MADSEN, M.C. and LUTTGES, M.W.   1963   1.29
Effect of electroconvulsive shock on extinction of an
approach response.
Psychol. Rep. 13: 225-226

MADSEN, M.C. and McGAUGH, J.L.   1961   1.28
The effect of ECS on one-trial avoidance learning.
J. comp. physiol. Psychol. 54: 522-523

MAGNUS, J.G. and LEE-TENG, E.   1971   1.171
The absence of residual memory consolidation following
transcranial current.
Physiol. and Behav. 7: 113-115

MAH, C.J., ALBERT, D.J. and JAMIESON, J.L.   1972   1.221
Memory storage: evidence that consolidation continues
following electroconvulsive shock.
Physiol. and Behav. 8: 283-286

MAHUT, H.   1962   1.86
Effects of subcortical electrical stimulation on
learning in the rat.
J. comp. physiol. Psychol. 55: 472-477

MALDONADO, H.   1968   1.204
Effect of electroconvulsive shock on memory
in Octopus vulgaris Lamarck.
Z. vergl. Physiol. 59: 25-37

MALDONADO, H.   1969   1.205
Further investigations on effect of electroconvulsive
shock (ECS) on memory in Octopus vulgaris.
Z. vergl. Physiol. 63: 113-118

MAYSE, J.F. and DeVIETTI, T.L.   1971   1.245
A comparison of state dependent learning induced by
electroconvulsive shock and pentobarbital.
Physiol. and Behav. 7: 717-721

McDONOUGH, J.H. Jnr. and KESNER, R.P.   1971   1.200
Amnesia produced by brief electrical stimulation of
amygdala or dorsal hippocampus in cats.
J. comp. physiol. Psychol. 77: 171-178

McGAUGH, J.L.   1966
Time-dependent processes in memory storage.
Science 153: 1351-1358

McGAUGH, J.L.   1972
Impairment and facilitation of memory consolidation
Activitas nerv. sup. 14: 64-74

McGAUGH, J.L. and ALPERN, H.P.   1966   1.33
Effects of electroshock on memory: Amnesia without
convulsions.
Science 152: 665-666

McGAUGH, J.L. and DAWSON, R.G.   1971
Modification of memory storage processes.
Behavl. Sci. 16: 45-63

McGAUGH, J.L., DAWSON, R.G., COLEMAN, R. and
RAWIE, J.   1971   1.51
Electroshock effects on memory in Diethyl Ether-treated
mice: analysis of the CER-incubation hypothesis of
retrograde amnesia.
Commun. Behavl. Biol. 6: 227-232

McGAUGH, J.L. and HERZ, M.J.   1972
Memory Consolidation.
San Francisco: Albion Pub. Co.

McGAUGH, J.L. and LANDFIELD, P.W.   1970   1.50
Delayed development of amnesia following electroconvulsive
shock.
Physiol. and Behav. 5: 1109-1113

McGAUGH, J.L. and LONGACRE, B.   1969   1.41
Effect of electroconvulsive shock on performance of a
well learned avoidance response: Contribution of the
convulsion.
Commun. Behavl. Biol. 4: 177-182

McGAUGH, J.L. and MADSEN, M.C.   1964   1.31
Amnesic and punishing effects of electroconvulsive shock.
Science 144: 182-183

McGAUGH, J.L. and PETRINOVICH, L.F.   1966
Neural consolidation and electroconvulsive shock
reexamined.
Psychol. Rev. 73: 382-387

McGAUGH, J.L. and ZORNETZER, S.   1970   1.44
Amnesia and brain seizure activity in mice: Effects of
diethyl ether anaesthesia prior to electroshock
stimulation.
Commun. Behavl. Biol. 5: 243-248

McINTYRE, D.C.   1970   1.228
Differential amnesic effect of cortical vs amygdaloid
elicited convulsions in rats.
Physiol. and Behav. 5: 747-753

McMICHAEL, J.S.   1966
Incubation of anxiety and instrumental behaviour.
J. comp. physiol. Psychol. 61: 208-211

MENDOZA, J.E. and ADAMS, H.E.   1969   1.75
Does electroconvulsive shock produce retrograde amnesia?
Physiol. and Behav. 4: 307-309

MILLER, A.J.   1968   1.194
Variations in retrograde amnesia with parameters of
electroconvulsive shock and time of testing.
J. comp. physiol. Psychol. 66: 40-47

MILLER, R.R.   1970   1.79
Effects of environmental complexity on amnesia induced
by electroconvulsive shock in rats.
J. comp. physiol. Psychol. 71: 267-275

MILLER, R.R. and MISANIN, J.R.   1969
Critique of electroconvulsive shock-induced retrograde
amnesia:analysis of the familiarization effect.
Commun. Behavl. Biol. 4: 255-256

MILLER, R.R., MISANIN, J.R. and LEWIS, D.J.   1969   1.76
Amnesia as a function of events during the learning-
ECS interval.
J. comp. physiol. Psychol. 67: 145-148

MILLER, R.R. and SPEAR, N.E.   1969   1.78
Memory and extensor phase of convulsions induced by
electroconvulsive shock.
Psychon. Sci. 15: 164-166

MILLER, R.R. and SPRINGER, A.D.   1971   1.81
Temporal course of amnesia in rats after
electroconvulsive shock.
Physiol. and Behav. 6: 229-234

MILLER, R.R. and SPRINGER, A.D.   1972a   1.83
Induced recovery of memory in rats following
electroconvulsive shock.
Physiol. and Behav. 8: 645-651

MILLER, R.R. and SPRINGER, A.D.   1972b   1.84
Recovery from amnesia following transcorneal
electroconvulsive shock.
Psychon. Sci. 28: 7-9

MISANIN, J.R.   1966   1.69
Role of fear in the facilitation and inhibitory
effects of electroconvulsive shock.
J. comp. physiol. Psychol. 61: 411-415

MISANIN, J.R.   1970   1.80
The effects of ECS on ECT: Implications for
behavioural research.
Psychon. Sci. 20: 159-161

MISANIN, J.R., MILLER, R.R. and LEWIS, D.J.   1968   1.73
Retrograde amnesia produced by ECS after reactivation
of a consolidated memory trace.
Science 160: 554-555

MISANIN, J.R. and SMITH, N.F.   1964   1.66
Role of response-linked fear on the effects of a
single ECS on an avoidance response.
J. comp. physiol. Psychol. 58: 212-216

MISANIN, J.R., SMITH, N.F. and MILLER, R.R.   1971   1.82
Memory of electroconvulsive shock as a function of
intensity and duration.
Psychon. Sci. 22: 5-7

NACHMAN, M.   1970   1.212
Limited effects of electroconvulsive shock on memory
of taste stimulation.
J. comp. physiol. Psychol. 73: 31-37

NACHMAN, M. and MEINECKE, R.O.   1969   1.211
Lack of retrograde amnesia effects of repeated ECS
and CO_2 treatments.

J. comp. physiol. Psychol. 68: 631-636

NAITOH, P.   1971   1.248
Selective impairment of pavlovian conditional responses
by electroconvulsive shock.
Physiol. and Behav. 7: 291-296

NIELSON, H.C.   1968   1.206
Evidence that electroconvulsive shock alters memory
retrieval rather than memory consolidation.
Expl Neurol. 20: 3-20

OLSON, G.H. and HAGSTROM, E.   1971   1.249
Recovery experiences and the source of aversive effects
of electroconvulsive shock.
Psychon. Sci. 22: 161-162

PAGANO, R.R., BUSH, D.F., MARTIN, G. and
HUNT, E.B.   1969   1.209
Duration of retrograde amnesia as a function of
electroconvulsive shock intensity.
Physiol. and Behav. 4: 19-21

PAOLINO, R.M., QUARTERMAIN, D. and LEVY, H.M.   1969   1.24
Effect of electroconvulsive shock duration on the
gradient of retrograde amnesia.
Physiol. and Behav. 4: 147-149

PAOLINO, R.M., QUARTERMAIN, D. and MILLER, N.E.   1966   1.22
Different temporal gradients of retrograde amnesia
produced by carbon dioxide anesthesia and electroconvulsive shock.
J. comp. physiol. Psychol. 62: 270-274

PEEKE, H.V.S. and HERZ, M.J.   1967   1.153
Permanence of electroconvulsive shock-produced
retrograde amnesia.
Proc. Am. psychol. Ass. 2: 85-86

PEEKE, H.V.S. and HERZ, M.J.   1971   1.158
Caudate nucleus stimulation retroactively impairs
complex maze learning in the rat.
Science 173: 80-82

PEEKE, H.V.S., McCOY, F. and HERZ, M.J.   1969   1.156
Drive consummatory response effects on memory
consolidation for appetitive learning in mice.
Commun. Behavl. Biol. 4: 49-53

PFINGST, B.E. and KING, R.A.   1967   1.118
A one-trial response-choice technique for the
biological study of memory.
Psychon. Sci. 8: 497-498

PFINGST, B.E. and KING, R.A.   1968   1.119
Time course of consolidation as measured by response
choice behaviour.
Proc. Am. psychol. Ass. 3: 327-328

PFINGST, B.E. and KING, R.A.   1969   1.120
Effects of post training electroconvulsive shock on
retention-test performance involving choice.
J. comp. physiol. Psychol. 68: 645-649

PINEL, J.P.J.   1968   1.95
Evaluation of the one-trial passive avoidance task as
a tool for studying ECS-produced amnesia.
Psychon. Sci. 13: 131-132

PINEL, J.P.J.   1969   1.96
A short gradient of ECS-produced amnesia in a one-trial
appetitive learning situation.
J. comp. physiol. Psychol. 68: 650-655

PINEL, J.P.J.   1970   1.97
Two types of ECS-produced disruption of one-trial
training in the rat.
J. comp. physiol. Psychol. 72: 272-277

PINEL, J.P.J. and COOPER, R.M.   1966a   1.91
Demonstration of the Kamin effect after one-trial
avoidance learning.
Psychon. Sci. 4: 17-18

PINEL, J.P.J. and COOPER, R.M.   1966b   1.92
Incubation and its implications for the interpretation
of the ECS gradient effect.
Psychon. Sci. 6: 123-124

PINEL, J.P.J. and COOPER, R.M.   1966c   1.93
The relationship between incubation and ECS gradient
effects.
Psychon. Sci. 6: 125-126

PINEL, J.P.J., CORCORAN, M.E. and MALSBURY, C.W.   1971
Incubation effect in rats: decline of footshock-
produced activation.
J. comp. physiol. Psychol. 77: 271-276

PINEL, J.P.J., MALSBURY, C.W. and CORCORAN, M.E.   1971a   1.98
The incubation effect in rats: Skin resistance changes
after footshock.
Physiol. and Behav. 6: 111-114

PINEL, J.P.J., MALSBURY, C.W. and CORCORAN, M.E.   1971b
The incubation effect produced in rats without footshock.
Psychon. Sci. 24: 109-110

PIRCH, J.H.   1969   1.213
Temporary improvement in shuttle box performance of
rats after repeated electroconvulsive shock treatment.
Physiol. and Behav. 4: 517-521

POSCHEL, B.P.H.   1957   1.18
Proactive and retroactive effects of electroconvulsive
shock on approach-avoidance conflict.
J. comp. physiol. Psychol. 50: 392-396

POSLUNS, D. and VANDERWOLF, C.H.   1970   1.229
Amnesic and disinhibitory effects of electroconvulsive
shock in the rat.
J. comp. physiol. Psychol. 73: 291-306

POTTS, W.J.   1971   1.250
The effect of different environments prior to electro-
convulsive shock on the gradient of retrograde amnesia.
Physiol. and Behav. 7: 161-164

PRYOR, G.T., PEACHE, S. and SCOTT, M.K.   1972
Escape response thresholds in rats following repeated
electroconvulsive shock seizures.
Physiol. and Behav. 8: 95-99

QUARTERMAIN, D., McEWAN, B.S. and
AZMITIA, E.C., Jnr.   1970   1.25
Amnesia produced by electroconvulsive shock or
cycloheximide: Conditions for recovery.
Science 169: 683-686

QUARTERMAIN, D., McEWAN, B.S. and
AZMITIA, E.C., Jnr.   1972   1.27
Recovery of memory following amnesia in the rat and
mouse.
J. comp. physiol. Psychol. 79: 360-370

QUARTERMAIN, D., PAOLINO, R.M. and BANUAZIZI, A.   1968   1.23
Effect of electroconvulsive shock on retention of a
one-trial approach and a one-trial-avoidance response
in a T-maze.
Commun. Behavl. Biol. 2: 121-127

QUARTERMAIN, D., PAOLINO, R.M. and MILLER, N.E.   1965   1.21
A brief temporal gradient of retrograde amnesia
independent of situational change.
Science 149: 1116-1118

RAY, O.S. and BARRETT, R.J.   1969a   1.177
Disruptive effects of ECS as a function of current
level and mode of delivery.
J. comp. physiol. Psychol. 67: 110-116

RAY, O.S. and BARRETT, R.J.   1969b   1.178
Step-through latencies in mice as a function of
ECS-test interval.
Physiol. and Behav. 4: 583-586

RAY, O.S. and BIVENS, L.W.   1968   1.176
Reinforcement magnitude as a determinant of performance
decrement after electroconvulsive shock.
Science 160: 330-332

RIDDELL, W.I.   1969   1.214
Effect of electroconvulsive shock: permanent or
temporary retrograde amnesia.
J. comp. physiol. Psychol. 67: 140-144

ROBBINS, J.M. and MEYER, D.R.   1970   1.231
Motivational control of retrograde amnesia
J. exp. Psychol. 84: 220-225

ROBUSTELLI, F., GELLER, A., ARON, C. and
JARVIK, M.E.   1969   1.144
The relationship between the amnesic effect of
electroconvulsive shock and strength of conditioning
in a passive avoidance task.
Commun. Behavl. Biol. 3: 233-239

ROBUSTELLI, F., GELLER, A. and JARVIK, M.E.   1968   1.138
Potentiation of the amnesic effect of ECS by detention.
Psychon. Sci. 12: 85-86

ROBUSTELLI, F., GELLER, A. and JARVIK, M.E.   1969   1.142
Extinction in a passive avoidance task and its
interaction with electroconvulsive shock.
Psychon. Sci. 15: 139-140

ROBUSTELLI, F., GELLER, A. and JARVIK, M.E. 1969b   1.145
Temporal gradient of 23 hours with electroconvulsive
shock and its implications.
Commun. Behavl. Biol. 4: 79-84

ROBUSTELLI, F., GELLER, A. and JARVIK, M.E.   1969c   1.146
Combined action of two amnesic treatments.
Commun. Behavl. Biol. 4: 221-229

ROBUSTELLI, F. and JARVIK, M.E.   1968   1.137
Retrograde amnesia from detention.
Physiol. and Behav. 3: 543-547

ROUTTENBERG, A. and KAY, K.E.   1965   1.123
Effect of one electroconvulsive seizure on rat behaviour.
J. comp. physiol. Psychol. 59: 285-288

ROUTTENBERG, A., ZECHMEISTER, E.B. and BENTON, C.   1970   1.124
Hippocampal activity during memory disruption of passive
avoidance by electroconvulsive shock.
Life Sci. 9: 909-918

ST. OMER, V.V. and KRAL, P.A.   1971   1.225
Electroconvulsive shock impedes the learning of taste
aversions: absence of blood-brain-barrier involvement.
Psychon. Sci. 24: 251-252

SCHILLER, P.H. and CHOROVER, S.L.   1967   1.105
Short-term amnesic effect of electroconvulsive shock
in a one-trial maze learning paradigm.
Neuropsychologia 5: 155-163

SCHNEIDER, A.M., KAPP, B., ARON, C., and
JARVIK, M.E.   1969   1.143
Retroactive effects of transcorneal and transpinnate
ECS on step-through latencies of mice and rats.
J. comp. physiol. Psychol. 69: 506-509

SCHNEIDER, A.M., MALTER, A. and ADVOKAT, C.   1969   1.140
Pretreatment effects of a single ECS and footshock plus
ECS on stepdown latencies of trained and untrained rats.
J. comp. physiol. Psychol. 68: 627-630

SCHNEIDER, A.M., and SHERMAN, W.   1968   1.139
Amnesia: a function of the temporal relation of
footshock to electroconvulsive shock.
Science 159: 219-221

SHINKMAN, P.G. and KAUFMAN, K.P.   1972   1.253
Time course of retroactive effects of hippocampal
stimulation on learning.
Expl Neurol. 34: 476-483

SPEVACK, A.A., RABEDEAU, R.G. and SPEVACK, M.E.   1967   1.187
A temporally graded ECS function following one trial
learning.
Psychon. Sci. 9: 153-154

SPEVACK, A.A. and SUBOSKI, M.D.   1967   1.188
A confounding of conditioned suppression in passive
avoidance: ECS effects.
Psychon. Sci. 9: 23-24

SPEVACK, A.A. and SUBOSKI, M.D.   1969
Retrograde effects of electroconvulsive shock on
learned responses.
Psychol. Bull. 72: 66-76

SPRINGER, A.D. and MILLER, R.R.   1972   1.85
Retrieval failure induced by electroconvulsive shock:
reversal with dissimilar training and recovery agents.
Science 177: 628-630

SPROTT, R.L.   1966   1.173
Retrograde amnesia in 2 strains of mice.
Psychol. Rep. 19: 1247-1250

SPROTT, R.L. and WALLER, M.B.   1966   1.174
The effects of electroconvulsive shock on the action
of a reinforcing stimulus.
J. exp. Analysis Behav. 9: 663-669

STEIN, D.G. and CHOROVER, S.L.   1968   1.106
Effects of post trial electrical stimulation of
hippocampus and caudate nucleus on maze learning in
the rat.
Physiol. and Behav. 3: 787-791

STEPHENS, G. and McGAUGH, J.L.   1968   1.37
Retrograde amnesia - effects of periodicity and degree
of training.
Commun. Behavl. Biol. 1: 267-275

STEPHENS, G.J. and McGAUGH, J.L.   1969   1.38
Retrograde amnesia in mice: Alteration in temporal
gradients with phase-shifting of the temperature rhythm.
Commun. Behavl. Biol. 3: 253-257

STEPHENS, G., McGAUGH, J.L. and ALPERN, H.P.   1967   1.36
Periodicity and memory in mice.
Psychon. Sci. 8: 201-202

SUBOSKI, M.D., BLACK, M., LITNER, J., GREENER, R.T.
and SPEVACK, A.A.   1969   1.189
Long and short-term effects of ECS following one-trial
discriminated avoidance conditioning.
Neuropsychologia 7: 349-356

SUBOSKI, M.D., SPEVACK, A.A., LITNER, J. and
BEAUMASTER, E.   1969   1.190
Effects of ECS following one-trial discriminated
avoidance conditioning.
Neuropsychologia 7: 67-78

SUBOSKI, M.D. and WEINSTEIN, L.   1969   1.191
An ECS-maintained Kamin effect in rats.
J. comp. physiol. Psychol. 69: 510-513

TENEN, S.S.   1965a   1.125
Retrograde amnesia from ECS in a one trial appetitive
learning task.
Science 148: 1248-1250

TENEN, S.S.   1965b   1.126
Retrograde amnesia.
Science 149: 1521

THOMPSON, C.I. and GROSSMAN, L.B.   1972   1.235
Loss and recovery of long-term memories after ECS in
rats: evidence for state-dependent recall.
J. comp. physiol. Psychol. 78: 248-254

THOMPSON, C.I. and NEELY, J.E.   1970   1.234
Dissociated learning in rats produced by
electroconvulsive shock.
Physiol. and Behav. 5: 783-786

THOMPSON, R.   1957a   1.11
The comparative effects of ECS and anoxia on memory.
J. comp. physiol. Psychol. 50: 397-400

THOMPSON, R.   1957b   1.12
The effect of ECS on retention in young and old rats.
J. comp. physiol. Psychol. 50: 644-646

THOMPSON, R.   1958a   1.15
The effects of degree of learning and problem difficulty
on perseveration.
J. exp. Psychol. 55: 496-500

THOMPSON, R.   1958b   1.16
The effect of intracranial stimulation on memory in cats.
J. comp. physiol. Psychol. 51: 421-426

THOMPSON, R. and DEAN, W.   1955   1.10
A further study on the retroactive effect of
electroconvulsive shock.
J. comp. physiol. Psychol. 48: 488-491

THOMPSON, R., HARAVEY, F., PENNINGTON, D.F.,
SMITH, J., Jnr., GANNON, D. and STOCKWELL, F.   1958   1.13
An analysis of the differential effects of ECS on memory
in young and adult rats.
Can. J. Psychol. 12: 83-96

THOMPSON, R. and PENNINGTON, D.F., Jnr.   1957   1.14
Memory decrement produced by ECS as a function of
distribution in original learning.
J. comp. physiol. Psychol. 50: 401-404

THOMPSON, R.W., ENTER, R. and RUSSELL, N.   1967   1.114
Effect of electroconvulsive shock (ECS) on retention
of a passive avoidance response in rats.
Psychol. Rep. 21: 150-152

VARDARIS, R.M. and GEHRES, L.D.   1970   1.236
Brain seizure patterns and ESB-induced amnesia
for passive avoidance.
Physiol. and Behav. 5: 1271-1276

VARDARIS, R.M. and SCHWARTZ, K.E.   1971   1.237
Retrograde amnesia for passive avoidance produced
by stimulation of dorsal hippocampus.
Physiol. and Behav. 6: 131-136

WEAVER, T. and MAGNUS, J.G.   1969   1.168
Effects of unconditioned stimulus linked subconvulsive
current in chicks.
Psychon. Sci. 16: 265-266

WEISSMAN, A.   1963   1.87
Effect of electroconvulsive shock intensity and
seizure pattern on retrograde amnesia in rats.
J. comp. physiol. Psychol. 56: 806-810

WEISSMAN, A.   1964   1.88
Retrograde amnesic effect of supramaximal electroconvulsive
shock on one trial acquisition in rats.
J. comp. physiol. Psychol. 57: 248-250

WEISSMAN, A.   1965   1.89
Effect of anticonvulsant drugs on electroconvulsive
shock induced retrograde amnesia.
Archs int. Pharmacodyn. Ther. 154: 122-130

WHISHAW, I.Q. and DEATHERAGE, G.   1971   1.230
The effects of hippocampal electrographic seizures
on one-way active avoidance and visual discrimination
in rats: state-dependent effects.
Psychon. Sci. 25: 129-133

WILBURN, M.W. and KESNER, R.P.   1972   1.201
Differential amnestic effects produced by electrical
stimulation of the caudate nucleus and nonspecific
thalamic system.
Expl Neurol. 34: 45-50

WINOCUR, G. and MILLS, J.A.   1970   1.238
Aversive consequences of electroconvulsive shock.
Physiol. and Behav. 5: 631-634

WYERS, E.J. and DEADWYLER, S.A.   1971   1.157
Duration and nature of retrograde amnesia produced by
stimulation of caudate nucleus.
Physiol. and Behav. 6: 97-104

WYERS, E.J., PEEKE, H.V.S., WILLISTON, J.S.
and HERZ, M.J.   1968   1.154
Retroactive impairment of passive avoidance learning
by stimulation of the caudate nucleus.
Expl Neurol. 22: 350-366

YAGINUMA, S. and IWAHARA, S.   1971   1.251
Retrograde effects of electroconvulsive shock on a
passive avoidance response and conditioned emotionality
(defecation) in rats.
A. Animal Psychol. (Japan) 21: 1-9

YARNELL, T.D.   1968   1.77
The effect of electroconvulsive shock on a socially
motivated instrumental response.
Psychon. Sci. 12: 297-298

YARNELL, T.D. and ADAMS, H.E. 1964   1.67
Electroconvulsive shock and competing responses:
Stimulus generalization.
J. comp. physiol. Psychol. 58: 470-471

YOUNG, A.G. and DAY, H.D. 1971   1.242
Effect of ECS on one-trial learning and on the
partial reinforcement effect.
Psychon. Sci. 24: 99-100

YOUNG, A.G. and GALLUSCIO, E.H. 1970   1.240
Failure of ECS to produce retrograde amnesia following
partial reinforcement training.
Psychon. Sci. 18: 175-176

YOUNG, A.G. and GALLUSCIO, E.H. 1971   1.243
Recovery from ECS-produced amnesia.
Psychon. Sci. 22: 149-150

ZERBOLIO, D.J. Jnr. 1969a   1.215
The proactive effect of electroconvulsive shock on
memory storage: with and without convulsions.
Commun. Behavl. Biol. 4: 23-27

ZERBOLIO, D.J. Jnr. 1969b   1.216
Memory storage: the first posttrial hour.
Psychon. Sci. 15: 57-58

ZERBOLIO, D.J. Jnr. 1971   1.217
Retrograde Amnesia: the first posttrial hour.
Commun. Behavl. Biol. 6: 25-29

ZINKIN, S. and MILLER, A.J. 1967   1.193
Recovery of memory after amnesia induced by ECS.
Science 155: 102-103

ZORNETZER, S.F. 1972   1.49
Brain stimulation and retrograde amnesia in rats:
a neuroanatomical approach.
Physiol. and Behav. 8: 239-244

ZORNETZER, S.F. and McGAUGH, J.L. 1969   1.43
Effects of electroconvulsive shock upon inhibitory
avoidance: The persistence and stability of amnesia.
Commun. Behavl. Biol. 3: 173-180

ZORNETZER, S.F. and McGAUGH, J.L. 1970   1.45
Effects of frontal brain electroshock stimulation on
EEG activity and memory in rats: Relationship to
ECS-produced retrograde amnesia.
J. Neurobiol. 1: 379-394

ZORNETZER, S.F. and McGAUGH, J.L.   1971a   1.46
Retrograde amnesia and brain seizures in mice.
Physiol. and Behav. 7: 401-408

ZORNETZER, S.F. and McGAUGH, J.L.   1971b   1.47
Retrograde amnesia and brain seizures in mice:
a further analysis.
Physiol. and Behav. 7: 841-845

ZORNETZER, S.F. and McGAUGH, J.L.   1972   1.48
Electrophysiological correlates of frontal cortex-
induced retrograde amnesia in rats.
Physiol. and Behav. 8: 233-238

References

ADAMS, H.E., HOBLIT, P.R. and SUTKER, P.B.   1969   2.11
Electroconvulsive shock, brain acetylcholinesterase
activity and memory.
Physiol. and Behav. 4: 113-116

BIVENS, L.W. and RAY, O.S.   1967   2.9
Effects of electroconvulsive shock and strychnine
sulphate on memory consolidation.
Neuropsychopharmacology, (Proc. V. Intern. Congr.
C.I.N.P., Washington, 1966) p. 1030-1034

BUCKHOLTZ, N.S. and BOWMAN, R.E.   1970   2.15
Retrograde amnesia and brain RNA content after TCAP.
Physiol. and Behav. 5: 911-914

DAVIS, J.W., THOMAS, R.K. Jr. and ADAMS, H.E.   1971   2.12
Interactions of scopolamine and physostigmine with
ECS and one trial learning.
Physiol. and Behav. 6: 219-222

DUNN, A.   1971
Brain protein synthesis after electroshock.
Brain Res. 35: 254-259

DUNN, A., GIUDITTA, A. and PAGLIUCA, N.   1971
The effect of electroconvulsive shock on protein synthesis
in mouse brain.
J. Neurochem. 18: 2093-2099

ESSMAN, W.B.   1966   2.2
The effect of tricyanoaminopropene on the amnesic effect
of electroconvulsive shock.
Psychopharmacologia 9: 426-433

ESSMAN, W.B.   1967a   2.3
Changes in memory consolidation with alterations in
neural RNA. Neuropsychopharmacology, (Proc. V. Intern.
Congr. C.I.N.P., Washington, 1966) p. 108-113

ESSMAN, W.B.   1967b   2.4
The temporal limits of memory consolidation as a
function of alterations in brain serotonin.
Proc. VII. Intern. Congr. Biochem., Tokyo, p.997

ESSMAN, W.B.   1968a   2.5
Changes in ECS-induced retrograde amnesia with DBMC:
Behavioural and biochemical correlates of brain
serotonim antagonism.
Physiol. and Behav. 3: 527-531

ESSMAN, W.B.   1968b   2.6
Electroshock-induced retrograde amnesia and brain
serotonin metabolism: Effects of several anti-depressant
compounds.
Psychopharmacologia 13: 258-266

ESSMAN, W.B.   1970
Some neurochemical correlates of altered memory consolidation.
Trans. N.Y. Acad. Sci. 32: 948-973

ESSMAN, W.B.   1972
Neurochemical changes in ECS and ECT.
Seminars in Psychiatry 4: 67-78

ESSMAN, W.B. and GOLOD, M.I.   1968   2.8
Reduction of retrograde amnesia by tricyanoaminopropene-
drug dosage and electroshock intensity.
Commun. Behavl. Biol. 1: 183-187

ESSMAN, W.B., STEINBERG, M.L. and GOLOD, M.I.   1968   2.7
Alterations in the behavioural and biochemical effects
of electroconvulsive shock with nicotine.
Psychon. Sci. 12: 107-108

KOPP, R., BOHDANECKY, Z. and JARVIK, M.E.   1967   2.10
Depressing effect of scopolamine on the temporal
gradient of retrograde amnesia to ECS in mice.
Neuropsychopharmacology, (Proc. V. Intern. Congr.
C.I.N.P., Washington, 1966) p. 1052-1054

LEWIS, D.J. and BREGMAN, N.J.   1972   2.18
The cholinergic system, amnesia and memory.
Physiol. and Behav. 8: 511-514

MILLER, R.R. and SPRINGER, A.D.   1972   2.19
Effects of strychnine on ECS-induced amnesia in the rat.
Psychon. Sci. 26: 289-290

MINARD, F.N. and RICHTER, D.   1968
Electroshock-induced seizures and the turnover of brain
proteins in the rat.
J. Neurochem. 15: 1463-1468

MUSACCHIO, J.M., JULOU, L. KETY, S.S.
and GLOWINSKI, J.   1969   2.13
Increase in rat brain tyrosine hydroxylase activity
produced by electroconvulsive shock.
Proc. natn. Acad. Sci. U.S.A. 63: 1117-1119

OTT, T. and MATTHIES, H.   1971   2.16
The influence of orotic acid on the retrograde
amnesia caused by ECS.
Psychopharmacologia 20: 16-21

RIEGE, W.H.   1971   2.17
One-trial learning and brain serotonin depletion
by para-chlorophenylalanine.
Int. J. Neuroscience 2: 237-240

STEIN, D.G. and BRINK, J.J.   1969   2.14
Prevention of RA by injection of magnesium pemoline
in dimethylsulfoxide.
Psychopharmacologia 14: 240-247

VESCO,C. and GIUDITTA, A.   1968
Disaggregation of brain polysomes induced by
electroconvulsive treatment.
J. Neurochem. 15: 81-85

WEISSMAN, A.   1965   2.1
Effect of anticonvulsant drugs on electroconvulsive
shock-induced retrograde amnesia.
Archs int. Pharmacodyn. Ther. 154: 122-130

TRANSMITTERS
References

BERGER, B.D. and STEIN, L. 1969   3.20
An analysis of learning deficits produced by scopolamine.
Psychopharmacologia 14: 271-283

BOHDANECKY, Z. and JARVIK, M.E. 1967   3.15
The effect of D-amphetamine and physostigmine upon
acquisition and retrieval in a single trial learning task.
Archs int. Pharmacodyn. Ther. 170: 58-65

BURKHALTER, A. 1963
Effect of puromycin on cholinesterase activity of
embryonic chick intestine in organ culture.
Nature, Lond. 199: 598-599

CHRIST, D.D. and NISHI, S. 1971
Effects of adrenaline on nerve terminals in the superior
cervical ganglion of the rabbit.
Brit. J. Pharmacol. 41: 331-338

DEUTSCH, J.A. 1966   3.4
Substrates of learning and memory.
Dis. Nerv. Syst. 27: 20-24

DEUTSCH, J.A. 1969   3.10
The physiological basis of memory.
Psychol. Rev. 20: 85-104

DEUTSCH, J.A. 1971
The cholinergic synapse and the site of memory.
Science 174: 788-794

DEUTSCH, J.A., HAMBURG, M.D. and DAHL, H. 1966   3.3
Anticholinesterase-induced amnesia and its temporal
aspects.
Science 151: 221-223

DEUTSCH, J.A. and LEIBOWITZ, S.F. 1966   3.5
Amnesia or reversal of forgetting by anticholinesterase,
depending simply on time of injection.
Science 153: 1017-1018

DEUTSCH, J.A. and LUTZKY, H. 1967   3.6
Memory enhancement by anticholinesterase as a function
of initial learning.
Nature, Lond. 213: 742

DEUTSCH, J.A. and ROCKLIN, K. 1967   3.7
Amnesia induced by scopolamine and its temporal variations.
Nature, Lond. 216: 89-90

DEUTSCH, J.A. and WIENER, N.I.   1969   3.12
Analysis of extinction through amnesia.
J. comp. physiol. Psychol. 69: 179-184

DILTS, S.L. and BERRY, C.A.   1967   3.16
Effect of cholinergic drugs on passive avoidance in mouse.
J. Pharm. Exptl. Ther. 158: 279-285

DISMUKES, R.K. and RAKE, A.V.   1972   3.33
Involvement of biogenic amines in memory formation.
Psychopharmacologia 23: 17-25

ENERO, M.A., LANGER, S.Z., ROTHLIN, R.P.
and STEPHANO, F.J.E.   1972
Role of the α-adrenoceptor in regulating noradrenaline
overflow by nerve stimulation.
Brit. J. Pharmacol. 44: 672-688

ESSMAN, W.B.   1972
Neurochemical changes in ECS and ECT.
Seminars in Psychiatry 4: 67-78

EVANS, H.L. and PATTON, R.A.   1968   3.18
Scopolamine effects on a one-trial test of fear
conditioning.
Psychon. Sci. 11: 229-230

GLICK, S.D. and ZIMMERBERG, B.   1971   3.26
Comparative learning impairment and amnesia by
scopolamine, phencyclidine, and ketamine.
Psychon. Sci. 25: 165-166

GLICK, S.D. and ZIMMERBERG, B.   1972   3.27
Amnesic effects of scopolamine.
Behavl. Biol. 7: 245-254

GOLDBERG, M.E., SLEDGE, K., HEFNER, M.
and ROBICHAUD, R.C.   1971   3.29
Learning impairment after three classes of agents
which modify cholinergic function.
Archs int. Pharmacodyn. Ther. 193: 226-235

HAMBURG, M.D.   1967   3.8
A retrograde amnesia produced by intraperitoneal
injections of physostigmine.
Science 156: 973-974

HARTMAN, B.K., ZIDE, D. and UDENFRIEND, S.   1972
The use of dopamine β-hydroxylase as a marker for the
central noradrenergic nervous system in rat brain.
Proc. natn. Acad. Sci. U.S.A. 69: 2722-2726

HUPPERT, F.A. and DEUTSCH, J.A. 1969   3.11
Improvement in memory with time.
Q. Jl exp. Psychol. 21: 267-271

KASA, P. 1971
Ultrastructural localisation of cholineacetyltransferase
and acetylcholinesterase in central and peripheral
nervous tissue.
In: Histochemistry of Nervous Transmission, edited by
O. Ëränko, Progress in Brain Research 34: 337-334

KETY, S.S. 1970
The biogenic amines in the central nervous system: their
possible roles in arousal, emotion and learning.
In: The Neurosciences Second Study Program, edited by
F.O. Schmitt, New York: The Rockefeller Uni. Press,p.324-336

KRAL, P.A. 1971   3.30
Effects of scopolamine injection during CS-US interval
on conditioning.
Psychol. Rep. 28: 690

MADDEN, T.C.,Jnr. and GREENOUGH, W.T. 1972   3.34
Adrenergic and cholinergic drug effects on retention
of a discriminated escape.
Psychon. Sci. 26: 133-134

MEYERS, B. 1965   3.2
Some effects of scopolamine on a passive avoidance
response in rats.
Psychopharmacologia 8: 111-119

MUSCHOLL, E. 1970
Cholinomimetic drugs and release of the adrenergic
transmitter.
In: Bayer Symposium II, New Aspects of Storage and
Release Mechanisms of the Catecholamines, edited by
H.S. Schumann and G. Kronenberg, Berlin, New York:
Springer-Verlag, p. 168-186

PAZZAGLI, A. and PEPEU, G. 1964   3.1
Amnesic properties of scopolamine and brain
acetylcholine in the rat.
Intern. J. Neuropharm. 4: 291-299

RANDT, C.T., QUARTERMAIN, D., GOLDSTEIN, M.
and ANAGNOSTE, B. 1971   3.32
Norepinephrine biosynthesis inhibition: effects on
memory in mice.
Science 172: 498-499

RUSSELL, R.W., WARBURTON, D.M., VASQUEZ, B.J.,
OVERSTREET, D.H. and DALGLISH, F.W.   1971   3.23
Acquisition of new responses by rats during chronic
depression of acetylcholinesterase activity.
J. comp. physiol. Psychol. 77: 228-233

SCHNEIDER, A.M., KAPP, B.S. and SHERMAN, W.M.   1970   3.28
The effects of centrally and peripherally acting
cholinergic drugs on the short-term performance
gradient following passive-avoidance training.
Psychopharmacologia 18: 77-81

SILVER, A.   1967
Cholinesterases of the central nervous system with
special reference to the cerebellum.
Int. Rev. Neurobiol. 10: 57-109

SILVER, A.   1971
The significance of cholinesterase in the developing
nervous system.
In: Histochemistry of Nervous Transmission, edited by
O. Eränko, Progress in Brain Research vol. 34: 345-355

SLATER, P.   1968   3.19
The effects of triethylcholine, hemicholinium-3 and
N-4-Diethylamino -2-butynyl -succinimide on maze
performance and brain acetylcholine in the rat.
Life Sci. 7: 833-837

SQUIRE, L.R.   1969
Effects of pretrial and post-trial administration of
cholinergic and anticholinergic drugs on spontaneous
alternation.
J. comp. physiol. Psychol. 69: 69-75

SQUIRE, L.R.   1970   3.24
Physostigmine: Effects on retention at different times
after brief training.
Psychon. Sci. 19: 49-50

SQUIRE, L.R., GLICK, S.D. and GOLDFARB, J.   1971   3.25
Relearning at different times after training as affected
by centrally and peripherally acting cholinergic drugs
in the mouse.
J. comp. physiol. Psychol. 74: 41-45

STAHL, S.M., ZELLER, E.A. and BOSCHES, B.   1971   3.31
On the effect of modulation of cerebral amine metabolism
on the learning and memory of goldfish (Carassius auratus).
Trans. Amer. Neurol. Assoc. p. 96

STARK, L.G.   1967   3.17
The inability of scopolamine to induce state-dependent
one-trial learning.
Fed. Proc. 26: 613

SUITS, E. and ISAACSON, R.L.   1969   3.21
Effects of scopolamine hydrobromide on passive avoidance
learning in rats.
Psychon. Sci. 15: 135-137

WARBURTON, D.M.   1969   3.22
Behavioural effects of central and peripheral changes
in acetylcholine systems.
J. comp. physiol. Psychol. 68: 56-64

WEISS, B. and HELLER, A.   1969
Methodological problems in evaluating the role of
cholinergic mechanisms in behaviour.
Fed. Proc. 28: 135-146

WIENER, N.I.   1970   3.13
Electroconvulsive shock induced impairment and
enhancement of a learned response.
Physiol. and Behav. 5: 971-974

WIENER, N.I. and DEUTSCH, J.A.   1968   3.9
Temporal aspects of anticholinergic and anticholinesterase
induced amnesia.
J. comp. physiol. Psychol. 66: 613-617

WIENER, N.I. and MESSER, J.   1972   3.14
Hemicholinium-3 induced amnesia: some temporal properties.
Psychon. Sci. 26: 129-130

References

ABT, J.P., ESSMAN, W.B. and JARVIK, M.E.   1961   4.8
Ether-induced retrograde amnesia for one-trial
conditioning in mice
Science 133: 1477-1478

AHLERS, R.H. and BEST, P.J.   1972   4.54
Retrograde amnesia for discriminated taste aversions:
a memory deficit.
J. comp. physiol. Psychol. 79: 371-376

AHMAD, A. and ACHARI, G.   1968   4.33
Effect of some tranquilizers on learning and memory
traces in rats.
Indian J. Physiol. Pharmacol. 12: 81-85

ALPERN, H.P. and KIMBLE, D.P.   1967   4.27
Retrograde amnesic effects of diethyl ether and
bis (trifluorethyl) ether.
J. comp. physiol. Psychol. 63: 168-171

ANGEL, C., BOUNDS, M.S.,Jnr. and PERRY, A.   1972   4.55
A comparison of the effects of halothane on blood-
brain barrier and memory consolidation.
Dis. Nerv. Syst. 33: 87-93

BALDWIN, B.A. and SOLTYSIK, S.S.   1969   4.42
The effect of cerebral ischaemia or intracarotid
injection of methohexitone on short term memory in goats.
Brain Res. 16: 105-120

BLACK, M., SUBOSKI, M.D. and FREEDMAN, N.L.   1967   4.29
Effects of cortical spreading depression and ether
following one-trial discriminated avoidance learning.
Psychon. Sci. 9: 597-598

BOHDANECKY, Z., KOPP, R. and JARVIK, M.E.   1968   4.11
Comparison of ECS and flurothyl-induced retrograde
amnesia in mice.
Psychopharmacologia 12: 91-95

BOOTH, D.A.   1970
Neurochemical changes correlated with learning and
memory retention.
In: Molecular Mechanisms in Memory and Learning, edited
by G. Ungar, New York: Plenum Press, pp 1-57

BOVET, D., McGAUGH, J.L. and OLIVERIO, A.   1966   4.25
Effects of post trial administration of drugs on
avoidance learning in mice.
Life Sci. 5: 1309-1315

BUREŠ, J. and BUREŠOVÁ, W.   1963   4.14
Cortical spreading depression as a memory
disturbing factor.
J. comp. physiol. Psychol. 56: 268-272

CHERKIN, A.   1968
Retrograde amnesia: role of temperature, dose and
duration of amnesic agent.
Psychon. Sci. 13: 255

CHERKIN, A.   1969   4.18
Kinetics of memory consolidation: role of amnesic
treatment parameters.
Proc. natn. Acad. Sci. U.S.A. 63: 1094-1101

CHERKIN, A.   1970   4.19
Retrograde amnesia: impaired memory consolidation
or impaired retrieval?
Commun. Behavl. Biol. 5: 183-190

CHERKIN, A.   1972   4.20
Retrograde amnesia in the chick: resistance to the
reminder effect.
Physiol. and Behav. 8: 949-955

CHERKIN, A. and LEE-TENG, E.   1965   4.17
Interruption by halothane of memory consolidation.
Fed. Proc. 24: 328

DOTY, B.A. and DOTY, L.A.   1964   4.16
Effect of age and chlorpromazine on memory consolidation.
J. comp. physiol. Psychol. 57: 331-334

ELIAS, M.F. and SIMMERMAN, S.J.   1971   4.49
Proactive and retroactive effects of diethyl ether
on spatial discrimination learning in inbred mouse
strains DBA/2J and C57BL/6J
Psychon. Sci. 22: 299-301

ESSMAN, W.B.   1968   4.12
Retrograde amnesia in seizure protected mice: behavioural
and biochemical effects of pentylenetetrazol.
Physiol. and Behav. 3: 549-552

ESSMAN, W.B. and JARVIK, M.E.   1960   4.6
The retrograde effect of ether anaesthesia on a
CAR in mice.
Amer. Psychologist 15: 498

ESSMAN, W.B. and JARVIK, M.E. 1961   4.9
Impairment of retention for a conditioned response by
ether anaesthesia in mice.
Psychopharmacologia 2: 172-176

FRANCHINA, J.J. and MOORE, M.H. 1968   4.34
Strychnine and the inhibition of previous experience.
Science 160: 903-904

FRECKLETON, W.C. and WAHLSTEN, D. 1968   4.35
Carbon dioxide-induced amnesia in the cockroach
Periplaneta americana
Psychon. Sci. 12: 179-180

GARG, M. and HOLLAND, H.C. 1968   4.36
Consolidation and maze learning: the effects of post-
trial injections of a depressant drug (Pentobarbital
Sodium).
Psychopharmacologia 12: 127-132

GLICK, S.D., NAKAMURA, R.K. and JARVIK, M.E. 1970   4.13
Stress-induced amnesia and potentiation by ether.
Psychon. Sci. 19: 259-260

GROSSMAN, S.P. 1969   4.43
Facilitation of learning following intracranial
injections of pentylenetetrazol.
Physiol. and Behav. 4: 625-628

GRUBER, R.P. 1971   4.50
Retrograde amnesic facilitative effects of ether on
learning and generalization gradients.
J. Gen. Psychol. 85: 285-293

HERZ, M.J. 1969   4.24
Interference with one-trial appetitive and aversive
learning by ether and ECS.
J. Neurobiol. 1: 111-122

HERZ, M.J., PEEKE, H.V.S. and WYERS, E.J. 1966   4.23
Amnesic effects of ether and electroconvulsive shock
in mice.
Psychon. Sci. 4: 375-376

IWAHARA, S., IWASAKI, T. and HASEGAWA, Y. 1968   4.38
Effects of chlorpromazine and homofenazine upon a
passive avoidance response in rats.
Psychopharmacologia 13: 320-331

IWASAKI, T., KATAYAMA, M. and IWAHARA, S.   1968   4.37
Differential effects of chlorpromazine upon passive
avoidance response in rats under two types of shock
treatment.
Jap. Psychol. Res. 10: 191-198

JOHNSON, F.N.   1969   4.44
The effects of chlorpromazine on the decay and
consolidation of short-term memory traces in mice.
Psychopharmacologia 16: 105-114

JOHNSON, F.N.   1970a   4.45
The effects of chlorpromazine on one-trial passive
avoidance learning in mice: further reexamination of
pre- and post- learning administration.
Psychopharmacologia 18: 11-18

JOHNSON, F.N.   1970b   4.46
The effects of chlorpromazine on the expression of an
acquired passive avoidance response in mice.
Psychopharmacologia 18: 333-345

JOHNSON, F.N.   1971   4.47
Stimulus significance and chlorpromazine effects on
the expression of avoidance learning in mice.
Neuropharmacol. 10: 267-272

KINCAID, J.P.   1967   4.32
Permanence of amnesia after single post-trial
treatments of metrazol or electroconvulsive shock.
Psychon. Sci. 9: 56-60

LEUKEL, F.   1957   4.2
A comparison of the effects of ECS and anaesthesia on
acquisition of the maze habit.
J. comp. physiol. Psychol. 50: 300-306

LEUKEL, F. and QUINTON, E.   1964   4.3
Carbon dioxide effects on acquisition and extinction
of avoidance behaviour.
J.comp. physiol. Psychol. 57: 267-270

MAYSE, J.F. and DeVIETTI, T.L.   1971   4.51
A comparison of state dependent learning induced by
electroconvulsive shock and pentobarbital.
Physiol. and Behav. 7: 717-721

McGAUGH, J.L. and ALPERN, H.   1966   4.26
Effects of electroshock on memory: amnesia without
convulsions.
Science 152: 665-666

NACHMAN, M. and MEINECKE, R.O.   1969   4.48
Lack of retrograde amnesic effects of repeated ECS and
CO_2 treatments.
J. comp. physiol. Psychol. 68: 631-636

OVERTON, D.A.   1964   4.15
State dependent or "dissociated" learning produced with
pentobarbital.
J. comp. physiol. Psychol. 57: 3-12

PALFAI, T. and CHILLAG, D.   1971   4.40
Time-dependent memory deficits produced by pentylene-
tetrazol (Metrazol)- the effect of reinforcement magnitude.
Physiol. and Behav. 7: 439-442

PALFAI, T. and CORNELL, J.M.   1968   4.39
Effect of drugs on consolidation of classically
conditioned fear.
J. comp. physiol. Psychol. 66: 584-589

PAOLINO, R.M., QUARTERMAIN, D. and MILLER, N.E.   1966   4.28
Different temporal gradients of retrograde amnesia
produced by carbon dioxide anaesthesia and electroconvulsive shock.
J. comp. physiol. Psychol. 62: 270-274

PEARLMAN, C.A.,Jnr.   1966   4.10
Similar retrograde amnesic effects of ether and
spreading cortical depression.
J. comp. physiol. Psychol. 61: 306-308

PEARLMAN, C.R.,Jnr., SHARPLESS, S.K. and JARVIK, M.E.1959 4.5
Effects of ether, pentobarbital and pentylenetetrazol
upon one-trial learning of an avoidance response.
Fed. Proc. 18: 432

PEARLMAN, C.A.,Jnr., SHARPLESS, S.K. and JARVIK, M.E.1961 4.7
Retrograde amnesia produced by anaesthetic and convulsant
agents.
J. comp. physiol. Psychol. 54: 109-112

PENROD, W.C. and BOICE, R.   1971   4.52
Effects of halothane anesthesia on the retention of
a passive avoidance task in rats.
Psychon. Sci. 23: 205-207

PORTER, A.L.   1972
An analytical review of the effects of non-hydrogen-
bonding anesthetics on memory processing.
Behavl. Biol. 7: 291-309

QUINTON, E.E.   1966   4.4
Retrograde amnesia induced by carbon dioxide inhalation.
Psychon. Sci. 5: 417-418

RANSMEIER, R.E. and GERARD, R.W.   1954   4.1
Effects of temperature, convulsion and metabolic
factors on rodent memory and EEG.
Am.J. Physiol. 179: 663-664

SCHMALTZ, L.W.   1971   4.53
Deficit in active avoidance learning in rats following
penicillin injection into hippocampus.
Physiol. and Behav. 6: 667-674

SUBOSKI, M.D., LITNER, J. and BLACK, M.   1968   4.30
Further on the effects of ether anaesthesia following
one-trial discriminated avoidance learning.
Psychon. Sci. 10: 161-162

TABER, R.I. and BANUAZIZI, A.   1965   4.21
CO_2- induced retrograde amnesia in a one-trial learning
situation.
Fed. Proc. 24: 329

TABER, R.I. and BANUAZIZI, A.   1966   4.22
CO_2-induced retrograde amnesia in a one-trial learning
situation.
Psychopharmacologia 9: 382-391

WEISSMAN, A.   1967   4.31
Drugs and retrograde amnesia.
Intern. Rev. Neurobiol. 10: 167-198

WIMER, R.E.   1968   4.41
Bases of a facilitative effect upon retention resulting
from posttrial etherization.
J. comp. physiol. Psychol. 65: 340-342

TEMPERATURE
References

BEITEL, R.E. and PORTER, P.B. 1968   5.10
Deficits in retention and impairments in learning
induced by severe hypothermia in mice.
J. comp. physiol. Psychol. 66: 53-59

CERF, J.A. and OTIS, L.S. 1957   5.4
Heat narcosis and its effect on retention of a
learned behaviour in the goldfish.
Fed. Proc. 16: 20-21

DAVIS, R.E., BRIGHT, P.J. and AGRANOFF, B.W. 1965   5.9
Effect of ECS and puromycin on memory in fish.
J. comp. physiol. Psychol. 60: 162-166

ESSMAN, W.B. and SUDAK, F.N. 1962   5.5
Sustained and temporary hypothermia as variables in
successful maze learning.
Psychol. Rep. 10: 551-557

ESSMAN, W.B. and SUDAK, F.N. 1963   5.6
Effect of hypothermia on the establishment of
a conditioned avoidance response in mice.
J. comp. physiol. Psychol. 56: 336-369

FRENCH, J.W. 1942
The effect of temperature on the retention of a
maze habit in fish.
J. exp. Psychol. 31: 79-87

GERARD, R.W. 1955   5.3
Biological roots of psychiatry.
Science 122: 225-230

GROSSER, G.S. and PERCY, H.E. 1971   5.17
Postshock immersion of mice without memory disruption.
J. comp. physiol. Psychol. 76: 119-122

JACOBS, B.L. and SORENSON, C.A. 1969   5.15
Memory disruption in mice by brief post-trial
immersion in hot or cold water.
J. comp. physiol. Psychol. 68: 239-244

JENSEN, R.A. and RICCIO, D. 1970   5.14
Effects of prior experience upon retrograde amnesia
produced by hypothermia.
Physiol. and Behav. 5: 1291-1294

JONES, M.R.   1943   5.1
The effect of hypothermia on retention.
J. comp. physiol. Psychol. 35: 311-316

KANE, J. and JARVIK, M.E.   1970   5.16
Amnesic effects of cooling and heating in mice.
Psychon. Sci. 18: 7-8

MISANIN, J.R. and HOOVER, M.   1971   5.18
Recovery rate as a determinant of the amnesic-like
effect of hypothermia.
Physiol. and Behav. 6: 689-693

MISANIN, J.R., NAGY, Z.M., KEISER, E.F.
and BOWEN, W.   1971   5.19
Emergence of long-term memory in the neonatal rat.
J. comp. physiol. Psychol. 77: 188-199

MROSOVSKY, N.   1963   5.8
Retention and reversal of conditioned avoidance
following severe hypothermia.
J. comp. physiol. Psychol. 56: 811-813

RANSMEIER, R.E. and GERARD, R.W.   1954   5.2
Effects of temperature, convulsion and metabolic
factors on rodent memory and EEG.
Am. J. Physiol. 179: 663-664

RICCIO, D.C., GAEBELEIN, C. and COHEN, P.   1968   5.11
Some behavioural aspects of retrograde amnesia
produced by hypothermia.
Physiol. and Behav. 3: 973-976

RICCIO, D.C., HODGES, L.A. and RANDALL, P.K.   1968   5.12
Retrograde amnesia produced by hypothermia in rats.
J. comp. physiol. Psychol. 66: 618-622

RICCIO, D.C. and STIKES, E.R.   1969   5.13
Persistent but modifiable retrograde amnesia
produced by hypothermia.
Physiol. and Behav. 4: 649-652

SMITH, S.L. and MISANIN, J.R.   1972   5.20
A reduction in ECS-produced amnesia through cooling.
Psychon. Sci. 26: 21-22

SUDAK, F.N. and ESSMAN, W.B.   1964   5.7
Retrograde retention deficit produced by body
temperature reduction in rats.
Fed. Proc. 23: 312

BALDWIN, B.A. and SOLTYSIK, S.S.   1966   6.6
The effect of cerebral ischaemia, resulting in loss
of EEG on the acquisition of conditioned reflexes in
goats.
Brain Res. 2: 71-84

BALDWIN, B.A. and SOLTYSIK, S.S.   1969   6.7
The effect of cerebral ischaemia or intracarotid
injection of methohexitone on short term memory in goats.
Brain Res. 16: 105-120

CHERKIN, A.   1971   6.10
Memory consolidation in the chick: Resistance to
prolonged post-training hypoxia.
Commun. Behavl. Biol. 5: 325-330

ERKERT, J.D. and VIERCK, C.J.,Jnr. 1971   6.11
The effect of hyperbaric oxygen on memory.
Psychon. Sci. 22: 151-152

GIURGEA, C., LEFEVRE, D., LESCRENIER, C.
and DAVID-REMACLE, M.   1971   6.12
Pharmacological protection against hypoxia induced
amnesia in rats.
Psychopharmacologia 20: 160-168

HAYES, K.J.   1953   6.1
Anoxic and convulsive amnesia in rats.
J. comp. physiol. Psychol. 46: 216-217

PENNINGTON, D.R.,Jnr. 1958   6.5
The effects of ECS on retention of a discrimination
habit in rats subjected to anoxia.
J. comp. physiol. Psychol. 51: 687-690

RANSMEIER, R.E. and GERARD, R.W.   1954   6.2
Effects of temperature, convulsion and metabolic
factors on rodent memory and EEG.
Am. J. Physiol. 179: 663-664

REICHELT, K.L.   1968
Chemical basis for intolerance of brain to anoxia.
Acta anaesth. scand. 29: 35-46

SARA, S.J. and LEFEVRE, D.   1972   6.13
Hypoxia-induced amnesia in one-trial learning and
pharmacological protection by piracetam
Psychopharmacologia 25: 32-40

TABER, R.I. and BANUAZIZI, A.   1966   6.8
CO_2 induced retrograde amnesia in a one-trial
learning situation.
Psychopharmacologia 9: 382-391

THOMPSON, R.   1957   6.4
The comparative effects of ECS and anoxia on memory.
J. comp. physiol. Psychol. 50: 397-400

THOMPSON, R. and PRYER, R.S.   1956   6.3
The effect of anoxia on the retention of a
discrimination habit.
J. comp. physiol. Psychol. 49: 297-300

VACHER, J.M., KING, R.A. and MILLER, A.T., Jnr.   1968   6.9
Failure of hypoxia to produce retrograde amnesia.
J. comp. physiol. Psychol. 66: 179-181

POTASSIUM CHLORIDE

References

ALBERT, D.J.   1966
The effect of spreading depression on the consolidation
of learning.
Neuropsychologia 4: 49-64

AVIS, H. and CARLTON, P.L.   1968   7.6
Retrograde amnesia produced by hippocampal spreading
depression.
Science 161: 73-75

BARONDES, S.H. and COHEN, H.D.   1966
Puromycin effect on successive phases of memory
storage.
Science 151: 594-595

BLACK, M., SUBOSKI, M.D. and FREEDMAN, N.L.   1967   7.5
Effects of cortical spreading depression and ether
following one-trial discriminated avoidance learning.
Psychon. Sci. 9: 597-598

BIVENS, L.W. and RAY, O.S.   1965
Memory trace disruption by cortical spreading depression.
Psychol. Rep. 17: 175-178

BRINLEY, F.J., KANDEL, E.R. and MARSHALL, W.H.   1960
Potassium outflux from rabbit cerebral cortex during
spreading depression.
J. Neurophysiol 23: 246-256

BUREŠ, J. and BUREŠOVÁ, W.   1963   7.3
Cortical spreading depression as a memory
disturbing factor.
J. comp. physiol. Psychol. 56: 268-272

COHEN, H.D. and BARONDES, S.H.   1967
Puromycin effect on memory may be due to occult
seizures.
Science 157: 333-334

COHEN, H.D., ERVIN, F. and BARONDES, S.H.   1966
Puromycin and cycloheximide: different effects on
hippocampal electrical activity.
Science 154: 1557-1558

COLLEWIJN, H. and VAN HARREVELD, A.   1966
Membrane potential of cerebral cortical cells
during spreading depression and asphyxia.
Expl Neurol. 15: 425-436

DAVIS, R.E. and KLINGER, P.D.   1969   7.7
Environmental control of amnesic effects of various
agents in goldfish.
Physiol. and Behav. 4: 269-271

FIFKOVA, E. and VAN HARREVELD, A.   1970
Glutamate effects in developing chicken.
Expl Neurol. 28: 286-298

GRAFSTEIN, B.   1956
Mechanism of spreading cortical depression.
J. Neurophysiol. 19: 154-171

HUGHES, R.A.   1969
Retrograde amnesia in rats produced by hippocampal
injections of potassium chloride.
J. comp. physiol. Psychol. 68: 637-644

KAPP, B.S. and SCHNEIDER, A.M.   1971   7.10
Selective recovery from retrograde amnesia produced
by hippocampal spreading depression.
Science 173: 1149-1151

KUPFERMANN, I.   1965   7.4
Failure of spreading depression to produce
retrograde amnesia.
Psychon. Sci. 3: 43-44

LEÃO, A.A.P.   1944
Spreading depression of activity in the cerebral
cortex.
J. Neurophysiol. 7: 359-390

LEÃO, A.A.P.   1947
Further observations on spreading depression of
activity in the cerebral cortex.
J. Neurophysiol. 10: 409-414

LEÃO, A.A.P. and FERREIVA, H.M.   1953
Anais. Acad. Brasil Gen. 25: 259
Quoted by A. Van Harreveld.
The extracellular space in the vertebrate nervous system.
In: Structure and Function of the Nervous System, edited by
G.H. Bourne, New York: Academic Press, vol. VI., p.447-511

MORLOCK, N.L., MORI, K. and WARD, A.A., Jnr.   1964
A study of single cortical neurones during spreading
depression.
J. Neurophysiol. 27: 1192-1198

PAOLINO, R.M. and LEVY, H.M.   1971   7.11
Amnesia produced by spreading depression and ECS:
evidence for time-dependent memory trace localization.
Science 172: 746-749

PEARLMAN, C.A., Jnr. 1966   7.2
Similar retrograde amnesic effects of ether and
spreading cortical depression.
J. comp. physiol. Psychol. 61: 306-308

PEARLMAN, C.A., Jnr.and JARVIK, M.E.   1961   7.1
Retrograde amnesia produced by spreading cortical
depression.
Fed. Proc. 20: 340

RAY, O.S. and EMLEY, G.   1964
Time factors in interhemispheric transfer of learning.
Science 144: 76-78

REED, V.G. and TROWILL, J.A.   1969   7.9
Stimulus control value of spreading depression
demonstrated without shifting depressed hemispheres.
J. comp. physiol. Psychol. 69: 40-43

RUSSELL, I.S. and OCHS, S.   1963
Localization of a memory trace in one cortical
hemisphere and transfer to the other hemisphere.
Brain 86: 37-54

SCHNEIDER, A.M.   1966
Retention under spreading depression: a generalization
decrement phenomenon.
J. comp. physiol. Psychol. 62: 317-319

SCHNEIDER, A.M.   1967
Control of memory by spreading cortical depression:
a case for stimulus control.
Psychol. Rev. 74: 201-215

VAN HARREVELD, A.
The extracellular space in the vertebrate central
nervous system.
In: Structure and Function of the Nervous System, edited by
G.H. Bourne, New York: Academic Press, vol. VI., p.447-511

VAN HARREVELD, A. and MALHOTRA, S.K.   1967
Extracellular space in the cerebral cortex of the
mouse.
J. Anat. 101: 197-207

ALLEN, D.W. and ZAMECNIK, P.C.   1962
The effect of puromycin on rabbit reticulocyte
ribosomes.
Biochim. biophys. Acta 55: 865-874

AGRANOFF, B.W.   1969
Protein synthesis and memory formation.
In: The Future of the Brain Sciences, edited by
S. Bogoch, New York: Plenum Press, p. 341-344

AGRANOFF, B.W.   1970a
Protein synthesis and memory formation.
In: Protein Metabolism in the Nervous System,
edited by A. Lajtha, New York: Plenum Press, p. 533-543

AGRANOFF, B.W.   1970b   8.36
Recent studies on the stages of memory formation in
the goldfish.
In: Molecular Approaches to Memory and Learning,
edited by W.L. Byrne, New York: Academic Press, p.35-39

AGRANOFF, B.W., DAVIS, R.E. and BRINK, J.J.   1965   8.28
Memory fixation in the goldfish.
Proc. natn. Acad. Sci. U.S.A. 54: 788-793

AGRANOFF, B.W., DAVIS, R.E. and BRINK, J.J.   1966   8.31
Chemical studies on memory formation in goldfish.
Brain Res. 1: 303-309

AGRANOFF, B.W., DAVIS, R.E., CASOLA, L.
and LIM, R.   1967   8.32
Actinomycin D blocks formation of memory of shock
avoidance in goldfish.
Science 158: 1600-1601

AGRANOFF, B.W. and KLINGER, P.D.   1964   8.26
Puromycin effect on memory formation in the goldfish.
Science 146: 952-953

AGRANOFF, B.W., DAVIS, R.E., LIM, R.
and CASOLA, L.   1968
Biological effects of antimetabolites used in
behavioral studies.
In: Psychopharmacology: A Review of Progress,
1957-1967, edited by D.H. Efron, Public Health Service
Publication no. 1836. 909-917

APPEL, S.H.   1965
Effect of inhibition of RNA synthesis on neural
information storage.
Nature, Lond. 207: 1163-1166

APPLEMAN, M.M. and KEMP, R.G.   1966
Puromycin: a potent metabolic effect independent
of protein synthesis
Biochem. biophys. Res. Comm. 24: 564-568

BARONDES, S.H.   1965
Relationship of biological regulatory mechanisms to
learning and memory.
Nature, Lond. 205: 18-22

BARONDES, S.H. and COHEN, H.D.   1966   8.42
Puromycin effect on successive phases of memory storage.
Science 151: 594-595

BARONDES, S.H. and COHEN, H.D.   1967a   8.45
Comparative effects of cycloheximide and puromycin on
cerebral protein synthesis and consolidation of
memory in mice.
Brain Res. 4: 44-51

BARONDES, S.H. and COHEN, H.D.   1967b   8.46
Delayed and sustained effect of acetoxycycloheximide
on memory in mice.
Proc. natn. Acad. Sci. U.S.A. 58: 157-164

BARONDES, S.H. and COHEN, H.D.   1968a   8.48
Memory impairment after subcutaneous injection of
acetoxycycloheximide.
Science 160: 556-557

BARONDES, S.H. and COHEN, H.D.   1968b   8.51
Arousal and the conversion of short term memory to
long term memory.
Proc. natn. Acad. Sci. U.S.A. 61: 923-929

BARONDES, S.H. and DUTTON, G.R.   1969
Acetoxycycloheximide effect on synthsis and metabolism
of glucosamine-containing macromolecules in brain and
in nerve endings.
J. Neurobiol. 1: 99-110

BARONDES, S.H. and JARVIK, M.E.   1964   8.40
The influence of actinomycin D on brain RNA
synthesis and on memory.
J. Neurochem. 11: 187-195

BOGOCH, S.   1968
The Biochemistry of Memory.
London: Oxford Univ. Press

BONDESON, C., EDSTRÖM, A. and BEVIZ, A.   1967
Effects of different inhibitors of protein synthesis
on electrical activity in the spinal cord of fish.
J. Neurochem. 14: 1032-1034

BONNER, J.   1966
Molecular biological approaches to the study of
memory.
In: Macromolecules and Behavior, edited by J. Gaito,
New York: Appleton-Century-Crofts, p. 158-164

BRIGGS, M.H. and KITTO, G.B.   1962
The molecular basis of memory and learning.
Psychol. Rev. 69: 537-641

BRINK, J.J., DAVIS, R.E. and AGRANOFF, B.W.   1966   8.30
Effects of puromycin, acetoxycycloheximide, and
actinomycin D on protein synthesis in goldfish brain.
J. Neurochem. 13: 889-896

CASOLA, L., LIM, R., DAVIS, R.E. and
AGRANOFF, B.W.   1968   8.33
Behavioural and biochemical effects of intracranial
injection of cytosine arabinoside in goldfish.
Proc. natn. Acad. Sci. U.S.A. 60: 1389-1395

CHAMBERLAIN, T.J., ROTHSCHILD, G.H. and
GERARD, R.W.   1963   8.25
Drugs affecting RNA and learning.
Proc. natn. Acad. Sci. U.S.A. 49: 918-924

CHOROVER, S.L.   1969
In: The Future of the Brain Sciences, edited by
S. Bogoch, New York: Plenum Press, p.351

CODISH, S.D.   1971   8.80
Actinomycin D injected into the hippocampus of chicks:
effects on imprinting.
Physiol. and Behav. 6: 95-96

COHEN, H.D.   1970
Learning, memory and metabolic inhibitors.
In: Molecular Mechanisms in Memory and Learning,
edited by G. Ungar, New York: Plenum Press, p. 59-70

COHEN, H.D. and BARONDES, S.H.   1966b   8.41
Further studies on learning and memory after
intracerebral actinomycin D.
J. Neurochem. 13: 207-211

COHEN, H.D. and BARONDES, S.H.   1967a   8.44
Puromycin effect on memory may be due to occult seizure.
Science 157: 333-334

COHEN, H.D. and BARONDES, S.H.   1967b   8.47
Relationship of degree of training to the effect of
acetoxycycloheximide on memory in mice.
Proc. Am. psychol. Ass. 2: 79-80

COHEN, H.D. and BARONDES, S.H.   1968a   8.49
Effect of acetoxycycloheximide on learning and memory
of a light-dark discrimination.
Nature, Lond. 218: 271-273

COHEN, H.D. and BARONDES, S.H.   1968b   8.50
Cycloheximide impairs memory of an appetitive task.
Commun. Behavl. Biol. 1: 337-340

COHEN, H.D., ERVIN, F. and BARONDES, S.H.   1966   8.43
Puromycin and cycloheximide: Different effects on
hippocampal electrical activity.
Science 154: 1557-1558

CORNING, W.C. and JOHN, E.R.   1961
Effect of ribonuclease on retention of conditioned
response in regenerated planarians.
Science 134: 1363-1365

DAHL, N.A.   1969
Nerve electrical activity; depressed by puromycin not
related to inhibited protein synthesis.
J. Neurobiol. 2: 169-180

DANIELS, D.   1971a   8.81
Effect of Actinomycin D on memory and brain RNA
synthesis in an appetitive learning task.
Nature, Lond. 231: 395-397

DANIELS, D.   1971b   8.82
Acquisition, storage, and recall of memory for
brightness discrimination by rats following
intracerebral infusion of acetoxycycloheximide.
J. comp. physiol. Psychol. 76: 110-118

DANIELS, D.   1972   8.83
Effects of acetoxycycloheximide on appetitive learning
and memory.
Q. Jl exp. Psychol. 24: 102-114

DARKEN, M.A.   1964
Puromycin inhibition of protein synthesis.
Pharmac. Rev. 16: 223-243

DAVIS, R.E.   1968   8.34
Environmental control of memory fixation in goldfish.
J. comp. physiol. Psychol. 65: 72-78

DAVIS, R.E. and AGRANOFF, B.W.   1966   8.29
Stages of memory formation in goldfish: Evidence for
an environmental trigger.
Proc. natn. Acad. Sci. U.S.A. 55: 555-559

DAVIS, R.E., BRIGHT, P.J. and AGRANOFF, B.W.   1965   8.27
Effect of ECS and puromycin on memory in fish.
J. comp. physiol. Psychol. 60: 162-166

DAVIS, R.E. and KLINGER, P.D.   1969   8.35
Environmental control of amnesic effects of various
agents in goldfish.
Physiol. and Behav. 4: 269-271

DINGMAN, W. and SPORN, M.B.   1961   8.1
The incorporation of 8-azaguanine into rat brain DNA
and its effect on maze-learning by the rat: An
inquiry into the biochemical basis of memory.
J. Psychiat. Res. 1: 1-11

DINGMAN, W. and SPORN, M.B.   1964
Molecular theories of memory.
Science 144: 26-29

ELUL, R.   1966
Dependence of synaptic transmission on protein
metabolism of nerve cells: A possible electrokinetic
mechanism of learning.
Nature, Lond. 210: 1127-1131

ENNIS, H.L. and LUBIN, M.   1964
Cycloheximide: Aspects of inhibition of protein
synthesis in mammalian cells.
Science 146: 1474-1476

FLEXNER, J.B. and   FLEXNER, L.B.   1967   8.10
Restoration of expression of memory lost after
treatment with puromycin.
Proc. natn. Acad. Sci. U.S.A. 57: 1651–1654

FLEXNER, J.B. and   FLEXNER, L.B.   1969a   8.15
Studies on memory: Evidence for a widespread memory
trace in the neocortex after the suppression of recent
memory by puromycin.
Proc. natn. Acad. Sci. U.S.A. 62: 729–732

FLEXNER, J.B. and   FLEXNER, L.B.   1969b   8.16
Puromycin: Effect on memory of mice when injected
with various cations.
Science 165:   1143–1144

FLEXNER, J.B. and FLEXNER, L.B.   1970a   8.17
Further observations on restoration of memory lost
after treatment with puromycin.
Yale J. Biol. Med. 42: 235–240

FLEXNER, J.B. and   FLEXNER, L.B.   1970b   8.18
Adrenalectomy and the suppression of memory by puromycin.
Proc. natn. Acad. Sci. U.S.A. 66: 48–52

FLEXNER, J.B. and   FLEXNER, L.B.   1971   8.22
Pituitary peptides and the suppression of memory by
puromycin.
Proc. natn. Acad. Sci. U.S.A. 68: 2519–2521

FLEXNER, J.B., FLEXNER, L.B. and   STELLAR, E.   1963   8.3
Memory in mice as affected by intracerebral puromycin.
Science 141: 57–59

FLEXNER, J.B., FLEXNER, L.B., STELLAR, E.,
de la HABA, G. and   ROBERTS, R.B.   1962   8.2
Inhibition of protein synthesis in brain and learning
and memory following puromycin.
J. Neurochem. 9: 595–605

FLEXNER, L.B. and   FLEXNER, J.B.   1966   8.7
Effect of acetoxycycloheximide and of an
acetoxycycloheximide-puromycin mixture on cerebral protein
synthesis and memory in mice.
Proc. natn. Acad. Sci. U.S.A. 55: 369–374

FLEXNER, L.B. and   FLEXNER, J.B.   1968a   8.11
Studies on memory: The long survival of peptidyl-
puromycin in mouse brain.
Proc. natn. Acad. Sci. U.S.A. 60: 923–927

FLEXNER, L.B. and FLEXNER, J.B.   1968b   8.12
Intracerebral saline: Effect on memory of trained mice
treated with puromycin.
Science 159: 330-331

FLEXNER, L.B., FLEXNER, J.B., de la HABA, G.
and ROBERTS, R.B.   1965   8.6
Loss of memory as related to inhibition of cerebral
protein synthesis.
J. Neurochem. 12: 535-541

FLEXNER, L.B., FLEXNER, J.B. and ROBERTS, R.B.   1966   8.8
Stages of memory in mice treated with acetoxycycloheximide
before or immediately after learning.
Proc. natn. Acad. Sci. U.S.A. 56: 730-735

FLEXNER, L.B., FLEXNER, J.B. and ROBERTS, R.B.   1967   8.9
Memory in mice analyzed with antibiotics.
Science 155: 1377-1383

FLEXNER, L.B., FLEXNER, J.B., ROBERTS, R.B.
and de la HABA, G.   1964   8.4
Loss of recent memory in mice as related to regional
inhibition of cerebral protein synthesis.
Proc. natn. Acad. Sci. U.S.A. 52: 1165-1169

FLEXNER, L.B., FLEXNER, J.B. and STELLAR, E.   1965   8.5
Memory and cerebral protein synthesis in mice as affected
by graded amounts of puromycin.
Expl Neurol. 13: 264-272

FLEXNER, L.B., GAMBETTI, P., FLEXNER, J.B.
and ROBERTS, R.B.   1971   8.20
Studies on memory: Distribution of peptidyl-puromycin
in subcellular fractions of mouse-brain.
Proc. natn. Acad. Sci. U.S.A. 68: 26-28

GAITO, J.   1961
A biochemical approach to learning and memory.
Psychol. Rev. 68: 288-292

GAITO, J.   1966
Molecular Psychobiology; a Chemical Approach to
Learning and Other Behavior.
Springfield Illinois: Charles C. Thomas

GAMBETTI, P., GONATAS, N.K. and FLEXNER, L.B.   1968a   8.13
The fine structure of puromycin-induced changes in
mouse entorhinal cortex.
J. Cell. Biol. 36: 379-390

GAMBETTI, P., GONATAS, N.K. and FLEXNER, L.B.   1968b   8.14
Puromycin: Action on neuronal mitochondria.
Science 161: 900-902

GELLER, A., ROBUSTELLI, F., BARONDES, S.H., COHEN, H.D.
and JARVIK, M.E.   1969   8.53
Impaired performance by post-trial injections of
cycloheximide in a passive avoidance task.
Psychopharmacologia 14: 371-376

GELLER, A., ROBUSTELLI, F. and JARVIK, M.E.   1970   8.57
A parallel study of the amnesic effects of cycloheximide
and ECS under different strengths of conditioning.
Psychopharmacologia 16: 281-289

GELLER, A., ROBUSTELLI, F. and JARVIK, M.E.   1971   8.58
Cycloheximide induced amnesia: its interaction with
detention.
Psychopharmacologia 21: 309-316

GIBBS, M.E., JEFFREY, P.L., AUSTIN, L. and MARK, R.F.   8.79
Biochemical aspects of drug inhibition of memory
formation in chickens.
In preparation.

GOLDBERG, I.H., RABINOWITZ, M., and REICH, E.   1962
Basis of actinomycin action. I. DNA binding and inhibition
of RNA-polymerase synthetic reactions by actinomycin.
Proc. natn. Acad. Sci. U.S.A. 48: 2094-2101

GOLDSMITH, L.J.   1967   8.60
Effect of intracerebral actinomycin D and of
electroconvulsive shock on passive avoidance.
J. comp. physiol. Psychol. 63: 126-132

GOLUB, M.S., CHEAL, M.L. and DAVIS, R.E.   1972   8.38
Effects of electroconvulsive shock and puromycin on
operant responding in goldfish.
Physiol. and Behav. 8: 573-578

GRIFFITH, J.S., and MAHLER, H.R.   1969
DNA ticketing theory of memory.
Nature, Lond. 223: 580-582

HECHTER, O., and HALKERSTON, I.D.K.   1964
On the nature of macromolecular coding in neuronal memory.
Perspect. Biol. Med. 7: 183-198

HUBER, H. and LONGO, N.   1970   8.72
The effect of puromycin on classical conditioning in the
goldfish.
Psychon. Sci. 18: 279-280

HYDÉN, H.   1959
Biochemical changes in glial cells and nerve cells at
varying activity.
In: Biochemistry of the Central Nervous System,
(Proc. 4th Intern. Congr. Biochem. Vienna, 1958),
London: Permagon. vol. 3, p. 64-89

HYDÉN, H.   1960
The Neuron.
In: The Cell: Biochemistry, Physiology and Morphology,
edited by J. Brachet and A.E. Mirsky, New York:
Academic Press, vol. 4, p. 215-323

HYDÉN, H. and LANGE, P.W.   1965
A differentiation in RNA response in neurones early
and late in learning.
Proc. natn. Acad. Sci. U.S.A. 53: 946-952

HYDÉN, H. and LANGE, P.W.   1966
A genetic stimulation with production of adenic-
uracil rich RNA in neurons and glia in learning.
Naturwissenschaften 53: 64-70

HYDÉN, H. and LANGE, P.W.   1970
S100 brain protein: Correlation with behavior.
Proc. natn. Acad. Sci. U.S.A. 67: 1959-1966

JEWETT, R.E., PIRCH, J.H. and NORTON, S.   1965
Effect of 8-azaguanine on learning of a fixed-
interval schedule.
Nature, Lond. 207: 277-278

JONES, C.T. and BANKS, P.   1969
Inhibition of respiration by puromycin in slices of
cerebral cortex.
J. Neurochem. 16: 825-828

KANFER, J.N. and RICHARDS, R.L.   1967
Effect of puromycin on the incorporation of radioactive
sugars into gangliosides in vivo
J. Neurochem. 14: 513-518

KATZ, J.J. and HALSTEAD, W.C.   1950
Protein organization and mental function.
Comp. Psychol. Monogr. 20: 1-38

KRYLOV, O.A.   1967   8.61
A study of the molecular basis of memory.
Neuropsychopharmacology, (Proc. V. Intern. Congr.
C.I.N.P., Washington, 1966), p.191-201

LANDAUER, T.K.   1964
Two hypotheses concerning the biochemical basis of
memory.
Psychol. Rev. 71: 167-179

LANDE, S., FLEXNER, J.B. and FLEXNER, L.B.   1972   8.24
Effect of corticotropin and desglycinamide-lysine
vasopressin on suppression of memory by puromycin.
Proc. natn. Acad. Sci. U.S.A. 69: 558-560

LIM, R., BRINK, J.J. and AGRANOFF, B.W.   1970   8.37
Further studies on the effects of blocking agents
on protein synthesis in goldfish brain.
J. Neurochem. 17: 1637-1648

LIVINGSTON, R.B.   1967
In: The Neurosciences, a Study Program, edited by
G.C. Quarton, T. Melnechnick and F.O. Schmitt,
New York: Rockefeller Univ. Press, p. 514

MAYOR, S.J.   1969   8.65
Memory in the Japanese Quail.   Effects of puromycin
and acetoxycycloheximide.
Science 166: 1165-1167

McCONNELL, J.V.   1964a
Cannibalism and memory in flatworms.
New Scient. 21: 465-468

McCONNELL, J.V.   1964b
Cannibals, chemicals and contiguity.
Anim. Behav. 13, suppl. 1, 61-68

MARK, R.F. and WATTS, M.E.   1971   8.77
Drug inhibition of memory formation in chickens.
I. Long-term memory.
Proc. R. Soc. B. 178: 439-454

NAKAJIMA, S.   1969   8.66
Interference with relearning in the rat after
hippocampal injection of actinomycin D.
J. comp. physiol. Psychol. 67: 457-461

NATHANS, D.   1964
Puromycin inhibition of protein synthesis: Incorporation
of puromycin into peptide chains.
Proc. natn. Acad. Sci. U.S.A. 51: 585-592

OTT, T., LÖSSNER, B. and MATTHIES, H.   1972   8.86
The effect of nucleotid-monophosphates on the
acquisition and extinction of conditioned reactions.
Psychopharmacologia 23: 261-271

OTT, T. and MATTHIES, H.   1972   8.87
Influence of 6-aza-uridine on facilitation of
relearning by precursors of ribonucleic acid.
Psychopharmacologia 23: 272-278

PAGGI, P. and TOSCHI, G.   1971
Inhibitors of protein synthesis involved in memory
disruption: A study of their effects on sympathetic
ganglion isolated in vitro.
J. Neurobiol. 2: 119-128

POTTS, A. and BITTERMAN, M.E.   1967   8.62
Puromycin and retention in goldfish.
Science 158: 1594-1596

PRIBRAM, K.H.   1966
Some dimensions of remembering: Steps towards a
neurophysiological model of memory.
In: Macromolecules and Behavior, edited by
J. Gaito, New York: Appleton-Century-Crofts, p.165-187

QUARTERMAIN, D. and McEWAN, B.S.   1970   8.73
Temporal characteristics of amnesia induced by protein
synthesis inhibitor: Determination by shock level.
Nature, Lond. 288: 677-678

QUARTERMAIN, D., McEWAN, B.S. and
AZMITIA, E.C.,Jnr.   1970   8.74
Amnesia produced by electroconvulsive shock or
cycloheximide: Conditions for recovery.
Science 169: 683-686

QUARTERMAIN, D., McEWAN, B.S. and
AZMITIA, E.C.,Jnr.   1972   8.76
Recovery of memory following amnesia in the rat and
mouse.
J. comp. physiol. Psychol. 79: 360-370

QUINTON, E.E.   1971   8.84
The cycloheximide-induced amnesia gradient of a
passive avoidance task.
Psychon. Sci. 25: 295-296

QUINTON, E.E.   1972   8.85
Memory retrieval, reactivation, and protein synthesis.
Presented at the meetings of the Rocky Mountain
Psychological Assn.

RANDT, C.T., BARNETT, B.M., McEWAN, B.S.
and QUARTERMAIN, D.   1971   8.75
Amnesic effects of cycloheximide on two strains of
mice with different memory characteristics.
Expl Neurol. 30: 467-474

REICH, E., FRANKLIN, R.M., SHATKIN, A.J.
and TATUM, E.L.   1962
Action of actinomycin-D on animal cells and viruses.
Proc. natn. Acad. Sci. U.S.A. 48: 1238-1245

REINIS, S.   1969   8.67
Indirect effect of puromycin on memory.
Psychon. Sci. 14: 44-45

REINIS, S.   1970   8.68
Delayed learning deficit produced by hydroxylamine.
Physiol. and Behav. 5: 253-256

REINIS, S.   1971a   8.69
Further study of the learning deficit produced by
hydroxylamine.
Physiol. and Behav. 6: 31-33

REINIS, S.   1971b   8.70
Effect of 5-iodouracil and 2,6-diaminopurine on
passive avoidance task.
Psychopharmacologia 19: 34-39

ROBERTS, R.B., FLEXNER, J.B. and FLEXNER, L.B.   1970   8.19
Some evidence for the involvement of adrenergic sites
in the memory trace.
Proc. natn. Acad. Sci. U.S.A. 66: 310-313

ROBERTS, R.B. and FLEXNER, L.B.   1969
The biochemical basis of long-term memory.
Q. Rev. Biophys. 2: 135-173

ROSENBAUM, M., COHEN, H.D. and BARONDES, S.H.   1968   8.52
Effect of intracerebral saline on amnesia produced
by inhibitors of cerebral protein synthesis.
Commun. Behavl. Biol. 2: 47-50

SCHMITT, F.O.   1962
Macromolecular Specificity and Biological Memory.
Massachusetts: M.I.T. Press, p. 1-6

SCHOEL, W.M. and AGRANOFF, B.W.   1972   8.39
The effect of puromycin on retention of conditioned
cardiac deceleration in the goldfish.
Behavl. Biol. 7: 553-565

SEGAL, D.S., SQUIRE, L.R. and BARONDES, S.H.   1971   8.56
Cycloheximide: Its effects on activity are dissociable
from its effects on memory.
Science 172: 82-84

SEROTA, R.G.   1971   8.21
Acetoxycycloheximide and transient amnesia in the rat.
Proc. natn. Acad. Sci. U.S.A. 68: 1249-1250

SEROTA, R.G., ROBERTS, R.B. and FLEXNER, L.B.   1972   8.23
Acetoxycycloheximide-induced transient amnesia:
protective effects of adrenergic stimulants.
Proc. natn. Acad. Sci. U.S.A. 69: 340-342

SHASHOUA, V.E.   1968   8.63
RNA changes in goldfish brain during learning.
Nature, Lond. 217: 238-240

SMITH, C.E.   1962
Is memory a matter of enzyme induction?
Science 138: 889-890

SQUIRE, L.R. and BARONDES, S.H.   1970   8.54
Actinomycin D: Effects on memory at different times
after training.
Nature, Lond. 225: 649-650

SQUIRE, L.R. and BARONDES, S.H.   1972   8.59
Variable decay of memory and its recovery in
cycloheximide-treated mice.
Proc. natn. Acad. Sci. U.S.A. 69: 1416-1420

SQUIRE, L.R., GELLER, A. and JARVIK, M.E.   1970   8.55
Habituation and activity as affected by cycloheximide.
Commun. Behavl. Biol. 5: 249-254

SWANSON, R., McGAUGH, J.L. and COTMAN, C.   1969   8.71
Acetoxycycloheximide effects on one trial inhibitory
avoidance learning.
Commun. Behavl. Biol. 4: 239-246

SZILARD, L.   1964
On memory and recall.
Proc. natn. Acad. Sci. U.S.A. 51: 1092-1099

UNGAR, G.   1968
Molecular mechanisms in learning.
Perspect. Biol. Med. 11: 217-232

WARBURTON, D.M. and RUSSELL, R.W.   1968   8.64
Effects of 8-azaguanine on acquisition of a temporal
discrimination.
Physiol. and Behav. 3: 61-63

WATTS, M.E. and MARK, R.F.   1971a   8.78
Separate actions of ouabain and cycloheximide on
memory.
Brain Res. 25: 420-423

WATTS, M.E. and MARK, R.F.   1971b   8.78
Drug inhibition of memory formation in chickens.
II. Short-term memory.
Proc. R. Soc. B. 178: 455-464

YARMOLINSKY, M. and de la HABA, G.L.   1959
Inhibition by puromycin of amino acid incorporation
into protein.
Proc. natn. Acad. Sci. U.S.A. 45: 1721-1729

CONCLUSIONS

References

BROADBENT, D.E.   1970
Psychological aspects of short-term and long-term
memory.
Proc. Roy. Soc. B.   175: 333-350

CHERKIN, A.   1966
Memory consolidation: probit analysis of retrograde
amnesia data.
Psychon. Sci. 4: 169-170

CRAIK, F.I.M. and LOCKHART, R.S.   1972
Levels of processing: a framework for memory research.
J. verb. learn. behav. 11: 671-684

MARK, R.F.   1973
Memory and Nerve Cell Connections.
London: Oxford University Press

STRUMWASSER, F.   1965
The demonstration and manipulation of a circadian
rhythm in a single neuron.
In: Circadian Clocks, edited by J. Aschoff,
Amsterdam: North-Holland Publ. Co., p 442-462

Author Index to References